Succeeding in your Medical School OSCES

First edition

By Bhoresh Dhamija

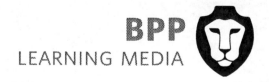

BPP
LEARNING MEDIA

First edition 2013

ISBN 9781 4453 7950 0
e-ISBN 9781 4453 9391 9

British Library Cataloguing-in-Publication Data
A catalogue record for this book is available from the British Library

Published by
BPP Learning Media Ltd
BPP House, Aldine Place
London W12 8AA

www.bpp.com/learning-media

Printed in the UK by
Ricoh
Ricoh House
Ullswater Crescent
Coulsdon
CR5 2HR

Your learning materials, published by BPP Learning Media Ltd, are printed on paper sourced from sustainable, managed forests.

A note about copyright

Dear Customer

What does the little © mean and why does it matter?

Your market-leading BPP books, course materials and e-learning materials do not write and update themselves. People write them on their own behalf or as employees of an organisation that invests in this activity. Copyright law protects their livelihoods. It does so by creating rights over the use of the content.

Breach of copyright is a form of theft – as well as being a criminal offence in some jurisdictions, it is potentially a serious breach of professional ethics.

With current technology, things might seem a bit hazy but, basically, without the express permission of BPP Learning Media:

- Photocopying our materials is a breach of copyright

- Scanning, ripcasting or conversion of our digital materials into different file formats, uploading them to Facebook or e-mailing them to your friends is a breach of copyright

You can, of course, sell your books, in the form in which you have bought them – once you have finished with them. (Is this fair to your fellow students? We update for a reason.) But the e-products are sold on a single user license basis: we do not supply 'unlock' codes to people who have bought them second hand.

And what about outside the UK? BPP Learning Media strives to make our materials available at prices students can afford by local printing arrangements, pricing policies and partnerships which are clearly listed on our website. A tiny minority ignore this and indulge in criminal activity by illegally photocopying our material or supporting organisations that do. If they act illegally and unethically in one area, can you really trust them?

BPP
LEARNING MEDIA

Contents

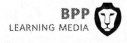

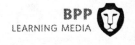

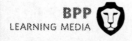

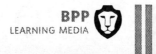

About the Publisher

BPP Learning Media is dedicated to supporting aspiring professionals with top quality learning material. BPP Learning Media's commitment to success is shown by our record of quality, innovation and market leadership in paper-based and e-learning materials. BPP Learning Media's study materials are written by professionally qualified specialists who know from personal experience the importance of top quality materials for success.

BPP
LEARNING MEDIA

About the Author

Mr Bhoresh Dhamija BSc MBChB MRCS is a Specialist Registrar in Neurosurgery currently completing higher surgical training in the West Midlands. He completed his Basic Surgical Training in West London with Imperial College, on rotation with the Hammersmith hospitals. He graduated from the University of St Andrews (BSc in Medical Science) and University of Manchester (MBChB). He has an active interest in medical education which has seen him work at Cambridge University, teaching undergraduate students a regional based anatomy syllabus. He has been a keen advocate of the use of OSCEs in undergraduate and postgraduate medical examinations and has been actively involved in preparing undergraduates to take this component of their final examination at Imperial College and the University of Birmingham medical schools.

He has also published several peer review papers in Neurosurgery along with books on Clinical Audit for Doctors and Healthcare Professionals, both as an author (1st edition) and editor (2nd edition).

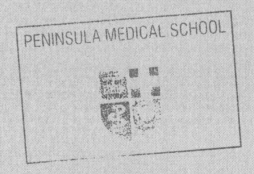

Acknowledgements

This book is a culmination of several years' work. Spanning two publishers, the author would like to thank several individuals who have played a fundamental role in the development and ultimate publication of the manuscript. From BPP, Matt Green, Akemi Hoe, Ruth D'Rozario, Jennifer Brookbanks, Lois Baily, from Keyline Consultancy, Jon Finegold and from Developmedica, Sarah Silvester, Jennifer Neal and Aidan Everett.

Thanks also to Mr Navneel Shahi and Mr Benjamin Fisher for their invaluable comments and suggestions.

BPP
LEARNING MEDIA

Dedication

For Shevata Dhamija.

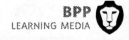

Preface

The objective structured clinical examination (OSCE) is a commonly used assessment tool in undergraduate medicine that is used to test a candidate's core skills, understanding, and attitudes in a variety of settings. These can include:

- Performing a physical examination

- Taking and presenting a history

- Performing clinical procedures

- Analysing and interpreting clinical data

- Communicating with patients and relatives in difficult and, often, highly charged situations

Over the past 15 to 20 years there has been a change in emphasis on the examination approaches employed by the various royal colleges in the United Kingdom, which is reflected in undergraduate curricula.

Previously, too much focus was placed on a candidate's achieving the correct level of factual knowledge with less focus put on understanding medical conditions, on the ability to interpret a set of data alongside the candidate's attitudes and beliefs, or on the ability to communicate with patients and colleagues. Because of this, the OSCE was introduced. This form of examination is now used as an adjunct to more traditional assessment methods in medical schools, including multiple-choice questions, extended matching questions, and essay writing. With the introduction of the OSCE, you are less likely to be faced with an assessment where chance seems to play an important role with respect to the types of patient encountered, or one in which inconsistencies exist in the way your performance is graded. These problems have been a flaw in previous clinical examination formats. The OSCE comprises a series of scenarios that vary in duration between 5 and 15 minutes, depending on the complexity of the task and the skills needed to show competence.

BPP LEARNING MEDIA

Many undergraduate curricula divide their OSCEs, so candidates are assessed according to the module recently completed. For example cardiac, respiratory and haematology scenarios might be assessed after a 'heart, lung and blood' module; or gastroenterology and endocrinology scenarios following completion of a 'nutrition, metabolism and excretion' module. Other medical schools choose to give candidates one longer OSCE examination at the end of the academic year to assess what has been learnt during the entire period. Regardless of the curriculum, you must be able to demonstrate the essential skills the examiner is looking for and successfully perform a task, or interpret an investigation, within the OSCE.

You are being assessed to determine whether you can competently and safely work as a trainee. You are not expected to achieve full competence in every scenario encountered; however, some stations do carry a pass or fail weighting, such as the ability to demonstrate basic life support skills on a mannequin. If, at this stage, a candidate cannot demonstrate basic resuscitation skills, there will be serious cause for concern as to whether they should be allowed to perform further clinical work on the wards.

Many OSCE texts available on the market today provide factual and detailed knowledge around the topic being assessed rather than providing candidates with true-life scenarios of what can be expected at each station and how best to answer some of the more common questions and hurdles the candidate will face. The aim of *Succeeding in your Medical School OSCEs* is to give an insight into the likely scenarios that will be encountered, the thought process of the examiners, as well as model answers to specific and general questions.

At the head of each scenario, a star rating is used to give an indication of its complexity:

- Basic   *
- Intermediate * *
- Advanced   * * *

The scenarios with a higher star rating may have a greater propensity to test you on 'real' patients with abnormal pathology; it does not, however, mean that they are worth more marks. It is the ability to carry out the task and interpret the results that you need to concentrate on. Where appropriate, suggestions for further reading are included to give candidates suitable texts for background reading on those topics.

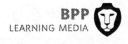

This book provides over 140 such clinical scenarios, divided into history taking, examination skills, clinical procedure, data interpretation and communication skills. It also includes some newly designed scenarios, detailing prescribing and writing skills, as well as medical ethics stations – which are both becoming more commonly assessed in UK medical schools. I hope that this book will be a useful addition to your bookshelf and provide a platform to achieve the skills necessary to function as a newly qualified doctor and, just as importantly, to succeed in the OSCE component of your examination!

Bhoresh Dhamija
September 2013

BPP
LEARNING MEDIA

Foreword

This book is a guide to the secrets of the OSCE – objective structured clinical examination – for medical students facing their final clinical examination. In a typical OSCE, students visit up to 20 stations, where they may encounter any of the following:

- An X-ray or scan, showing a common medical condition

- A patient with physical signs, such as a thyroid swelling or groin hernia or a facial nerve palsy

- The request to obtain a history, interpret the results of an investigation or carry out a simple practical procedure on a model

In many medical schools in the United Kingdom, OSCEs have largely replaced long and short clinical cases; in others, they are used as adjuncts to these traditional formats. Their advantage is that the candidate can be tested on his/her ability to address many different clinical scenarios rather than just a few, while the exam offers a degree of uniformity for candidates tackling the same set of problems in front of the same set of examiners. Thus the OSCE is indeed designed to be both objective and structured.

Mr Bhoresh Dhamija, an excellent surgical trainee who worked for me whilst completing his basic surgical rotation with Imperial College (Hammersmith hospitals), London, and currently a neurosurgical registrar with the West Midlands Deanery, presents over 140 different stations to illustrate many of the clinical scenarios that the student is likely to encounter in an OSCE. Clearly the full list of potential topics would be enormous. The selection for this book is not meant to be exhaustive, but it does cover a very large number of situations that students are likely to meet while being examined for their medical degree – as well as several peripheral topics that examiners may select in order to distinguish the better candidate from one less prepared. A good deal of thought has gone into the selection, as well as the way in which each topic is covered succinctly, yet in detail. The question-and-answer format allows the student to sample the way in which the exam is likely to be conducted in practice.

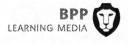

Examinations! The very thought still sets my pulse racing, though when I was a candidate myself the prospect of an exam caused more of a fright than a frisson. In my day, the basic entry examination for a surgical career – Primary FRCS – required an in-depth knowledge of anatomy, physiology and pathology. Each diet in London was held at the examination halls in Queen Square, a bleak building with a good deal of green paint on the walls and plentiful toilet facilities for last-minute visits by those contemplating the forthcoming inquisition. In the Primary you did not pass or fail: you were approved or referred, referral meaning a return visit. Candidates entered the halls from a rear basement door approached via a slope at the side of the building. Some years later, I joined a board of eight examiners conducting the conjoint examination in pathology as a representative of the Royal College of Surgeons. I can still remember the shock of walking in through the front door of Queen Square at ground level, while the unhappy candidates continued to trudge down the slope for their tryst with the examiners. In the old conjoint pathology station, each clinician was paired with a pathologist. My own appointment lowered both the average age and the IQ of the board. My venerable co-examiners sometimes forgot that I was a colleague rather than a candidate. I learned the memorable fact that leprosy is one of the commonest causes of blindness worldwide, because it rotates the eyeball upwards to gaze at the roof of the orbit; even in the early 1980s I had a suspicion that this fact was a few years out of date. I do not remember a single candidate in six years who answered the question to the examiner's satisfaction, although most of them managed to obtain an overall pass mark.

For students, it is worth remembering that all your examiners were once candidates in their turn and that, despite what you might believe, they would much prefer to pass you than to fail you. Once the terror subsides, and with a modicum of knowledge, one can almost enjoy the tussle with the examiner. Common sense tends to fly out of the window under the stress of an exam, which is why it is so useful to have seen a similar case to the one you are given. In the preparation for a clinical exam, therefore, there is no adequate substitute for seeing as many patients as you can on the ward, in the emergency department and in the outpatient clinic. I strongly believe that every examination represents a teaching experience: it brings together a treasure house of physical signs, some of which may be exotic. Nowhere outside an examination hall have I seen a patient with Volkmann's ischaemic contracture of the forearm, a lipoma of the thyroid, a Charcot's elbow joint or pulsatile metastases to the skull from a renal cell carcinoma.

I thoroughly commend Mr Dhamija's book to all students preparing to face the dreaded OSCE. If you can remember even a fraction of the know-how offered here, you are bound to have a better chance of coming through the exam triumphantly. Good reading – and good luck.

Professor Robin Williamson, MA MD MChir FRCS (Eng) FRCS (Ed)

Chairman, The London Clinic (2012–Current position)

Professor of Surgery and Consultant Surgeon, Hammersmith Hospital, London (1987–2009)

Former President, Association of Surgeons of Great Britain and Ireland (1998–1999)

Former President, Royal Society of Medicine, London UK (2008–2010)

Disclaimer

All medical information is provided in good faith and reflects current thinking and standard medical practice, but is not offered as a diagnostic or treatment manual. No responsibility can be accepted for the use of any information for purposes other than the OCSEs.

BPP
LEARNING MEDIA

Chapter 1

History taking

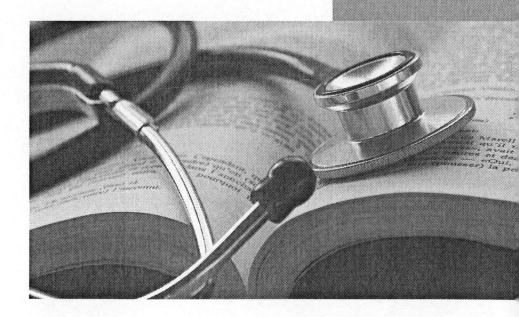

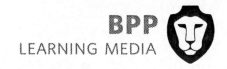

BPP
LEARNING MEDIA

History taking 1:   Level: *

Performing a general medical history

You are a medical student attached to an A&E placement. You have been asked by your consultant to elicit a full history on the next patient in cubicle 10. Mr Anderson is a 43-year-old male.

Describe how you would go about doing this and the salient questions you need to ask.

RESPONSE:

- INTRODUCTION: To begin with I would introduce myself. I would check I am speaking to the right patient by verifying his name and date of birth. At this stage I would try to establish a rapport and make him feel at ease.

- PERSONAL DETAILS: In addition to patient's name and age, I would identify his occupation and ethnic origin.

- PRESENTING COMPLAINT (PC): In his own words, I would invite him to let me know what has brought him into hospital today.

- HISTORY OF PRESENTING COMPLAINT (HPC): This relates to asking direct and specific questions about the PC. I would ask the following questions:

    - Does the patient have any risk factors which could be contributing to his problem, eg if he is complaining of shortness of breath, is he known to be a smoker, or does he have any cardiovascular complaints such as a history of angina?

    - Is this the first time this has occurred or have these symptoms happened previously?

    - If so, what if any investigations and management options have been undertaken?

With regards to regional pain, a useful mnemonic to remember is **SOCRATES**:

- **Site & Severity**: Please point on your abdomen where, exactly, you feel the pain. Also, please indicate how severe pain is, on a scale of 1 to 10, 10 being the worst pain you have ever felt, 1 being the least.

- **Onset**: When did you first notice the pain and what were you doing at that time?

- **Character**: Can you describe what the pain feels like? Is it sharp, stabbing in nature? A dull, aching sensation? Is it constantly there or does it come and go?

- **Radiation and Relieving factors**: Is the pain localised or does it radiate elsewhere, for example, to your back, to either shoulder or even down towards your groin? Have you noticed anything that improves the pain, for example, sitting or lying in a certain position?

- **Aggravating factors**: Have you noticed anything that makes the pain worse, for example, eating certain foods or drinking alcohol?

- **Timing**: How long does the pain last? Is it episodic or constant?

- **Exercise**: What effect does exercise have, if any, on the pain? How far can you walk before the pain comes on?

- **(Associated) Symptoms**: Have you noticed any other symptoms, for example, a change in bowel or urine habit, change in appetite, weight loss, nausea and/or vomiting, pale stools, dark stools, jaundice?

- PAST MEDICAL HISTORY (PMH): I would ask whether he has any medical problems. I would have my **MJ THREADS** checklist at hand, and ask whether he suffers from, or has had in the past, any of the following: **M**yocardial infarction, **J**aundice, **T**uberculosis, **H**ypertension, **R**heumatic fever, **E**pilepsy, **A**sthma, **D**iabetes, **S**troke.

  In addition to any medical complaints, I would also ask if he has had any previous surgical history, as well as any previous problems or reactions when given an anaesthetic.

- DRUG HISTORY AND ALLERGIES: I would ask the patient if he is taking any medication, or if he has any allergies that he is aware of.

- SOCIAL HISTORY: I would check the patient's use of smoking, alcohol and drug usage by asking:
    - 'Do you smoke, or have you in the past? If so, how many a day and for how long?' (I remember that 20 cigarettes a day for one year equates to one pack year.)
    - 'Do you drink alcohol? If so, roughly how much?' and then calculate the number of units in an average week.
    - 'Do you have any history of recreational drug use?'
    - I would also check the patient's marital status and occupation; if not elicited earlier, I may need to ask if there has been any exposure to industrial toxins such as asbestos.
    - Finally, in terms of standard questions, I would check his accommodation type, ie house/flat, and if there were any problems with access; and also if he were able to carry out his activities of daily living (ADLs) such as washing, cooking, cleaning, shopping etc. on an independent basis.
    - Depending on the relevance to the presentation, I may need to enquire about any recent history of foreign travel, or household pets.
- FAMILY HISTORY: I would ask if the patient has any family members with similar problems, or if there is a history of any inherited disorders running in the family including heart problems or diabetes.

Systems review

At this stage you should go through each of the body systems, to ensure you have not missed anything that could give you important clues to the diagnosis – see History taking 2: Performing a systems review.

Key points

- Have your own systematic approach for taking a general medical history; a commonly used approach is outlined above.

- Patients may not always remember their complete past medical history, so it is often useful to prompt them using a checklist; remember the mnemonic: MJ THREADS.

- Do not concentrate only on the presentation of the current complaint. Marks will be awarded for asking about the patient's family and social histories.

- Once you have more of an idea of what pathology is involved, you can target and tailor your questions accordingly.

- Remember to perform a systems review. Whether you will have time to complete this will depend on the complexity of the scenario and the allocated time you have. However, aim to ask the most relevant questions first to give you the best chance of scoring highly, just in case you run out of time.

- When practising history taking, also practise giving a summary of your findings to the examiner.

Further reading

Swash, M (2012) *Hutchison's Clinical Methods.* 23rd edition. Oxford: Saunders Ltd.

BPP
LEARNING MEDIA

History taking 2:   Level: *

Performing a systems review

After taking a targeted history from any patient, can you state the questions you would ask to complete a systems review?

Please describe the systems involved and the questions you should ask.

RESPONSE:

- **Cardiovascular**

  Do you ever experience any chest pain, shortness of breath (SOB), general difficult or laboured breathing (dyspnoea), difficult or laboured breathing when lying flat, eg when sleeping (orthopnoea), ankle swellings, palpitations?

- **Respiratory**

  Do you ever experience any dyspnoea, paroxysmal nocturnal dyspnoea (severe attacks of SOB or coughing which generally occur at night and may wake the patient up from sleep), chest pain, wheeze, coughing non-productive or productive, fever or hoarseness of voice?

- **Gastrointestinal**

  Do you have any history of weight loss (if so, roughly how much and over what time duration?), change in appetite recently/ dietary regime, change in bowel habit (is it tending towards constipation or diarrhoea?), abdominal pain, nausea or vomiting, any per rectal bleeding noted, increased flatulence, problems with swallowing, ie dysphagia (difficulty with swallowing), or odynophagia (pain on swallowing), features suggestive of jaundice (eg yellowing of sclera, mucous membranes or skin)?

- **Metabolic system**

  Goes hand in hand with the gastrointestinal system, ie has there been a recent change in appetite or weight (perhaps best quantified by measuring the BMI and comparing with previous values, if known)? Any notable change in physical appearance or build?

- **Urogenital**

  Any problems with micturition such as increased frequency, or pain (dysuria), urgency, large amounts being passed (polyuria), notable change in colour of urine, smell, blood mixed with urine (haematuria), need to get up in the night to pass urine (nocturia), sensation of incomplete voiding, abdominal pain; in males, ask about impotence?

- **Central and peripheral nervous system**

  Any change in personality or behaviour, alteration in sensation such as pins and needles in fingers or toes, or paraesthesia?

  Any muscle weakness; if present, which limb(s) are affected? Any changes in the senses (sight, hearing, or smell)? Any new onset funny turns, fits, fainting episodes including previous loss of consciousness, any complaints of headache?

- **Musculoskeletal system**

  Any recent complaints of muscle, joint or bone pain, body swelling, stiffness or decreased range of movements? On inspection are there any deformities or have you noted any functional loss?

Key points

- A systems review performed after a general medical or surgical history helps to ensure no vital clues to diagnosis are missed.

- Practise with colleagues and devise your own method of learning what to ask patients to encompass a systems review.

- Depending on the length of your OSCE scenario you may not have the time (and may not be expected) to ask all the questions at the end of your history; practice and fluency are the key.

Further reading

Swash, M (2012) *Hutchison's Clinical Methods*. 23rd edition. Oxford: Saunders Ltd.

History taking 3:   Level: * *

Abdominal pain

You are a Foundation Year doctor in a General Surgery firm.
Mr Maynard is a 29-year-old male who has presented to A&E with
abdominal pain.

Please take a history from him, with a view to making a diagnosis.

RESPONSE:

- **INTRODUCTION:** To begin with I would introduce myself and
  check I am speaking to the right patient by verifying his name
  and date of birth. At this stage I would try to establish a rapport
  and make him feel at ease.

- **PERSONAL DETAILS:** In addition to his name and age, I would
  identify his occupation and ethnic origin.

- **PRESENTING COMPLAINT (PC):** I would invite the patient to let
  me know, in his own words, what has brought him into hospital
  today.

- **HISTORY OF PRESENTING COMPLAINT (HPC):** This relates
  to asking direct and specific questions about the PC. I would use
  the SOCRATES mnemonic to ensure I touched on all aspects.

- **PAST MEDICAL HISTORY:** I would go through my checklist,
  using the mnemonic MJ THREADS.

- **DRUG HISTORY AND ALLERGIES:** I would check this, as many
  drugs are known to have abdominal pain as a side effect.

- **SOCIAL HISTORY:**

  - Smoking, number a day and for how many years

  - Alcohol consumption, number of units a week

  - Travel, any recent history of travel, particularly foreign
    travel

- **FAMILY HISTORY:** Is there any history of first-degree relatives
  with any inherited gastrointestinal disorders?

- SYSTEMS REVIEW: I would perform a systems review, as detailed in History taking 2:
  - Cardiovascular
  - Respiratory
  - Gastrointestinal
  - Metabolic
  - Urogenital
  - Central and peripheral nervous system
  - Musculoskeletal

- **Right lower quadrant (RLQ):** Appendicitis, mesenteric adenitis, Meckel's diverticulitis, inflammatory bowel disease (IBD), stones (renal/ureteric), perforated bowel (caecal), psoas abscess, pancreatitis, gynaecological causes (ectopic pregnancy/ endometriosis, ovarian cyst, pelvic inflammatory disease (PID), period pain) hernia, irritable bowel syndrome (IBS), neoplasia.

- **Left lower quadrant (LLQ):** Diverticulitis, IBD, perforated bowel (sigmoid), stones (renal), gynaecological causes (ectopic pregnancy/endometriosis, ovarian cyst, PID, period pain), hernia, IBS, hernia, colorectal carcinoma.

- **Right upper quadrant (RUQ):** Cholecystitis, hepatitis, appendicitis, duodenal ulcer, hepatomegaly, pneumonia (right sided), pyelonephritis.

- **Left upper quadrant (LUQ):** Stomach ulcer, splenic rupture, perforation (transverse/descending colon), abdominal aortic aneurysm, pneumonia (left sided), pyelonephritis.

Table 1.1: Differential diagnosis of abdominal pain

Key points

- Ensure you have a systematic way to cover all of the patient's presenting symptoms for abdominal pain; remember the mnemonic SOCRATES.

- There are many factors that could contribute to abdominal pain; these should be elicited by completing a thorough history taking.

- The location of the pain in the abdomen will give clues to and help narrow down the differential diagnosis.

Further reading

Logan, R et al (2012) *ABC of the Upper Gastrointestinal Tract (ABC Series)*. Oxford: Wiley-Blackwell.

History taking 4:   Level: * *

Chest pain

 You are a FY2 doctor in a General Medical firm. Mr Booker is a 60-year-old male who has presented to A&E with chest pain.

Please take a history from him, with a view to making a diagnosis.

RESPONSE:

*   INTRODUCTION: To begin with I would introduce myself, and check I am speaking to the right patient by verifying his name and date of birth. At this stage I would try to establish a rapport and make him feel at ease.

*   PERSONAL DETAILS: In addition to his name and age, I would identify his occupation and ethnic origin.

*   PRESENTING COMPLAINT (PC): In his own words, I would invite the patient to let me know what has brought him into hospital today.

*   HISTORY OF PRESENTING COMPLAINT (HPC): This relates to asking direct and specific questions about the PC. With regards to regional pain, a useful mnemonic to remember is SOCRATES:

    –   **S**ite & Severity: Can you point on your chest where exactly you feel the pain? Also how severe is the pain, on a scale of 1 to 10 (with 10 being the worst pain you have ever felt, 1 being the least)?

    –   **O**nset: When did you first notice the pain and what were you doing at that time?

    –   **C**haracter: Can you describe what the pain feels like, is it sharp, stabbing in nature? A dull aching sensation? Does it feel like pressure? A burning sensation? Is it constantly there or does it come and go?

    –   **R**adiation and Relieving factors: Is the pain localised or does it radiate elsewhere, for example, to your back, to either arm, shoulder or even to your jaws?

    –   Have you noticed anything that improves the pain, for example, on resting in a certain position. Have you taken any glyceryl trinitrate (GTN) spray, if so, does this help?

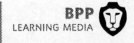

- **A**ggravating factors: Have you noticed anything that makes the pain worse, for example, walking or any other exercise, exposure to cold weather, violent coughing, deep inspiration, or even eating a heavy meal?

- **T**iming: How long does the pain last? Is it episodic or constant?

- **E**xercise: Does exercise make the pain worse? How far can you walk roughly before you notice the pain?

- (Associated) **S**ymptoms: Have you noticed any other symptoms with the pain, for example, difficulty in breathing/shortness of breath, problems breathing when lying flat (Orthopnoea – if so, ask how many pillows do you use to sleep with)? Have you noticed any dizziness or palpitations?

- PAST MEDICAL HISTORY: I would go through my checklist, using the mnemonic MJ THREADS.

- DRUG HISTORY AND ALLERGIES: Common drug groups given to people with cardiovascular disease include anti-hypertensives, such as ACE inhibitors and beta blockers, aspirin and statins.

- SOCIAL HISTORY:

  - Smoking, number a day and for how many years

  - Alcohol consumption, number of units a week

  - Travel, any recent history of travel, particularly foreign travel

- FAMILY HISTORY: Is there any history of first-degree relatives with diabetes or of myocardial infarction (before 50 years of age)?

- SYSTEMS REVIEW: I would perform a systems review:

  - Cardiovascular
  - Respiratory
  - Gastrointestinal
  - Metabolic
  - Urogenital
  - Central and peripheral nervous system
  - Musculoskeletal

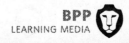

- Heart: Angina, IHD, MI, pericarditis, myocarditis, post-MI Dressler's syndrome, left ventricular hypertrophy (LVH), hypertrophic obstructive cardiomyopathy (HOCM)

- Lungs: Pneumonia, pneumothorax, pleurisy, pulmonary embolus, localised trauma with rib injuries

- Aorta: thoracic aortic aneurysm

- Gastrointestinal: Pancreatitis, gastric ulcer, cholecystitis, oesophageal spasm/oesophagitis

- Others: localised trauma causing rib injuries/spinal fractures, shingles

Table 1.2: Differential diagnosis of chest pain

Key points

- Ensure you have a systematic way to cover all of the patient's presenting symptoms for chest pain; remember, for example, the mnemonic SOCRATES.

- There are many factors that could contribute to chest pain; these should be elicited by completing a thorough history.

- The location of the pain in the chest will give clues to, and help narrow down, the differential diagnosis.

Further reading

Albarran, J and Tagney, J eds. (2007) *Chest Pain: Advanced Assessment and Management Skills*. Oxford: Wiley-Blackwell.

History taking 5:   Level: * * *

Leg weakness

Mr Horne is a 37-year-old male who has come to your clinic with a several-week history of progressive right-leg weakness.

Please take a history from him, with a view to making a diagnosis.

RESPONSE:

- INTRODUCTION: To begin with I would introduce myself and check I am speaking to the right patient by verifying his name and date of birth. At this stage I would try to establish a rapport and make him feel at ease.

- PERSONAL DETAILS: In addition to his name and age, I would identify his occupation and ethnic origin.

- PRESENTING COMPLAINT (PC): In his own words, I would invite the patient to let me know what has brought him into the clinic today.

- HISTORY OF PRESENTING COMPLAINT (HPC): This relates to asking direct and specific questions about the PC.

    - Onset: When did you first notice the symptoms and what were you doing at that time? Did the weakness come on suddenly or gradually?

    - Duration of weakness: is it acute or chronic in nature?

    - Frequency of weakness: is it episodic or continuous?

    - Are there any things you have noticed that aggravate the weakness?

    - Have you noticed anything which relieves the weakness?

    - Since it has occurred, have you noticed any progression – ie is it improving or deteriorating?

    - How severe is the weakness? Is it causing a paralysis? If this is the case, is it partial or complete?

With regards to any pain, ie in the legs or lower back, I would use the mnemonic SOCRATES and would also ask:

– Have you noticed any sensory problems such as numbness? If this is present try to identify a sensory level.

– Has there been any sphincteric disturbance of bladder or bowel function such as incontinence?

– What other associated features are present? I'd look out for:

- Leg swelling

- Loss of movement and function in the leg or any other joints; where this exists how it impacts on activities of daily living (ADLs) such as walking distances, washing, cooking, cleaning etc

- Visible deformity

- Joint stiffness

- I would identify what investigations and treatments, if any, have been performed up to this point.

- PAST MEDICAL HISTORY (PMH): I would go through my checklist, using the mnemonic MJ THREADS; I would also include conditions which may be contributory to leg weakness:

– History of neurological disorders.

– Any musculoskeletal deformity.

– Sciatica or known vertebral disc problems.

– Previous history of tumours/malignancy, if so, which body systems are affected.

– Where malignancy is known, any radiotherapy or chemotherapy.

– Any recent infections.

- DRUG HISTORY AND ALLERGIES: What analgesics is the patient taking?

- SOCIAL HISTORY: I would ask the patient about his:

– Smoking, number a day and for how many years
– Alcohol consumption, number of units a week

- FAMILY HISTORY: Is there any history of first-degree relatives with neurological or musculoskeletal disorders?

- SYSTEMS REVIEW: I'd perform a systems review:
    - Cardiovascular
    - Respiratory
    - Gastrointestinal
    - Metabolic
    - Urogenital
    - Central and peripheral nervous system
    - Musculoskeletal

- **Spinal cord pathology:** disc bulge/prolapse, spinal cord tumour, secondary malignancy eg from prostate, breast, lung, subdural or extradural haematoma, vertebral fracture or subluxation causing nerve root impingement

- **Autoimmune disorders:** Guillain-Barré syndrome, Multiple Sclerosis (MS)

- **Hereditary, familial, genetic disorders:** Duchenne muscular dystrophy, Friedreich's ataxia,

- **Infectious disorders:** Osteomyelitis, spinal/lumbar epidural abscess

- **Causes of a foot drop:** Diabetes mellitus, MS, common peroneal nerve injury, cerebrovascular disease, lumbo-sacral prolapsed disc

---

Table 1.3: Differential diagnosis of leg weakness

Key points

- There are many causes for leg weakness; a thorough history is essential to help narrow down your differential diagnosis.

- Examiners will want to know you are considering the patient as a whole. Remember to ask how the condition is impacting on the patient's ADLs.

- For the rarer causes, such as Duchenne muscular dystrophy, remember to ask if there is a family history of genetic/hereditary disorders.

Further reading

Lindsay, K et al (2010) *Neurology and Neurosurgery Illustrated.* 5th edition. Oxford: Churchill Livingstone.

History taking 6:   Level: *

Gynaecological history

Miss Clarke is a 33-year-old female presenting to the gynaecology ward with a recent history of vaginal discharge; as the FY2 doctor you have been asked to take a history from her, with a view to making a diagnosis.

How would you approach this?

RESPONSE:

- INTRODUCTION: To begin with, I would introduce myself. Check I am speaking to the right patient by verifying her name and date of birth. At this stage I would try to establish a rapport and make her feel at ease. I would sit directly opposite her, ensure good eye contact and explain that I am going to take a history.

- PERSONAL DETAILS: In addition to name and age, I would also identify her ethnic origin and occupation.

- PRESENTING COMPLAINT (PC): In her own words, I would invite the patient to let me know what has brought her to the ward today.

- HISTORY OF PRESENTING COMPLAINT (HPC): This relates to asking direct and specific questions about the PC.

  – Onset: When did you first notice the problem? Did it come on suddenly or gradually?

  – Duration: Has this been going on for a while, or is it a short-lived concern ie is the problem acute or chronic?

  – Frequency of discharge.

  – Are there any things you have noticed which aggravate the problem?

  – Have you noticed anything which relieves the problem?

  – How does the problem affect your activities of daily living (ADLs)?

  – Have you had any investigations and/or treatments performed up until now?

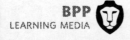

- SPECIFIC QUESTIONS FOR A GYNAECOLOGICAL HISTORY:
    - Date of the last menstrual period (LMP)?
    - In this case, the patient is a 33-year-old, so she is unlikely to be post-menopausal, but always bear in mind this is a possibility. Check if this is the case, and if so, at what age did the menopause commence?
    - Do you have any children, and at what age did you have your first child?
    - Is there a history of painful periods (menses), (aka dysmenorrhoea)?
    - Is your menstrual cycle regular or irregular? What is the frequency and duration of menses?
    - Are your menses heavy (menorrhagia), or light? (This can be gauged by asking the number of tampons or pads used, or the number of clots passed).
    - Is there any post-coital bleeding?
    - What colour is the vaginal discharge – is it clear, purulent or bloodstained? Does it smell of anything or is it odourless?
    - Have you had any cervical smears? If so, when was the last and what was the result of the previous tests?
    - Sexual history including contraceptive use: number of sexual partners, is there any pain on intercourse (aka dyspareunia); methods of contraception used currently and previously?
- GENITO-URINARY HISTORY: This will follow hand-in-hand with the gynaecology history:
    - Is there pain on micturition (aka dysuria)? If so, does it occur during or after voiding?
    - Frequency of micturition, is there any nocturia (waking up at night to pass urine)?
    - Is there any history of urinary incontinence; if so, is it stress or urge incontinence?
    - Is there any history of blood in the urine, (aka haematuria)?
    - Is there any history of vaginal prolapse?

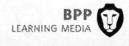

- **OBSTETRIC HISTORY:** I would ask:
    - How many children do you have?
    - How many pregnancies, any history of abortions or miscarriages?
    - Were the deliveries all normal vaginal; if not, how were your children delivered?
    - Any complications during the pregnancy or labour either to child or mother?
- **PAST MEDICAL HISTORY (PMH):** Go through the checklist, using the mnemonic MJ THREADS; also ask about:
    - History of previous hospital admissions
    - Any previous gynaecological or other surgical operations performed
- **DRUG HISTORY AND ALLERGIES:** Specifically ask if the patient is taking contraception, either in the form of an oral contraceptive pill, a depot injection or a fitted coil (eg Mirena)?
- **SOCIAL HISTORY:** I would ask the patient about:
    - Smoking, number a day and for how many years
    - Alcohol consumption, number of units a week
    - Marital status
- **FAMILY HISTORY:** Check to see:

    Is there any history of first-degree relatives with gynaecological disorders?

    Were there problems during pregnancy, eg pre-eclampsia or gestational diabetes?
- **SYSTEMS REVIEW:** Perform a systems review:
    - Cardiovascular
    - Respiratory
    - Gastrointestinal
    - Metabolic
    - Central and peripheral nervous system
    - Musculoskeletal

Key points

- Do not concentrate on the presentation alone of 'history of vaginal discharge': the intention should be to take a thorough history looking for a background of gynaecological disorders.

- You will be also assessed on how tactful you are when taking your history but do not shy away from asking pertinent questions relating to problems with menses, post-coital bleeding and sexual history.

- Leave time to cover the patient's PMH, along with the other facets of a general medical history.

Further reading

Bain, C et al (2011) *Gynaecology Illustrated*. 6th edition. Oxford: Churchill Livingstone.

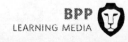

History taking 7: Level: *

Paediatric history

Paul is a 14-year-old male presenting to the paediatric ward with a several-month history of feeling generally lethargic and unwell. As the Foundation Trainee in the department you have been asked to take his history by speaking to him and his mother who has accompanied him today.

How do you proceed?

RESPONSE:

- INTRODUCTION: To begin with I would introduce myself. Check I am speaking to the right patient by verifying his name and date of birth. At this stage I would try to establish a rapport and make him feel at ease. I would sit directly opposite him, ensure good eye contact and explain that I am going to take a history.

- PERSONAL DETAILS: In addition to his name and age, I'd identify his weight and height.

- PRESENTING COMPLAINT (PC): In their own words, I would invite the patient and his mother to let me know what has brought them to the ward today.

- HISTORY OF PRESENTING COMPLAINT (HPC): This relates to asking direct and specific questions about the PC.

    - Onset: When did you first notice the problem? Did it come on suddenly or gradually?

    - Duration: Has this been going for a while or is it a short-lived concern, ie is the problem acute or chronic?

    - Was the child well before all these problems started?

    - Is there anything that you have noticed which may have precipitated the problem, eg exposure to other unwell children, including siblings?

    - Are there any things you have noticed which aggravate the problem?

    - Have you noticed anything which relieves the problem?

    - Ask about any associated symptoms, such as any recent change in appetite; general noticeable reduction or increase in activity levels or problems at school, academic and behavioural

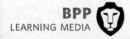

- Have you had any investigations and or treatments performed up until now?

- Ask if the child has met all their developmental milestones during the first few years of life, or has there been a noticeable delay in meeting some of these?

Tell the examiner you would like to look at a growth/height chart and plot the patient's measurements on this.

- **PAST MEDICAL HISTORY:** I'd go through my checklist, using the mnemonic MJ THREADS; I'd also ask the mother about the very early years.

  - I'd ask about the pregnancy:

    - problems in pregnancy

    - prematurity of delivery

    - problems during labour, was it prolonged?

    - mode of delivery, normal vaginal, assisted or caesarean section

    - weight at birth, under or overweight

  - As a newborn, or in the early years of childhood, has there been any concern regarding:

    - fits or convulsions
    - fevers
    - feeding problems
    - jaundice
    - bleeding disorders

- **DRUG HISTORY AND ALLERGIES:** Specifically ask:

  - Where allergies exist, not only identify the offending drug(s), but also the adverse reaction it is associated with

  - Are there known allergies to types of food, pets, pollen etc?

- **IMMUNISATIONS:** Is the child up to date with all immunisations?

- **SOCIAL HISTORY:**

  - Smoking: this should be asked about, even if the child is under age.

  - Alcohol intake: ditto

  - Any learning difficulties

  - Any history of disruptive behaviour

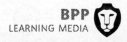

- Type of residential accommodation: enquire about location, type and with whom. Both family and non-family members living there should be noted.

- FAMILY HISTORY: Is there any history of first-degree relatives with inherited disorders such as cerebral palsy or cystic fibrosis?

- SYSTEMS REVIEW: Perform a systems review:

  - Cardiovascular
  - Respiratory
  - Gastrointestinal
  - Metabolic
  - Urogenital
  - Central and peripheral nervous system
  - Ear, nose and throat
  - Musculoskeletal

Key points

- In a station like this, where information is required from more than one individual (mother and son), aim to engage with both parties.

- You will need to ask questions about problems in and around the pregnancy to complete your history and score full marks, not just concentrate on the immediate presentation.

- Question if there have been any problems in school, either of an academic or behavioural nature.

- Leave time to perform a systems review.

Further reading

Lissauer, T and Clayden, G (2011) *Illustrated Textbook of Paediatrics*. 4th edition. Oxford: Mosby.

History taking 8:   Level: * * *

Expressive dysphasia

> You are a FY2 doctor in a General Medical firm; Mr Briggs is a
> 50-year-old male who has presented to A&E with a recent history of
> difficulty in verbally expressing speech. Please take a history from
> him, with a view to making a diagnosis.

RESPONSE:

- INTRODUCTION: To begin with I would introduce myself. Check
  I am speaking to the right patient by verifying his name and date
  of birth. At this stage I would try to establish a rapport and make
  him feel at ease.

- PERSONAL DETAILS: In addition to his name and age, I would
  identify his occupation and hand dominance.

- PRESENTING COMPLAINT (PC): In his own words, I would
  invite the patient to let me know what has brought him into
  hospital today.

- HISTORY OF PRESENTING COMPLAINT (HPC): This relates to
  asking direct and specific questions about the PC. With regards
  to this, I would try to identify:

  - Onset: When did you first notice this problem and what were
    you doing at that time? Did it come on suddenly or gradually?

  - Duration: How long has this been going on for? (ie is this
    an acute or a chronic problem)?

  - Periodicity: Is it constant whenever you speak (ie continuous)
    or is it a problem that comes and goes, (ie episodic)?

  - Have you noticed it to be deteriorating or actually getting
    better?

  - Are there any predisposing events?

  - Relieving factors: Have you noticed anything that improves
    your speech?

  - Aggravating factors: Have you noticed anything that makes
    your speech worse?

- Whilst communicating with the patient, I would ask direct
  questions to determine:

  - Ability to comprehend: ask the patient to perform a three-
    step command, eg 'take the paper in your left hand, fold it
    in half and put it on the table'.

- Repetition: state a sentence, eg 'I live on 27 West Street, on the south side of the city'; then ask the patient to repeat this.

- During my conversation, I would assess the patient's fluency and grammar along with the general content of the words spoken.

- I would ask the patient to write a sentence on a piece of paper, as general writing skills can also be affected.

- (Associated) Symptoms: I would ask if the patient had noticed any other symptoms along with the difficulty in expressing speech, particularly looking out for:
  - Headache
  - Loss of consciousness
  - Faints, fits or 'funny turns'
  - Weakness in one or more limbs
  - Paraesthesia/sensory disturbance
  - Problems or changes with the sense of smell, vision or hearing
  - Any behavioural or personality change.

- What investigations or treatment methods have been performed up until now?

- PAST MEDICAL HISTORY: I would go through my checklist, and use the mnemonic MJ THREADS. Also, I would remember to ask about:

  - History of neurological disorders

  - History of cardiac rhythm disorders, such as atrial fibrillation, and check hypercholesterolemia (raised cholesterol levels)

- DRUG HISTORY AND ALLERGIES:

  - Is the patient on any anticoagulation medication including, aspirin, clopidogrel or warfarin?

  - Is he taking medication for hypertension or diabetes, if applicable?

- SOCIAL HISTORY:

  - Smoking, number a day and for how many years
  - Alcohol consumption, number of units a week
  - Marital status
  - Accommodation type, specific aids in the home, do you have any home help?

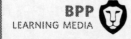

- FAMILY HISTORY: Is there any history of first-degree relatives with a history of vascular disease including stroke, any other neurovascular disorders or malignancy?

- SYSTEMS REVIEW: I would perform a systems review:
    - Cardiovascular
    - Respiratory
    - Gastrointestinal
    - Metabolic
    - Urogenital
    - Central and peripheral nervous system
    - Musculoskeletal

- **Broca's (expressive) dysphasia.** Broca's area is the part of the cerebral cortex that is responsible for the motor control of speech. It is usually located on the inferior frontal lobe on the left side. Damage to this area can produce an expressive dysphasia whereby speech becomes non-fluent; vocabulary may appear limited, with errors in grammar and syntax.

- **Wernicke's (receptive) dysphasia:** Wernicke's area is the part of the cerebral cortex that is responsible for the understanding of written and spoken language. It is usually located on the superior temporal lobe on the left side. Damage to this area can produce a receptive dysphasia, namely problems with the comprehension of speech. Speech itself retains a natural sounding and fluent rhythm, but appears nonsensical with abnormal letters and words used.

- **Conductive dysphasia:** Repetition of words and phrases is poor. Speech is nonsensical but fluent, yet comprehension is normal.

- **Global dysphasia:** Non-fluent speech with impaired comprehension. This often results from damage to large parts of the dominant (usually left-sided) hemisphere. There will be a combination of Broca's and Wernicke's dysphasia.

Table 1.4: Differential diagnosis of dysphasia

Key points

- From your history and communication with a patient try to identify the type of dysphasia he or she has. You will be given higher marks if you can relate this to the anatomical location in the brain the problem arises from.

- Broca's area is that part of the cerebral cortex that is responsible for the motor control of speech. It is usually located on the inferior frontal lobe on the left side. Problems here result in an expressive dysphasia.

- Wernicke's area is that part of the cerebral cortex that is responsible for the understanding of written and spoken language. It is usually located on the superior temporal lobe on the left side. Problems here result in a receptive dysphasia.

Further reading

Lindsay, K et al (2011) *Neurology and Neurosurgery Illustrated.* 5th edition. Oxford: Churchill Livingstone.

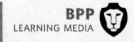

History taking 9:   Level: * *

Thyroid disease

You are a foundation trainee attached to an endocrine clinic. The next patient is Mrs Lynch, a 56-year-old woman, who has been referred by her GP to this outpatient clinic with a recent history of weight gain, hoarseness of voice, constipation, and generally feeling tired.

Please take a history from her, with a view to making a diagnosis.

RESPONSE:

- INTRODUCTION: To begin with I would introduce myself and check I am speaking to the right patient by verifying her name, date of birth and hospital number. At this stage I would try to establish a rapport and make her feel at ease. I would sit directly opposite her, ensure good eye contact and explain that I am going to take a history

- PERSONAL DETAILS: In addition to name and age, I would also identify her occupation and ethnic origin.

- PRESENTING COMPLAINT (PC): In her own words, I would invite her to let me know what has brought her to the clinic today.

- HISTORY OF PRESENTING COMPLAINT (HPC): This relates to asking direct and specific questions about the PC. From the background information, the patient has some of the features of hypothyroidism (an underactive thyroid gland), hence my questions would be directed at determining the nature of the symptoms she has presented with, and also if the patient has other features related to this disorder.

    – Weight gain: I understand you have gained some weight recently; could you tell me roughly how much weight you have put on and in what length of time?

    – Hoarse voice: When did you first notice problems with your voice?

    – Bowel habit: Have you noticed any change in your bowel habit recently (constipation in this case)? If so, over what length of time?

    – Lethargy and concentration: have you noticed any changes to your general energy levels and ability to concentrate?

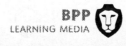

- Cold intolerance: Do you feel an unusual discomfort when in a cold (seen in hypothyroidism) or hot (seen in hyperthyroidism) environment?

- Hair changes: Have you noted any changes in the feeling of your hair (dry, thinning, coarse hair in hypothyroidism)?

- Skin changes: Have you noted any changes in the feeling of your skin (cold, dry, pale, yellowing of skin on the palms of the hands and soles of the feet. Also depigmented skin patches – vitiligo, all features seen in hypothyroidism).

- Do you have a history of any autoimmune diseases such as diabetes or anaemia?

- How does the problem affect your activities of daily living (ADLs)?

- Have you had any investigations or treatments performed up until now?

- PAST MEDICAL HISTORY: I would go through my checklist, using the mnemonic MJ THREADS.

- DRUG HISTORY AND ALLERGIES: Many drugs are known to have an effect on thyroid function as a side effect. Some of the more commonly used ones include lithium, propranolol, corticosteroids, iron tablets and amiodarone.

- SOCIAL HISTORY: I would check:

  - Smoking, number a day and for how many years
  - Alcohol consumption, number of units a week

- FAMILY HISTORY: Is there any history of first-degree relatives with any autoimmune disorders including problems with thyroid function?

- SYSTEMS REVIEW: I'd perform a systems review:

  - Cardiovascular
  - Respiratory
  - Gastrointestinal
  - Metabolic
  - Urogenital
  - Central and peripheral nervous system
  - Musculoskeletal

- Heat intolerance. Hands hot and sweaty.

- Increase in physiological tremor

- Onycholysis (nail separation from its bed)

- Thyroid acropachy (another nail sign associated with pseudo clubbing, swelling of the distal phalanges and periosteal bone formation)

- Weight loss

- Diarrhoea

- Proximal myopathy/weakness

- Palpitations, this may be an indication of atrial fibrillation. All patients with newly diagnosed atrial fibrillation should have a thyroid function test.

- Tachycardia and high pulse pressure

- Lid lag

Table 1.5: Symptoms and signs associated with hyperthyroidism (thyrotoxicosis)

Graves' disease

This is an autoimmune disease of the thyroid in which the patient's own immune system attacks the thyroid gland causing it to produce too much thyroxine. It is the most common cause of hyperthyroidism. It is characterised by pretibial myxoedema (localised lesions in the skin most commonly in the pretibial area), thyroid acropachy (characterised by subperiosteal new bone formation, commonly manifesting as clubbing of the fingers and toes and soft tissue swelling) and Graves' eye disease.

Graves' eye disease

- Exophthalmos – both eyelids move away from the centre of the iris, so that the sclera is visible all around the iris.

- Proptosis – when examining the patient from behind, looking over their head, the eye has protruded so far forward that it can be seen beyond the level of the supraorbital ridge.

- Other signs of Graves' eye disease are those associated with complications of proptosis:

    – Conjunctivitis

    – Corneal ulceration

    – Chemosis – here the venous and lymphatic drainage is so distorted by the proptosis that the eye appears oedematous

    – Ophthalmoplegia

You must be able to distinguish the features of an underactive thyroid gland from that of an overactive gland.

Key points

- You are likely to be given a hypothyroid or hyperthyroid patient to take a history from; be able to distinguish the common symptoms and signs associated with each condition.

- Graves' disease is an autoimmune disease of the thyroid in which the patient's own immune system attacks the thyroid gland causing it to produce too much thyroxine. It is the most common cause of hyperthyroidism.

Further reading

Todd, CH. Management of thyroid disorders in primary care: challenges and controversies. *Postgraduate Medical Journal.* Dec 2009; 85 (1010): 655–9.

BPP
LEARNING MEDIA

History taking 10:

Level: *

Constipation

You are a FY2 doctor in a General Surgery firm; Mr Barlow is a 57-year-old male who has presented to the outpatient clinic with a background of constipation. You have been asked by your consultant to see him.

Please take a history from him, with a view to making a diagnosis.

RESPONSE:

- INTRODUCTION: To begin with I would introduce myself. Check I am speaking to the right patient by verifying his name and date of birth. At this stage I would try to establish a rapport and make him feel at ease.

- PERSONAL DETAILS: In addition to his name and age, I would identify his occupation and ethnic origin.

- PRESENTING COMPLAINT (PC): In his own words, I would invite the patient to let me know what has brought him into the clinic today.

- HISTORY OF PRESENTING COMPLAINT (HPC): This relates to asking direct and specific questions about the PC.

    - Time and onset: When did you first notice the constipation; did it come on gradually?

    - Duration: How long has it been going on for (an acute or a chronic problem?)

    - Frequency: How often do you open your bowels? Identify average number of times over a certain period, eg 'once every 4 to 5 days.'

    - Aggravating factors: Have you noticed anything that makes the constipation worse, for example, eating certain foods or drinking alcohol?

    - Relieving factors: Have you noticed anything that relieves the constipation?

    - Progression: Is it getting worse or improving?

    - Blood in stool: Ask if he has noticed any blood mixed with his stool.

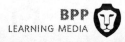

- Colour of stool: Does it appear particularly light or dark in colour? Also identify if there is any associated evident yellow/green mucus or pus.
- Consistency of stool: Does it appear soft, solid, semi-solid, unformed or watery in nature?
- Ask for presence of flatulence.
- Is there tenesmus: 'Is there often an urge to evacuate the bowel with straining which results in passage of little or no stool?' Tenesmus is a characteristic feature in cases of bacillary dysentery.
- Presence of straining to defecate?
- Quantity of stool: small or large volume each time?
- Pain: Any associated rectal, abdominal or anal pain?
- Incontinence: any urinary or bowel incontinence?
- Abdominal mass/distension: Have you noticed any abdominal lumps? Do you feel your abdomen appears distended?
- (Associated) symptoms: Have you noticed any other symptoms, for example, dysphagia or odynophagia (difficulty in, or pain on, swallowing), change in appetite, weight loss, nausea and/or vomiting, haematemesis, jaundice, gastro-oesophageal reflux?
- Investigations and treatments to date: Ask what, if any, have been implemented along with the results known.

- PAST MEDICAL HISTORY: I would go through a checklist, using the mnemonic MJ THREADS. In this station it would also be prudent to include:

  - Childhood conditions associated with constipation, such as Hirschsprung's disease, cystic fibrosis and cerebral palsy.
  - I would remember to ask for any past history of gastrointestinal or neurological conditions.
  - Any previous surgery.

- DRUG HISTORY AND ALLERGIES: Many drugs are known to have constipation as a side effect; these include:
  - Opiate analgesia
  - Anticonvulsant drugs
  - Antidepressants
  - Iron tablets
  - Diuretics

- SOCIAL HISTORY: I would check:
  - Smoking, number a day and for how many years
  - Alcohol consumption, number of units a week
  - Exercise (poor mobility can be a contributory factor)
  - Dietary habits (ask about fibre and level of fluid intake)
  - Occupation

- FAMILY HISTORY: Is there any history of first-degree relatives with any inherited gastrointestinal disorders?

- SYSTEMS REVIEW: I would perform a systems review:
  - Cardiovascular
  - Respiratory
  - Metabolic
  - Urogenital
  - Central and peripheral nervous system
  - Musculoskeletal

- Organic pathology: Colon cancer, adenocarcinoma, bowel obstruction, intestinal pseudo-obstruction, diverticulitis, diverticular disease, Crohn's disease.

- Painful disorders: Painful haemorrhoids, anal fissures.

- Drugs: opiate analgesics, iron tablets, antidepressants, anticonvulsants, diuretics.

- Psychological disorders: Depression, anxiety disorders.

- Poor dietary intake & exercise: Often secondary to a lack of dietary fibre combined with poor mobility.

Table 1.6: Differential diagnosis of constipation

Key points

- There are many drugs that have constipation as a side effect; these include opiate-based analgesics, anti-depressants and iron tablets.

- Particularly be aware of elderly patients presenting with constipation (alteration in bowel habit) along with blood mixed with stool, weight loss and poor appetite. These features should trigger a high possibility of colorectal carcinoma.

- Poor dietary intake and a lack of exercise can cause constipation in otherwise-healthy individuals.

- Certain childhood conditions show an increased propensity to develop constipation, eg Hirschsprung's disease.

BPP LEARNING MEDIA

History taking 11:   Level: *

Diarrhoea

You are a FY2 doctor in a General Surgery firm; Mrs Quirk is a 36-year-old female who has presented to the outpatient clinic with a recent background of diarrhoea. You have been asked by your consultant to see her.

Please take a history from her, with a view to making a diagnosis.

RESPONSE:

- INTRODUCTION: To begin with I would introduce myself. Check I am speaking to the right patient by verifying her name and date of birth, and at this stage I would try to establish a rapport and make her feel at ease.

- PERSONAL DETAILS: In addition to her name and age, I would identify her occupation and ethnic origin.

- PRESENTING COMPLAINT (PC): In her own words, I would invite her to let me know what has brought her into the clinic today.

- HISTORY OF PRESENTING COMPLAINT (HPC): This relates to asking direct and specific questions about the PC.

    - Time and onset: When did you first notice the diarrhoea; did it come on gradually?

    - Duration: How long has it been going on for (an acute or a chronic problem?)

    - Frequency: How often do you open your bowels? Identify average number of times over a certain period eg 'six times every day'.

    - Aggravating factors: Have you noticed anything that makes the diarrhoea worse, for example, eating certain foods or drinking alcohol?

    - Relieving factors: Have you noticed anything that relieves the diarrhoea?

    - Progression: Is it getting worse or improving?

    - Blood in stool: Ask if she has noticed any blood mixed with her stool.

- Colour of stool: Does it appear particularly light or dark in colour? Identify if there is any associated evident yellow/green mucus or pus?

- Consistency of stool: Does it appear soft, solid, semi-solid, unformed or watery in nature?

- Ask for presence of flatulence.

- Is there tenesmus is there often an urge to evacuate the bowel with straining which results in passage of little or no stool? (Tenesmus is a characteristic feature in cases of bacillary dysentery.)

- Presence of straining to defecate?

- Quantity of stool: small or large volume each time?

- Pain: Any associated rectal, abdominal or anal pain?

- Incontinence: any urinary or bowel incontinence?

- Abdominal mass/distension: Have you noticed any abdominal lumps? Do you feel your abdomen appears distended?

- Has there been any recent history of foreign travel?

- (Associated) symptoms: Have you noticed any other symptoms? For example, dysphagia or odynophagia (difficulty in, or pain on, swallowing), change in appetite, weight loss, nausea and/or vomiting, excess thirst, haematemesis, jaundice, gastro-oesophageal reflux.

- Investigations and treatments to date: Ask what if any have been implemented, along with the results known.

- PAST MEDICAL HISTORY: I'd go through a checklist, using the mnemonic MJ THREADS; in this station it would also be prudent to include:

  - History of coeliac disease (aka gluten-sensitive enteropathy)
  - Irritable bowel syndrome
  - Inflammatory bowel disease, namely Crohn's disease and ulcerative colitis
  - Diverticular disease
  - Colorectal cancer
  - Any past history of gastrointestinal disorders

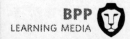

- – Any previous radiotherapy
- – Any previous surgery
- DRUG HISTORY AND ALLERGIES: Many drugs are known to have diarrhoea as a side effect; these include:
  - – Antibiotics as well as antibiotic overuse (aka antibiotic-associated diarrhoea)
  - – Laxatives
  - – Statins
  - – Antacid medications containing magnesium such as cimetidine
  - – Non-steroidal anti-inflammatory drugs (NSAIDs)
  - – Some antidepressant drugs
  - – Some chemotherapy drugs
- SOCIAL HISTORY: I would check:
  - – Smoking, number a day and for how many years
  - – Alcohol consumption, number of units a week
  - – History of any recreational drug usage
  - – Sexual history
  - – Dietary habits (consider fibre and quantity of fluid intake)
  - – Any recent contact history with other persons having diarrhoea
  - – Occupation
- FAMILY HISTORY: Is there any history of first-degree relatives with inherited gastrointestinal disorders, such as familial adenomatous polyposis (FAP) or hereditary non-polyposis colorectal cancer (HNPCC)?
- SYSTEMS REVIEW: I would perform a systems review:
  - – Cardiovascular
  - – Respiratory
  - – Metabolic
  - – Urogenital
  - – Central and peripheral nervous system
  - – Musculoskeletal

- Gastroenteritis.

- Organic disorders: Inflammatory bowel disease, colorectal carcinomas, pancreatitis, enteritis.

- Previous surgery: eg history of gastrectomy.

- Drugs: antibiotics including over-usage, laxatives, statins, some antacids.

- Endocrine disorders: thyrotoxicosis, thyroid cancer, carcinoid syndrome, Zollinger-Ellison syndrome.

- Congenital causes: Coeliac disease, cystic fibrosis.

Table 1.7: Differential diagnosis of diarrhoea

Key points

- There are many drugs which have diarrhoea as a side effect; these include: antibiotics, laxatives, statins, NSAIDs, magnesium containing antacids.

- Other factors which may contribute to developing diarrhoea (and hence should be asked about) include: a recent history of foreign travel, recreational drug abuse and sexual history.

- Certain congenital and genetic conditions show an increased propensity to developing diarrhoea such as coeliac disease, cystic fibrosis, FAP, HNPCC.

BPP
LEARNING MEDIA

History taking 12:   Level: * *

Headache

You are a FY2 doctor in a General Medical firm; Mr Dardis is a 54-year-old male who has presented to A&E with a headache.

Please take a history from him, with a view to making a diagnosis.

RESPONSE:

- INTRODUCTION: To begin with I would introduce myself. Check I am speaking to the right patient by verifying his name and date of birth. At this stage I would try to establish a rapport and make him feel at ease.

- PERSONAL DETAILS: In addition to his name and age, I would identify his occupation, hand dominance (whether he is left or right-handed) and ethnic origin.

- PRESENTING COMPLAINT (PC): In his own words, I would invite the patient to let me know what has brought him into hospital today.

- HISTORY OF PRESENTING COMPLAINT (HPC): This relates to asking direct and specific questions about the PC. I'd use the mnemonic for pain, **SOCRATES**:

    - Site & Severity: Can you point on your head where exactly you feel the pain? Also how severe on a scale of 1 to 10 is the pain, with 10 being the worst pain you have ever felt, 1 being the least?

    - Onset: When did you first notice the headache and what were you doing at that time?

    - Character: Can you describe what the headache feels like? Is it sharp, stabbing in nature? Or a dull, aching sensation? Does it feel like pressure? Is it constantly there, or does it come and go?

    - Radiation and Relieving factors: Is the headache localised or does it radiate elsewhere – for example, to your neck, shoulder or even to your jaws? Have you noticed anything that improves the headache, for example, lying on a flat surface?

    - Aggravating factors: Have you noticed anything that makes the headache worse, for example, light exposure, walking or any other exercise?

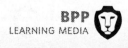

- Timing: How long does the headache last? Is it episodic or constant? Is it worse or better at any particular time of day, eg on waking up in the morning?

- Exercise: Does exercise make the headache worse?

- (Associated) Symptoms: Have you noticed any other symptoms with the headache, such as nausea or vomiting, neck stiffness, problems with bright light (photophobia), or blurring of vision, rash, fevers or rigors, generally feeling lethargic with problems with concentration? Have you noticed any weakness in your limbs or any pins and needles? How about any facial pain when you chew food or brush your teeth (jaw claudication), or any pain when brushing/combing your hair (scalp tenderness)? Have you had any recent weight loss?

- HEAD INJURY: Have you had any head injuries or falls recently?

- PAST MEDICAL HISTORY: Go through my checklist, use the mnemonic MJ THREADS.

- DRUG HISTORY AND ALLERGIES: Common drugs which are known to have headache as a side effect include:

  - Asthma medication
  - Contraceptive pills or any other type of hormone therapy
  - Drugs which contain nitrates, such as anti-hypertensives
  - Anticoagulant drugs

- SOCIAL HISTORY: I would check:

  - Smoking, number a day and for how many years

  - Alcohol consumption, number of units a week

  - Travel, any recent history of travel, particularly foreign travel

  - Recent stressful events or longstanding psychosocial stresses from work or family scenarios

  - Diet (including calorie intake)

  - Lifestyle factors contributing to headache, eg a lack of sleep.

- FAMILY HISTORY: Is there any history of first-degree relatives with a history of migraines?

BPP
LEARNING MEDIA

- SYSTEMS REVIEW: I would perform a systems review:
  - Cardiovascular
  - Respiratory
  - Gastrointestinal
  - Metabolic
  - Urogenital
  - Central and peripheral nervous system
  - Musculoskeletal

- Intracranial: migraine, meningitis (or other intracranial infections), CVA (stroke), tumours, intracranial haemorrhage including subarachnoid haemorrhage, hydrocephalus.

- Extracranial: temporal arteritis, sinusitis, arthritic disorders of the cervical spine along those affecting the temperomandibular joint, dental abscess.

Table 1.8: Differential diagnosis of headache

Key points

- Headache is a very common complaint and seen daily in many GP practices; pay particular attention to the associated features which often give a clue to the diagnosis, eg when photophobia and neck stiffness is present, meningitis must be high amongst the differentials.

- Remember that non-organic pathology, particularly stress can contribute/be responsible for headache.

- Be able to reel off a list of possible intracranial and extra cranial causes for headache.

Further reading

Lindsay, K et al (2010) *Neurology and Neurosurgery Illustrated*. 5th edition. Oxford: Churchill Livingstone.

History taking 13:   Level: *

Per rectal bleeding

You are a Foundation Year doctor in a General Surgery firm; Mr Khan is a 67-year-old male who has presented to the outpatient clinic with a recent history of rectal bleeding. You have been asked by your consultant to see him.

Please take a history from him, with a view to making a diagnosis.

RESPONSE:

- INTRODUCTION: To begin with I would introduce myself. Check I am speaking to the right patient by verifying his name and date of birth. At this stage I would try to establish a rapport and make him feel at ease.

- PERSONAL DETAILS: In addition to his name and age, I would identify his occupation and ethnic origin.

- PRESENTING COMPLAINT (PC): In his own words, I would invite the patient to let me know what has brought him into the clinic today.

- HISTORY OF PRESENTING COMPLAINT (HPC): This relates to asking direct and specific questions about the PC.

  - Time and Onset: When did you first notice the rectal bleeding, did it come on gradually or was it sudden?

  - Duration: How long has it been going on for (acute or chronic problem?)

  - Frequency: How often does it occur? Identify average number of times over a certain period eg 'once every 3 to 4 days'.

  - Precipitating events: eg any history of trauma?

  - Aggravating factors: Have you noticed anything that makes the problem worse, for example, when straining to open your bowels?

  - Relieving factors: Have you noticed anything that relieves the problem?

- – Progression: Is it getting worse, remaining constant or improving?

- – Blood in stool: Ask if he has noticed any blood mixed with his stool? Does the blood appear to lie on the surface of the stool eg bleeding from haemorrhoids or an anal fissure? Or is blood only noted after stool has been passed, ie on the toilet paper or in the toilet pan?

- – Colour of blood: Does it appear:

  - - black, 'tarry' in colour (malaena) (this is associated with gastrointestinal haemorrhage)

  - - bright red in colour (this is often fresh blood and implies bleeding from the anus or low down in the rectum)

  - - darker red (this often occurs when there is bleeding from the colon eg in diverticular disease, or from a bowel tumour)?

- – Estimate of the amount of blood noted.

- Gastrointestinal symptoms:

  - – Any abdominal pain, if so does it occur before or after opening your bowels, or is it unrelated to this?

  - – Any tenesmus?

  - – Presence of straining to defecate?

  - – History of constipation?

  - – Have you noticed any change in your bowel habit recently?

  - – Have you noticed any mass, lump over your abdomen, or do you think your abdomen feels distended?

  - – Any haematemesis?

  - – (Associated) Symptoms: Have you noticed any other symptoms, for example; dysphagia or odynophagia (difficulty in or pain on swallowing), change in appetite, weight loss, nausea and/or vomiting, haematemesis, jaundice, dizziness or shortness of breath?

  - – Investigations and treatments to date: Ask what, if any, have been implemented, along with the results known.

- PAST MEDICAL HISTORY: I'd go through my checklist, using the mnemonic MJ THREADS; in this station it would also be prudent to include:
  - Any history of inflammatory bowel disease, ie Crohn's disease or ulcerative colitis
  - Infective colitis
  - Anal fissures
  - Haemorrhoids
  - Diverticular disease
  - Familial adenomatous polyposis
  - Colorectal carcinoma
  - Anaemia
  - Any previous surgery

- DRUG HISTORY AND ALLERGIES: Some drugs may increase the propensity to develop per rectal bleeding:
  - Anticoagulants including aspirin and warfarin
  - Non-steroidal anti-inflammatory drugs (NSAIDs)

- SOCIAL HISTORY: I'd check:
  - Smoking, number a day and for how many years
  - Alcohol consumption, number of units a week
  - Occupation
  - Sexual history

- FAMILY HISTORY: Is there any history of first-degree relatives with any inherited gastrointestinal disorders, particularly colorectal carcinoma, familial adenomatous polyposis, or inflammatory bowel disease?

- SYSTEMS REVIEW: I'd perform a systems review:
  - Cardiovascular
  - Respiratory
  - Metabolic
  - Urogenital
  - Central and peripheral nervous system
  - Musculoskeletal

- **Organic pathology:** Colon cancer, adenocarcinoma, diverticulitis, diverticular disease, inflammatory bowel disease (Crohn's disease or ulcerative colitis), infective or radiation induced colitis, angiodysplasia

- **Localised trauma**

- **Painful disorders:** Painful haemorrhoids, anal fissures

- **Drugs:** anticoagulants, eg aspirin and warfarin, non-steroidal anti-inflammatory drugs

- **Bleeding disorders,** eg haemophilia

Table 1.9: Differential diagnosis of per rectal bleeding

Key points

- Remember per rectal bleeding can be a sign of a systemic problem such as a malignant cancer, or it may be a localised problem such as haemorrhoids or an anal fissure.

- Some drugs can increase the likelihood of developing per rectal bleeding; always ask about a history of anticoagulants or NSAID usage.

- Important clues to the diagnosis can be obtained by asking about the relationship of the blood with the stool and the colour of the blood.

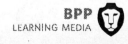

History taking 14:

Level: *

Cough

You are a FY2 doctor in a General Medical firm. Mr Ferguson is a 52-year-old male who has presented to the clinic with a long history of cough.

You have been asked to take a history from him by your consultant.

RESPONSE:

- INTRODUCTION: To begin with I would introduce myself. Check I am speaking to the right patient by verifying his name and date of birth. At this stage I would try to establish a rapport and make him feel at ease.

- PERSONAL DETAILS: In addition to his name and age, I would identify his occupation and ethnic origin.

- PRESENTING COMPLAINT (PC): In his own words, I would invite the patient to let me know what has brought him into the clinic today.

- HISTORY OF PRESENTING COMPLAINT (HPC): I'd use the mnemonic SOCRATES:

  - Severity: How severe, on a scale of 1 to 10, is the cough? (10 being the worst cough you have ever had, 1 being the least.)

  - Onset: When did you first notice the cough, and what were you doing at that time?

  - Character: Is it a productive cough – wet or dry?

  - Relieving factors: Have you noticed anything that improves the cough?

  - Aggravating factors: Have you noticed anything that makes the cough worse, for example, walking or any other exercise, or exposure to cold weather?

  - Timing: How long does the cough last? Is it episodic or constant? Does it vary according to the time of day?

  - Exercise: Does exercise make the cough worse? If so, which activities make it worse?

- (Associated) Symptoms: Have you noticed any other symptoms with the cough, such as difficulty in breathing or shortness of breath? Have you noticed any wheezing? Do you have any problems breathing when lying flat (orthopnoea – if so ask how many pillows the patient uses to sleep with). Do you have any chest pain or pain on inspiration?

  - Is there any sputum production, and if so, what is the colour, estimated quantity and how does it smell?

  - Have you ever coughed up blood (haemoptysis)?

  - Systemic symptoms: Have you had any fever, rigor or night sweats? Have you noticed any change in your appetite, bowel habit and weight loss recently?

  - Identify what, if any, investigations have been performed and their results.

- PAST MEDICAL HISTORY: I'd go through my checklist, using the mnemonic MJ THREADS; I'd specifically also ask about any congenital disorders which could be contributing, such as cystic fibrosis. Any history of pertussis (whooping cough) in childhood?

- DRUG HISTORY AND ALLERGIES: Common drug groups which can precipitate a cough include anti-hypertensives such as ACE inhibitors and beta blockers, and also some types of analgesia such as NSAIDs. Ask the patient if they have been given any anti-coughing drugs such as chlorpromazine (which belongs to a group of drugs called phenothiazines, also used as anti-emetics), or even tried codeine (also used as an analgesic).

- SOCIAL HISTORY: I'd check:

  - Smoking, number a day and for how many years

  - Alcohol consumption, number of units a week

  - Travel, any recent history of travel, particularly foreign travel

  - Verify the occupational history – has there been any exposure to asbestos, animals, dust or pollen?

  - Any pets at home?

  - Type of accommodation?

- FAMILY HISTORY: Is there any history of first-degree relatives with cardiac or respiratory problems? Is there any history of inherited genetic disorders eg cystic fibrosis secondary to α-1-antitypsin deficiency? Any history of immuno-deficient disorders?

- SYSTEMS REVIEW: I'd perform a systems review:
  - Cardiovascular
  - Respiratory
  - Gastrointestinal
  - Metabolic
  - Urogenital
  - Central and peripheral nervous system
  - Musculoskeletal

ACUTE

- An acute cough is often secondary to a respiratory tract infection caused by a virus; this will either be an upper respiratory tract infection (URTI), implying the virus has affected the trachea, pharynx or larynx. Examples of URTIs causing cough include laryngitis, the common cold, influenza (flu).

- If the cough is caused by a lower respiratory tract infection (LRTI), the virus has affected your airways lower down, or your lungs.

  Examples of LRTIs causing a cough are pneumonia and bronchitis.

CHRONIC

- Common causes of a persistent cough include smoking, post-nasal drip (where mucus drips down the throat from the back of the nose, caused by a condition such as rhinitis), bronchiectasis, asthma, bronchitis, emphysema, interstitial fibrosis, gastro-oesophageal disease.

- Others: less common causes include pulmonary oedema (often secondary to heart failure), pulmonary embolism, lung or throat cancer, tuberculosis, cystic fibrosis.

Table 1.10: Differential diagnosis of a common cough

Key points

- On identifying if a cough is acute or chronic, this should allow a narrowing of the differential diagnosis.

- Smoking along with occupational history must be verified.

- Where there are features to suggest immunodeficiency in the history, consider tuberculosis in addition to lung cancer high in the differential.

History taking 15:   Level: * *

Shortness of breath

You are a FY2 doctor in a General Medical firm. Mr Woo is a 64-year-old male who has presented to clinic with a long history of shortness of breath (SOB).

You have been asked to take a history from him by your consultant.

RESPONSE:

- **INTRODUCTION:** To begin with I would introduce myself. Check I am speaking to the right patient by verifying his name and date of birth. At this stage I would try to establish a rapport and make him feel at ease.

- **PERSONAL DETAILS:** In addition to his name and age, I would identify his occupation and ethnic origin.

- **PRESENTING COMPLAINT (PC):** In his own words, I would invite the patient to let me know what has brought him into the clinic today.

- **HISTORY OF PRESENTING COMPLAINT (HPC):** I'd use the mnemonic SOCRATES:

  - Severity: How severe on a scale of 1 to 10 is the SOB? (Is it something that leaves you just trying to catch your breath on occasion or has it left you gasping for air frequently?)

  - Onset: When did you first notice the SOB and what were you doing at that time? Are there any predisposing events that could have triggered this?

  - Character: Is there any associated noise production when you are SOB, if so, what is the character of this? Are there grunting or wheezing sounds produced, for example?

  - Relieving factors: Have you noticed anything that improves the SOB?

  - Aggravating factors: Have you noticed anything that makes the SOB worse, for example, exposure to cold weather?

  - Timing: How long does the SOB last? Is it episodic or constant? Does it vary according to the time of day? (Think of orthopnoea and paroxysmal nocturnal dyspnoea.)

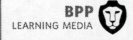

- Exercise and functional effect: Does exercise make the SOB worse? If so, which activities make it worse?

    - What activities does the SOB prevent you from doing?

    - What effect does it have on your Activities of Daily Living (ADLs), ie indication of exercise tolerance?

    - How far can you walk on a flat surface before feeling breathless, also how many steps up a flight of stairs are you able to climb?

    - Does washing and dressing, for example, lead to SOB?

    - Do you ever feel breathless when talking normally?

    - Do you ever get breathless at rest?

- (Associated) Symptoms: Have you noticed any other symptoms with the SOB, for example, coughing: is there any sputum production? If so, what is the colour, quantity and how does it smell? Have you noticed any wheezing? Do you have any problems breathing when lying flat? (Orthopnoea – if so, ask how many pillows they use to sleep with). Do you have any chest pain or pain on inspiration (suggesting it is pleuritic in nature)?

- Have you ever coughed up blood (haemoptysis)?

- Systemic symptoms: Have you had any fever, rigor or night sweats? Have you noticed any change in your appetite, bowel habit and weight loss recently?

- Smoking history: current or ex-smoker? Quantify in number of pack years, where 1 pack year equates to 20cpd for 1 year.

- Identify what, if any, investigations have been performed and their results.

- PAST MEDICAL HISTORY: I'd go through this, using the mnemonic MJ THREADS.

- DRUG HISTORY AND ALLERGIES: Relevant drugs to ask for include history of steroid usage, either in the form of oral drugs or inhaled. I'd check use of other inhalers or nebulisers acting as bronchodilators (eg in asthma). Any history of home oxygen therapy – do you have oxygen cylinders for use at home?

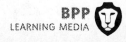

- SOCIAL HISTORY: I'd check:

  - Alcohol consumption, number of units a week

  - Verify the occupational history – has there been any exposure to asbestos, animals, coal, dust or pollen?

  - Any pets at home

  - Type of accommodation

  - Any recent travel abroad (think of the possibility of tuberculosis)?

- FAMILY HISTORY: Is there any history of first-degree relatives with cardiac or respiratory problems? Is there any history of inherited genetic disorders eg cystic fibrosis secondary to α-1-antitrypsin (A1AT) deficiency? Any history of any immuno-deficient disorders?

- SYSTEMS REVIEW: I'd perform a systems review:

  - Cardiovascular
  - Respiratory
  - Gastrointestinal
  - Metabolic
  - Urogenital
  - Central and peripheral nervous system
  - Musculoskeletal

- **Pulmonary disorders:** Asthma, bronchitis, emphysema, fibrosing alveolitis, cystic fibrosis, hookworm disease, pneumonia, pleural effusion, pneumothorax, lung cancer, tuberculosis, sarcoidosis.

- **Cardiac disorders:** Left ventricular failure (LVF) causing pulmonary oedema, mitral valve stenosis, Cardiomyopathy.

- **Causes of restriction in chest volume:** Ankylosing spondylitis, trauma causing fractured ribs, kyphosis or scoliosis of the spine, obesity, neuromuscular disorders causing respiratory muscle weakness or paralysis such as myasthenia gravis.

- **Other causes:**

  - Obstruction of the airway secondary to cancer of the larynx or pharynx, pulmonary aspiration, epiglottitis, laryngeal oedema.

  - Immobilisation of the diaphragm secondary to a lesion of the phrenic nerve, diaphragmatic tumour, polycystic liver disease.

  - Pharmacological disorders, eg aspirin poisoning.

  - Psychological disorders, eg anxiety, panic attack, hyperventilation.

Table 1.11: Differential diagnosis of shortness of breath

Key points

- The most likely scenarios associated with shortness of breath will be related to individuals with the more common respiratory (asthma, bronchitis, pleural effusion, lung cancer) and cardiac (LVF causing pulmonary oedema, cardiomyopathy) complaints.

- Be aware of the possibility of TB or sarcoidosis in individuals with a background of some immunocompromise or recent history of foreign travel.

- It is unlikely that a patient will have a history of primary lung cancer in the absence of a smoking history.

- If no obvious organic cause comes to mind, remember that some psychological disorders such as anxiety and panic attacks can be etiological reasons for SOB.

Further reading

Davis, R et al (2006) *ABC of Heart Failure (ABC series)*. 2nd edition. Oxford: Churchill Livingstone.

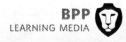

History taking 16:

Level: * *

Pyrexia of unknown origin (PUO)

You are a FY1 doctor who has been asked by your consultant to take a history from Mr Watt. He is a 44-year-old male presenting to the clinic with a recent history of feeling generally unwell and has noticed that he has had a raised temperature when he checks manually by himself at home.

Please take a history from him, with a view to making a diagnosis.

RESPONSE:

- INTRODUCTION: To begin with I would introduce myself. Check I am speaking to the right patient by verifying his name and date of birth. At this stage I would try to establish a rapport and make him feel at ease.

- PERSONAL DETAILS: In addition to his name and age, I would identify his occupation and ethnic origin.

- PRESENTING COMPLAINT (PC): In his own words, I would invite the patient to let me know what has brought him into the clinic today.

- HISTORY OF PRESENTING COMPLAINT (HPC): This relates to asking direct and specific questions about the PC. I would use the mnemonic SOCRATES:

  - Severity: How severe, on a scale of 1 to 10, are your symptoms, 1 being the lowest?

  - Onset: When did you first notice these symptoms and what were you doing at the time? Are there any predisposing events that could have triggered this?

  - Character: Do you feel the same symptoms each time the problem occurs or have you noticed any variability?

  - Relieving factors: Have you noticed anything that improves things?

  - Aggravating factors: Have you noticed anything that makes things worse?

  - Timing: How long do the symptoms last when they occur? Is it episodic or constant? Is there any diurnal variation?

  - Exercise: Does doing any exercise or physical activities have any effect?

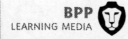

- – (Associated) Symptoms: Have you noticed any other symptoms with this problem, for example, feeling feverish/ having rigors or night sweats; diarrhoea, nausea or vomiting, recent change in appetite or weight loss, headache, or development of a body rash?

- Identify what, if any, investigations have been performed up to this point and their results.

- PAST MEDICAL HISTORY (PMH): I'd use the mnemonic MJ THREADS; In addition to any medical complaints, also ask if the patient has had any previous surgical history, as well as any previous problems or reactions when given an anaesthetic.

  - – Ask about any other history of immunosuppressive disorders including cancer

  - – Sexual history

  - – Recreational drug usage

- DRUG HISTORY AND ALLERGIES: I'd ask the patient if he is taking any medications including history of recent antibiotic usage; and if he has any allergies that he is aware of.

- SOCIAL HISTORY: I'd check:

  - – Smoking history
  - – Alcohol history
  - – Marital status
  - – Occupational history
  - – Accommodation type
  - – Recent history of foreign travel
  - – If there are any pets at home, or if they remember having been bitten by their pet or any other animal

- FAMILY HISTORY: I would ask if there are any family members with similar problems, or if there is a history of immunosuppressive illness or a haematological disorder.

- SYSTEMS REVIEW: I'd perform a systems review:

  - – Cardiovascular
  - – Respiratory
  - – Gastrointestinal
  - – Metabolic
  - – Urogenital
  - – Central and peripheral nervous system
  - – Musculoskeletal

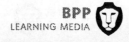

- **Infection:** eg abscess, tuberculosis, endocarditis, urinary tract infection, virus (including HIV), fungal.

- **Tumours:** eg lymphomas, leukaemias.

- **Connective tissue diseases:** eg systemic lupus erythematosus, rheumatoid arthritis, Still's disease, temporal arteritis, polymyalgia rheumatica.

- **Others:** eg pulmonary embolism, transfusion reactions, thyroiditis, alcohol/drug withdrawal, pancreatitis, acalculous cholecystitis.

Table 1.12: Differential diagnosis of pyrexia of unknown origin (PUO)

Key points

- Remember that PUO is not always secondary to an infectious cause; it can be a subtle presentation of, for example, a tumour or pulmonary embolism.

- When taking a PMH, remember to ask about sexual history and a recent history of foreign travel.

- Where immunosuppression exists, remember to consider tuberculosis.

History taking 17:

Level: * * *

Rash

You are the FY2 doctor in A&E; you have been asked to take the history of a 38-year-old female, who has come to hospital with a rash.

How do you proceed?

RESPONSE:

- INTRODUCTION: To begin with I would introduce myself. Check I am speaking to the right patient by verifying her name and date of birth. At this stage I would try to establish a rapport and make her feel at ease.

- PERSONAL DETAILS: In addition to her name and age, I would identify her occupation and ethnic origin.

- PRESENTING COMPLAINT (PC): In her own words, I would invite the patient to let me know what has brought her into hospital today.

- HISTORY OF PRESENTING COMPLAINT (HPC): This relates to asking direct and specific questions about the PC.

    - When did you first notice the rash, did it come on suddenly or gradually? Has it been there a while (chronic), or only recently (acute)?

    - Are there any factors that may have precipitated the rash, eg have you commenced any new medication or has there been a change in diet?

    - Have you been exposed to anything different recently, eg a pet, or been to a new environment – increasing exposure to substances such as industrial fumes or pollen?

    - Note the location and general appearance of the rash:

        - Is it flat (macular) or raised (papular)?

        - What colour is it?

        - How large is it and describe its shape (is it regular or irregular?)

        - Ask if it is tender, then assess to see if it blanches or not under pressure.

- Is the rash spreading or reducing in size?

- Is it episodic (comes and goes), or is it persistent?

- Have you noticed any aggravating or relieving factors?

- Are there any associated features:

  - Warmth over the rash site
  - Pruritus (itching)
  - Joint pain

- Is this the first time this kind of rash has occurred, or has there been any previous episodes?

- Any history of recent travel, abroad or otherwise?

- What methods of treatment, if any, have been tried up to now?

- PAST MEDICAL HISTORY: I would go through my checklist, using MJ THREADS.

  - Also ask about any history of skin disorders such as psoriasis, eczema and dermatitis.

- DRUG HISTORY AND ALLERGIES: Drugs which are well known to cause a rash include:

  - Steroids
  - Antibiotics, eg penicillin, doxycycline
  - Some anticonvulsants, including phenytoin

  I would also consider contact dermatitis secondary to contact of skin with agents such as copper, nickel and latex.

- SOCIAL HISTORY:

  - Smoking, number a day and for how many years

  - Alcohol consumption, number of units a week

  - Patient's occupation, note particularly any exposure to industrial chemicals and toxins

  - Pets

  - Marital status

- FAMILY HISTORY: Is there any history of first-degree relatives with any skin disorders or atopy?

- SYSTEMS REVIEW: I would perform a systems review:
  - Cardiovascular
  - Respiratory
  - Metabolic
  - Urogenital
  - Central and peripheral nervous system
  - Musculoskeletal

Key points

- Have your own systematic approach for taking a history from someone with a rash.

- You should try to identify the aetiology of a rash, namely is it secondary to a change in the environment, medication or could there be an element of genetic inheritance.

- Be able to describe a rash in relation to its location, size, colour, regularity and elevation.

- Note that social factors can also be contributory, such as occupational history, alcohol consumption and exposure to pets.

Further reading

Buxton, PK and Morris-Jones, R (2009) *ABC of Dermatology (ABC Series)*. 5th edition. Oxford: Wiley-Blackwell.

History taking 18: Level: * * *

Weight loss

You are a FY2 doctor in a General Surgery firm. Mr Campbell is a 68-year-old male who has presented to the outpatient clinic as a referral from his GP with a recent history of unintentional weight loss.

You have been asked by your consultant to take a history from him, with a view to making a diagnosis.

RESPONSE:

- INTRODUCTION: To begin with I would introduce myself. Check I am speaking to the right patient by verifying his name and date of birth. At this stage I would try to establish a rapport and make him feel at ease.

- PERSONAL DETAILS: In addition to his name and age, I would identify his occupation (or main occupation before retirement if appropriate) and ethnic origin.

- PRESENTING COMPLAINT (PC): In his own words, I would invite him to let me know what has brought him into the clinic today.

- HISTORY OF PRESENTING COMPLAINT (HPC): This relates to asking direct and specific questions about the PC.

    - . Quantity of weight loss: How much weight have you lost?

    - Timing: Over what length of time has this occurred?

    - Persistence: Has the weight loss persisted despite you taking your normal regular diet?

    - Predisposing factors: Have you noticed any increased levels of stress or anxiety in your life recently?

    - Aggravating factors: Have you noticed anything that makes the weight loss worse or more pronounced?

    - Relieving factors: Have you noticed anything that helps increase weight?

    - Progression: Is it getting worse or does it appear to be improving?

    - (Associated) Symptoms: Have you noticed any other symptoms, for example:

        - poor or loss of appetite

        - deliberate change in your regular diet

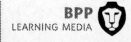

- dysphagia or odynophagia (difficulty in or pain on swallowing)

- nausea and/or vomiting

- haematemesis

- jaundice (yellowing of your skin)

- gastro-oesophageal reflux

- abdominal pain

- recent changes in bowel habit (eg are your bowels tending more towards constipation or becoming looser in nature)

- any increased flatulence

- rectal bleeding or blood mixed with stool

  – Investigations and treatments to date: Ask what, if any, have been implemented along with the results known.

- PAST MEDICAL HISTORY: I would go through my checklist, using the mnemonic MJ THREADS; in this station it would also be prudent to include:

  – Any history of gastrointestinal or neurological conditions

  – Any previous surgery

- DRUG HISTORY AND ALLERGIES: I must ask about specific medications the patient is taking (or has previously been taking) in an effort to lose weight, either prescription diet medication or over the counter weight reduction aids. Also ask about the use of drugs that can alter the fluid balance, such as the use of diuretics and laxatives.

- SOCIAL HISTORY: I'd check:

  – Smoking, number a day and for how many years

  – Alcohol consumption, number of units a week

  – Exercise (poor or increased levels of mobility)

  – Occupation

  – Factors including work, family and social life that may be contributing to increased levels of stress and anxiety, ie psychological factors

  – Recent major life events, such as death of a family member

  – Marital status

  – Accommodation type

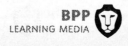

- FAMILY HISTORY: Is there any history of first-degree relatives with any inherited gastrointestinal or neurological disorders?

- SYSTEMS REVIEW: I would perform a systems review:
  - Cardiovascular
  - Respiratory
  - Metabolic
  - Urogenital
  - Central and peripheral nervous system
  - Musculoskeletal

- Poor appetite along with conditions that restrict or prevent food consumption eg dysphagia, odynophagia, loss of teeth, mouth sores.

- Malabsorption syndromes eg coeliac disease, inflammatory bowel disease (Crohn's disease or ulcerative colitis), chronic pancreatitis.

- Malignancy eg gastric cancer, lung cancer, lymphoma, leukaemia, sarcoma.

- Systemic disease eg cardiac failure, chronic respiratory disease (such as bronchitis or emphysema), chronic renal failure, rheumatoid arthritis, systemic lupus erythematosus.

- Endocrine disorders eg diabetes mellitus, Addison's disease, hyperthyroidism.

- Acute infections.

- Chronic infections eg HIV and TB.

- Psychological disorders eg anorexia nervosa, depression.

Table 1.13: Differential diagnosis of weight loss

Key points

- Be particularly suspicious of a diagnosis of some type of malignancy if you are faced with a weight loss scenario in your OSCE, particularly when this occurs in an elderly patient with poor appetite.

- This scenario also often occurs with patients having some kind of psychological disorder – watch out for the young girl with anorexia nervosa or some kind of depressive illness!

- If there is an infective element to the weight loss, consider HIV and TB high amongst your differentials.

History taking 19:   Level: *

Vision loss

You are a FY2 doctor in A&E; Mr Mannering is a 77-year-old male who has presented to hospital with transient visual loss.

Please take a history from him, with a view to making a diagnosis.

RESPONSE:

- INTRODUCTION: To begin with I would introduce myself. Check I am speaking to the right patient by verifying his name and date of birth. At this stage I would try to establish a rapport and make him feel at ease.

- PERSONAL DETAILS: In addition to his name and age, I would identify his occupation (or most recent occupation before retiring), hand dominance (whether they are left or right- handed) and ethnic origin.

- PRESENTING COMPLAINT (PC): In his own words, I would invite him to let me know what has brought him into hospital today.

- HISTORY OF PRESENTING COMPLAINT (HPC): This relates to asking direct and specific questions about the PC.

   – Onset: When did you first notice the visual loss, did it come on suddenly or gradually and what were you doing at that time?

   – Predisposing factors: Is there any event(s) that could have led to the visual loss, eg a stroke, malignancy, trauma or recent infection?

   – Duration: Have you had this problem for a long time (chronic) or only noticed it recently (acute problem)?

   – Frequency: Is the visual loss episodic or continuous in nature when it occurs?

   – Progressiveness: Is it improving or getting worse?

   – Relieving factors: Have you noticed anything that improves the visual loss?

   – Aggravating factors: Have you noticed anything that makes it worse?

   – Pain: Are your eyes painful, or do you have any associated headache?

- Aids to vision: Have you needed any specific aids to deal with the visual loss, eg a guide dog or braille?

- Characteristics associated with the visual loss:

  - photophobia
  - diplopia (double vision)
  - blurring of vision
  - any associated floaters, specks or halos noted

- What investigations or treatment methods have been performed up to now?

- PAST MEDICAL HISTORY: I would go through my checklist, using the mnemonic MJ THREADS.

- DRUG HISTORY AND ALLERGIES: Some drugs are known to have been implicated in visual loss or disturbance of vision, these include:

  - Antiarrhythmia drugs, such as digoxin and amiodarone

  - Corticosteroids, such as prednisolone

  - Tamsulosin (an alpha blocker used in the treatment of benign prostatic hypertrophy)

  - Tamoxifen (used in the treatment of breast cancer)

- SOCIAL HISTORY: I'd check:

  - Smoking, number a day and for how many years
  - Alcohol consumption, number of units a week
  - Occupation
  - Marital status
  - Type of living accommodation

- FAMILY HISTORY: Is there any history of first degree relatives with visual problems?

- SYSTEMS REVIEW: I would perform a systems review:

  - Cardiovascular
  - Respiratory
  - Gastrointestinal
  - Metabolic
  - Urogenital
  - Central and peripheral nervous system
  - Musculoskeletal

Causes of *sudden* loss of vision

- Amaurosis Fugax
- Central and peripheral retinal artery occlusion
- Central and peripheral vein occlusion
- Temporal arteritis
- Endophthalmitis secondary to bacterial or fugal cause
- Optic neuritis
- Corneal ulcer
- Retinal detachment

Causes of *gradual* loss of vision

- Cataract
- Age-related macular degeneration
- Toxic, drug related
- Late stage glaucoma
- Diabetic retinopathy
- Refractive error

Table 1.14: Differential diagnosis of visual loss

Key points

- Visual loss as an OSCE is often encountered when taking a history in diabetic patients. Retinopathy occurring in patients with long-standing and poorly controlled diabetes.

- Note that some drugs have an increased propensity to causing visual loss or disturbance of vision, these include digoxin, amiodarone, corticosteroids, tamsulosin and tamoxifen.

Further reading

Khaw, P et al (2004) *ABC of Eyes (ABC series)*. 4th edition. Oxford: Wiley-Blackwell.

BPP LEARNING MEDIA

History taking 20:   Level: * *

Swollen knee

Mr State is a 27-year-old male who has come to your clinic with a several-week history of a swollen right knee.

Please take a history from him, with a view to making a diagnosis.

RESPONSE:

- INTRODUCTION: To begin with I would introduce myself. Check I am speaking to the right patient by verifying his name and date of birth. At this stage I would try to establish a rapport and make him feel at ease.

- PERSONAL DETAILS: In addition to his name and age, I would identify his occupation and ethnic origin.

- PRESENTING COMPLAINT (PC): In his own words, I would invite the patient to let me know what has brought him into the clinic today.

- HISTORY OF PRESENTING COMPLAINT (HPC): This relates to asking direct and specific questions about the PC.

    - Onset: When did you first notice the swelling and what were you doing at that time? Did the swelling come on suddenly or gradually?

    - Predisposing factors, eg any history of trauma, also timing between any injury to the onset of swelling?

    - Duration of swelling, is it acute or chronic in nature?

    - Frequency of swelling, is it episodic or continuous?

    - Are there any things you have noticed which aggravate the swelling?

    - Have you noticed anything which relieves the swelling?

    - Since it has occurred, have you noticed any progression in the swelling, namely is it improving or deteriorating?

- What other associated features are present, look out for:

    - fever

    - tenderness and pain

    - joint deformity

    - knee-locking or giving way on movement, implying possibility of meniscal (cartilage) tear

    - restriction in the range of movement, including presence of stiffness.

  - Where there is loss of movement and function in the knee or any other joints, how does it impact on activities of daily living (ADLs), such as walking, exercise, etc?

- Identify what investigations and treatments, if any, have been performed up to this point.

- PAST MEDICAL HISTORY: I would go through my checklist, using the mnemonic MJ THREADS; I would also include features which may also be contributory to general leg swelling:

  - History of traumatic injury and particularly fractures

  - Any musculoskeletal deformity

  - Any previous orthopaedic surgery

  - History of neurological disorders

  - History of haematological disorders, such as clotting abnormalities, haemophilia and sickle-cell disease

  - Previous history of tumours/malignancy; if so, which body systems are affected

  - Any recent infections

- DRUG HISTORY AND ALLERGIES: What analgesics is the patient taking? Is he on antibiotics and is there any history of usage of aspirin, warfarin or any other anticoagulants?

- SOCIAL HISTORY: I'd check:

  - Smoking, number a day and for how many years
  - Alcohol consumption, number of units a week
  - Marital status
  - Occupational history
  - Hobbies, particularly in relation to sports activities

- FAMILY HISTORY: Is there any history of first-degree relatives with neurological, musculoskeletal, or haematological disorders?

- SYSTEMS REVIEW: I would perform a systems review:
    - Cardiovascular
    - Respiratory
    - Gastrointestinal
    - Metabolic
    - Urogenital
    - Central and peripheral nervous system
    - Musculoskeletal

This occurs as a result of fluid or mass accumulation in the knee joint cavity, ie synovial fluid, blood, pus or tumour (as well as the presence of surrounding oedema)

- Infection, eg septic arthritis of the knee

- Arthritis, eg osteoarthritis, rheumatoid arthritis

- Trauma causing haemarthrosis

- Gout and pseudogout

- Cysts

- Tumours eg osteochondroma

- Kneecap bursitis

Table 1.15: Differential diagnosis of knee swelling

Key points

- There are many causes for knee swelling; trauma will often lead to the presence of blood, haemarthrosis, to accumulate into the joint cavity.

- Where there is a suspicion of infection, think about a septic arthritis of the knee.

- Think laterally: it may be that a coagulation abnormality has manifested as a blood clot giving rise to knee swelling.

- Where some time has passed since the onset of symptoms (in a non-traumatic setting) giving rise to knee swelling, this should increase the suspicion of a malignancy.

Further reading

Dorling Kindersley (2010) *The BMA Guide to Sports Injuries.* London: Dorling Kindersley.

History taking 21:   Level: * *

Haematemesis

You are a FY2 doctor in a General Surgery firm. Mr Eaton is a 68-year-old male who has presented to A&E with a recent history of haematemesis (vomiting of blood).

You have been asked by your consultant to see and take a history from him, with a view to making a diagnosis.

RESPONSE:

- **INTRODUCTION:** To begin with, I would introduce myself. Check I am speaking to the right patient by verifying his name and date of birth. At this stage I would try to establish a rapport and make him feel at ease.

- **PERSONAL DETAILS:** In addition to his name and age, I would identify his occupation and ethnic origin.

- **PRESENTING COMPLAINT (PC):** In his own words, I would invite the patient to let me know what has brought him into hospital today.

- **HISTORY OF PRESENTING COMPLAINT (HPC):** This relates to asking direct and specific questions about the PC.

    - Time and onset: When did you first notice the haematemesis, did it come on gradually or was it sudden?

    - Duration: How long has it been going on for (acute or chronic problem?)

    - Frequency: How often does it occur? Identify average number of times over a certain period eg 'two times a day'.

    - Precipitating events: eg anything that you think may have brought this on, such as a history of trauma?

    - Aggravating factors: Have you noticed anything that makes the haematemesis worse, eg drinking alcohol or smoking?

    - Relieving factors: Have you noticed anything that relieves the problem?

    - Progression: Is it getting worse, remaining constant or improving?

- Colour and volume of the vomitus: for example, does it look coffee ground in colour (suggesting bleeding in the oesophagus, stomach or duodenum, ie bleeding proximal to the duodenal-jejunal junction) or bright red, frank blood (eg secondary to a Mallory-Weis tear of the oesophageal lining).

- Colour and volume of stool: Have you noticed any blood mixed with the stool?

- Does it appear:

    - black, 'tarry' in colour (malaena) (this is associated with gastrointestinal haemorrhage)

    - bright red in colour (this is often fresh blood and implies bleeding from the anus or low down in the rectum)

    - darker red (this often occurs when there is bleeding from the colon eg in diverticular disease, or from a bowel tumour)

- Gastrointestinal symptoms:

    - Any abdominal pain?

    - Any tenesmus?

    - Have you noticed any change in your bowel habit recently?

    - Have you noticed any mass, lump over your abdomen, or do you feel your abdomen feels distended?

    - Any history of weight loss?

    - Any history of appetite loss?

    - Any nausea or vomiting?

    - Any history of dysphagia or odynophagia?

    - Any history of indigestion or heartburn?

    - Any history of jaundice?

    - Investigations and treatments to date: Ask what, if any, have been implemented along with the results known.

- PAST MEDICAL HISTORY: I would go through my checklist, using the mnemonic MJ THREADS; in this station it would also be prudent to include:

    - History of abdominal ulcers
    - Liver disease
    - Jaundice

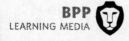

- – Blood clotting (or any other haematological) abnormalities
  - – Any previous surgery
- **DRUG HISTORY AND ALLERGIES:** I would remember to ask about the usage of:
  - – Anticoagulants including aspirin and warfarin
  - – Non-steroidal anti-inflammatory drugs (NSAIDs), as well as other analgesia
- **SOCIAL HISTORY:** I'd check:
  - – Smoking, number a day and for how many years
  - – Alcohol consumption, number of units a week
  - – Occupation
  - – Living accommodation
  - – Marital status
- **FAMILY HISTORY:** Is there any history of first-degree relatives with any inherited gastrointestinal disorders?
- **SYSTEMS REVIEW:** I would perform a systems review:
  - – Cardiovascular
  - – Respiratory
  - – Gastrointestinal
  - – Metabolic
  - – Urogenital
  - – Central and peripheral nervous system
  - – Musculoskeletal

- Mallory-Weiss syndrome: bleeding tears in the lining of the oesophageal mucosa, often secondary to prolonged retching.
- Peptic ulcer or severe peptic ulceration (Zollinger-Ellison Syndrome).
- Vomiting of ingested blood following bleeding into the oral cavity, nose or throat.
- Severe gastroenteritis or gastritis.
- Tumours of the stomach or oesophagus.
- Vascular malformations of the GI tract, eg bleeding gastric varices or intestinal varices.
- Colitis: ulcerative, radiation induced, ischaemic or infective.
- Leukaemia.
- Bleeding disorders such as thrombocytopenia and haemophilia.

Table 1.16: Differential diagnosis of haematemesis

Key points

- Remember that haematemesis can occur secondary to a wide spectrum of gastrointestinal pathology, in the acute setting it can be very severe indeed and even life-threatening.

- Bleeding disorders can manifest as haematemesis. In your list of subsequent investigations, tell the examiner you would perform a full set of blood tests including FBC, clotting screen, LFTS (and Us & Es) and also request a group and save.

- Less commonly, this can be a manifestation of a malignant disorder; remember to ask about the general features that might suggest this, such as recent weight loss, change in appetite and bowel habit.

Further reading

Logan, R et al (2002) *ABC of the Upper Gastrointestinal Tract (ABC Series)*. Oxford: Wiley-Blackwell.

BPP
LEARNING MEDIA

History taking 22:

Level: * *

Leg ulcers

Mr Gupta is a 68-year-old male presenting to the outpatient clinic as a referral from his GP with a history of leg ulceration. As the FY2 medical trainee, you have been asked by your consultant to see him.

Please take a history from him, with a view to making a diagnosis.

RESPONSE:

- INTRODUCTION: To begin with I would introduce myself. Check I am speaking to the right patient by verifying his name and date of birth. At this stage I would try to establish a rapport and make him feel at ease.

- PERSONAL DETAILS: In addition to their name and age, I would identify his occupation and ethnic origin.

- PRESENTING COMPLAINT (PC): In his own words, I would invite the patient to let me know what has brought him into the clinic today.

- HISTORY OF PRESENTING COMPLAINT (HPC): This relates to asking direct and specific questions about the PC.

    – Onset: When did you first notice the leg ulcers and what were you doing at that time? Did the ulceration come on suddenly or gradually?

    – Predisposing factors, eg any history of trauma?

    – Duration of the ulceration, is it acute or chronic in nature?

    – Are there any things you have noticed which aggravate the problem?

    – Have you noticed anything which relieves the problem?

    – Since it has occurred, have you noticed any progression, namely is it improving or deteriorating?

    – Have you noticed ulcers anywhere else on your body?

    – Do they come and go, namely have you noticed periods where they have healed?

- Dressing of ulcers, what are you using to dress the ulcers (if applicable), who is responsible for this and how frequently are they being changed?

- How does the ulceration impact on the activities of daily living?

- What other associated symptoms are present, look out for:
  - fever
  - pain
  - swelling
  - discharge

- What investigations and treatments have you had to date?

- PAST MEDICAL HISTORY: I would go through my checklist, using the mnemonic MJ THREADS; I would also include features which may also be contributory to leg ulcers:

  - History of atherosclerotic disease, Buerger's disease, vasculitis and renal failure which can be contributory to arterial ulcers

  - Varicose veins or deep vein thrombosis associated with venous ulcers

  - Peripheral neuropathy, diabetes or syphilis in neuropathic ulcers

  - Malignant melanoma, basal carcinoma, squamous cell carcinoma, Marjolin's ulcer or Bowen's disease, all possible contributory factors in neoplastic ulcers

  - Tuberculosis, sarcoidosis or pyoderma gangrenosum in infective ulceration.

- DRUG HISTORY AND ALLERGIES: Does the patient require analgesics, if so which ones are they using?

- SOCIAL HISTORY: I'd check:

  - Smoking, number a day and for how many years
  - Alcohol consumption, number of units a week
  - Marital status
  - Type of living accommodation
  - Occupational history

- FAMILY HISTORY: Is there any history of first-degree relatives with vascular or musculoskeletal disease?

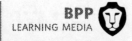

- SYSTEMS REVIEW: I would perform a systems review:

  - Cardiovascular
  - Respiratory
  - Gastrointestinal
  - Metabolic
  - Urogenital
  - Central and peripheral nervous system
  - Musculoskeletal

- Venous ulcers
- Arterial (ischaemic) ulcers
- Neuropathic ulcers
- Neoplastic ulcers
- Infective ulcers
- Hypertensive ulcers
- Pyoderma gangrenosum.

Table 1.17: Differential diagnosis of leg ulceration

Key points

- There are many aetiologies associated with leg ulceration, have a systematic method for a thorough history to pick up clues to the likely cause.

- The most common type of leg ulcers are venous ulcers, remember to consider a past or present history of varicose veins and deep vein thrombosis.

Further reading

Donnelly, R and London, N (2009) *ABC of Arterial and Venous Disease (ABC series).* 2nd edition. Oxford: Wiley-Blackwell.

History taking 23: Level: *

Per vaginal bleeding

Miss Cohen is a 37-year-old female presenting to the gynaecology ward with a recent history of vaginal bleeding; as the foundation trainee, you have been asked to take a history from her.

RESPONSE:

- INTRODUCTION: To begin with I would introduce myself. Check I am speaking to the right patient by verifying her name and date of birth. At this stage I would try to establish a rapport and make her feel at ease. I would sit directly opposite her, ensure good eye contact and explain that I am going to take a history.

- PERSONAL DETAILS: In addition to her name and age, I would also identify her occupation and ethnic origin.

- PRESENTING COMPLAINT (PC): In her own words, I would invite the patient to let me know what has brought her to the ward today.

- HISTORY OF PRESENTING COMPLAINT (HPC): This relates to asking direct and specific questions about the PC.

    - Onset: When did you first notice the bleeding, did it come on suddenly or gradually?

    - Duration: Has this been going for a while or is it a more recent problem, ie is the bleeding acute or chronic?

    - Frequency and timing of per vaginal bleeding (eg does it occur post-coital or intermenstrual)?

    - Volume of bleeding each time (rough estimation), including clot formation?

    - Progression: is it improving, worsening or constant?

    - Are there any predisposing events you can think of?

    - Are there any things you have noticed which aggravate the problem?

    - Have you noticed anything which relieves the problem?

    - Look out for symptoms associated with blood loss, such as breathlessness, dyspnoea, lethargy, palpitations and anaemia.

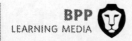

- Look out for symptoms associated with hypotension, such as headache, faints, fits and 'funny turns', numbness, other sensory disturbances, muscle weakness or transient paralysis.

- Look out for symptoms associated with infection, such as night sweats, fever and rigors, dysuria, productive cough and diarrhoea.

- Look for symptoms associated with malignancy such as change in bowel habit, loss of appetite and weight loss.

- How does the problem affect your activities of daily living (ADLs)?

- Have you had any investigations or treatments performed up until now?

- SPECIFIC QUESTIONS FOR A GYNAECOLOGICAL HISTORY:

  - Date of the last menstrual period (LMP)?

  - In this case the patient is 37 years old, so is unlikely to be post-menopausal, but always bear in mind this is a possibility; ask if this is the case, and if so, at what age did the menopause commence?

  - Any history of post-menopausal bleeding?

  - Is there a history of painful periods (menses), aka dysmenorrhoea?

  - Is your menstrual cycle regular or irregular; accordingly, what is the frequency and duration of menses?

  - Are your menses heavy (menorrhagia), or light? (This can be gauged by asking the number of tampons or pads used, or the number of clots passed)

  - Is there any history of vaginal discharge; if so, what colour is the vaginal discharge? Is it clear, purulent or bloodstained. Is it odorous?

  - Have you had any cervical smears, and if so, when was the last and what was the result of the previous tests?

  - Sexual history, including contraceptive use:

    - number of sexual partners, is there any pain on intercourse, aka dyspareunia

    - methods of contraception currently and previously

    - do you have any children, what age did you have your first child?

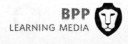

- GENITO-URINARY HISTORY: this will follow hand-in-hand with the gynaecology history:

    – Is there pain on micturition; if so, does it occur during or after voiding?

    – Frequency of micturition, is there any nocturia (waking up at night to pass urine)?

    – Is there any history of urinary incontinence; if so, is it stress or urge incontinence?

    – Any history of blood in the urine, aka haematuria?

    – Any pain on micturition, aka dysuria?

    – Any history of vaginal prolapse?

- OBSTETRIC HISTORY:

    – How many children do you have?

    – How many pregnancies; any history of abortions or miscarriages?

    – Were the deliveries all normal vaginal; if not, how were your children delivered?

    – Any complications during the pregnancy or labour either to child or mother?

- PAST MEDICAL HISTORY: I would go through my checklist, using the mnemonic MJ THREADS; I would also ask about:

    – History of previous hospital admissions

    – Any previous gynaecological or other surgical operations performed

    – Any haematological/coagulation abnormalities

    – Any background of thyroid disorder

- DRUG HISTORY AND ALLERGIES: Specifically ask if the patient is taking:

    – Contraception, either in the form of an oral contraceptive pill, a depot injection or a fitted coil (eg Mirena).

    – Any hormone replacement therapy (HRT)

    – Any anticoagulants

- **SOCIAL HISTORY:** I'd check:

    – Smoking, number a day and for how many years
    – Alcohol consumption, number of units a week
    – Marital status
    – Type of living accommodation

- **FAMILY HISTORY:** Is there any history of first-degree relatives with gynaecological disorders including gynaecological cancers including breast, ovaries and endometrial?

- **SYSTEMS REVIEW:** I would perform a systems review:

    – Cardiovascular
    – Respiratory
    – Gastrointestinal
    – Metabolic
    – Central and peripheral nervous system
    – Musculoskeletal

- **Traumatic causes:** Uterine cervix laceration or tear, abortion – criminal or traumatically induced.

- **Neoplastic causes:** Cervical carcinoma, adenocarcinoma of the uterus or vagina, choriocarcinoma.

- **General causes:** Coagulation disorders, eg von Willebrand's disease, thyroid abnormalities or use of anticoagulant medication.

- **Anatomic and structural disorders:** Ectopic pregnancy as well as ectopic pregnancy haemorrhage, placenta praevia, uterine fibroids and polyps, endometriosis.

Table 1.18: Differential diagnosis of per vaginal bleeding

Key points

- Be aware of the systemic symptoms and signs associated with blood loss per se including features associated with hypotension.

- You will be also assessed on how tactful you are when taking your history; however, do not shy away from asking pertinent questions relating to problems with menses, post-coital bleeding and sexual history.

- This scenario can lead to discussion on a variety of topics ranging from specific coagulation disorders, thyroid abnormalities and gynaecological cancers.

Further reading

Bain, C et al (2011) *Gynaecology Illustrated.* 6th edition. Oxford: Churchill Livingstone.

History taking 24:   Level: * *

Psychiatry history

Miss Willetts is a 43-year-old female presenting to the psychiatry outpatient department as a referral from her GP with a several-month history of generalised low mood.

As the foundation trainee you have been asked to assess her.

QUESTION A:

Please perform a psychiatric assessment of her, with a view to making a diagnosis.

RESPONSE A:

- I would divide my psychiatric assessment of the patient in to a few individual sections: history taking, performing a mental state examination, assessing a patient's clinical risk of self-harm including suicide and devising a management plan.

- INTRODUCTION: To begin with I would introduce myself. Check I am speaking to the right patient by verifying her name and date of birth. At this stage I would try to establish a rapport and make her feel at ease. I would sit directly opposite her, ensure good eye contact and explain that I am going to take a history.

- PERSONAL DETAILS: In addition to her name and age, I would also identify her occupation and ethnic origin.

- PRESENTING COMPLAINT (PC): In her own words, I would invite the patient to let me know what has brought her to the clinic today.

- HISTORY OF PRESENTING COMPLAINT (HPC): This relates to asking direct and specific questions about the PC.

    - Onset: When did you first notice the symptoms, did they come on suddenly or gradually?

    - Duration: Has this been going for a while or is it a short-lived concern, ie is the problem acute or chronic?

    - Progression over time: Are the symptoms improving or deteriorating?

    - Are there any precipitating factors (eg life events such as recent break-up with a partner/spouse, unemployment, death in the family etc)?

- How do the symptoms impact on your daily life including activities of daily living?

- Associated symptoms, Do you have any:

  - suicidal thoughts, any actions taken or plans made
  - depression
  - mania
  - psychosis (such as hallucinations or delusions)

- Do you use any recreational drugs?

- Risk factors during childhood development. While growing up are you aware of, or can you recall:

  - parental neglect

  - did you suffer any abuse, physical emotional or sexual

  - any developmental delay

  - behavioural problems

  - poor relationships with your peers leading to bullying

- Risk factors during the neonatal period. Has your mother or anyone related to you told you about:

  - problems during childbirth, such as any trauma

  - prenatal problems

  - genetic factors

  - a history of any medical problems that runs in the family?

- Have you noticed anything which relieves the problem?

- Are there any things you have noticed which aggravate the problem?

- Have you had any investigations or treatments performed up until now?

- Could you tell me if you are under the care of any doctor responsible for managing your mental health? If so, what is their name?

- PAST PSYCHIATRIC HISTORY: (also include medical and surgical history)

  - Note all previous episodes, their date, duration, nature of the concern and treatment received.

- – Any hospital admissions, if so, were they voluntary or involuntary sectioning under the Mental Health Act?
- – I would go through my checklist to identify any past medical history, using the mnemonic MJ THREADS.
- – Any previous surgical operations performed?

- DRUG HISTORY AND ALLERGIES: Note any:
  - – Medication, prescription and non-prescription drugs along with dosage
  - – Duration of treatment
  - – Allergies
  - – Recreational drug usage

- SOCIAL HISTORY:
  - – Smoking, number a day and for how many years
  - – Alcohol consumption, number of units a week
  - – Marital status and sexual history
  - – Occupation and financial concerns
  - – Accommodation type, and who else lives there
  - – Members of social network (family and friends)
  - – External support structure (social worker, mental health liaison nurse)

- FAMILY HISTORY: Is there any history of first-degree relatives with psychiatric problems such as schizophrenia, depression or mania?

- PREMORBID PERSONALITY TRAITS:
  - – Premorbid character: Any history of criminal behaviour/ trouble with the law?
  - – General interests suggesting perverse behaviour?

ASSESSMENT OF MENTAL STATE: Assess the state of the mind of the patient at the time of the assessment (perform in conjunction with scenario on mini-mental state examination to assess cognitive state).

OBSERVATION: Appearance, Behaviour and Activity

- – Appearance: Inspect the patient's clothes, is she well and appropriately dressed or are there signs of self-neglect (unkempt appearance) and inappropriate dress? (Observe the patient's posture and facial expression.)

- Behaviour: Is the patient behaving, does she appear withdrawn and apathetic. Does she look irritable or agitated?

- Activity: Does she appear overactive or underactive? Is she fidgety and restless? Does she appear tearful?

SPEECH: Articulation, Rate and Tone

- Articulation: Are there any problems with speech articulation, ie dysarthria?

- Rate: Does the speech appear slow and with long pauses showing retardation or does it appear pressured and accelerated?

- Tone & volume: Are words and sentences monotonous or spontaneous? Is the volume of speech increased and incoherent (flight of ideas) or is there restricted speech (poverty of speech)?

AFFECT (objective and subjective) AND MOOD:

- Objectively how does the patient's mood appear? Is it blunt or flat, does she appear depressed, anxious or angry?

- Subjectively: How do you feel? Is your mood low, or do you feel high and excited?

- Biological: Have you noticed any recent change (increase or decrease) in your appetite, weight, sleep pattern or sexual desire?

- Anxiety: Do you feel anxious? Have you experienced any recent panic attacks, any palpitations, feeling sweaty, headaches, or feeling of pins and needles in your arms or legs?

- Cognitive: How do you view your situation? Do you feel hopeless and helpless? How do you view yourself? Do you feel worthless, have low self-esteem? Do you feel happy and on top of the world?

SUICIDAL INTENT: Assessment of risk:

- Ideas: Have you ever thought about killing yourself?

- Intent: Did you ever plan it out?

- Previous attempts & self-harm: Have you ever previously attempted to take your own life? Have you ever previously harmed yourself?

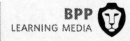

Classify the level of suicidal risk as:

- High
- Medium
- Low

- Male patient

- Old age (>75 years old)

- Previous attempts

- History of self harm

- History of mental illness

- Divorced, single or widowed

- Socially isolated

- Recent bereavement

- Living in a city

- Unemployment

- Physical illness (resulting in chronic pain and disability, or life-threatening/terminal illness).

Table 1.19: Factors associated with a higher suicidal risk

THOUGHT CONTENT AND PERCEPTIONS:

- Ideas: Are there any ideas which pre-occupy your head and that you can't stop constantly thinking about?

- Phobias: Are there any circumstances, places or objects that you would rather not be near to or in the presence of? When you are in their presence does it cause you to have panic attacks or experience palpitations?

- Obsessions: Are there any actions which you find yourself repeating throughout the day? This can include activities such as constantly checking, cleaning, counting or dressing. What is the impact of this on your activities of daily living (ADLs)? Obsessional thoughts are intrusive and repetitive thoughts.

- Delusions: Do you feel you have special powers? Do you think you are a god? (Delusions of grandeur). Do you get the feeling that people are talking to you from the TV or radio? Delusions are false beliefs that are firmly held by the patient, even in the face of clear evidence to the contrary?

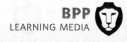

- Hallucinations: A hallucination is a perception that occurs in the absence of a stimulus. Hallucinations can occur in any sensory modality, visual, olfactory, auditory, gustatory or tactile. Ask the patient, 'Do you hear voices from persons that you cannot see or from objects?'. Where there are auditory hallucinations, ask the number of voices heard and if they are in the 1st, 2nd or 3rd person (eg I …; You …; He/she …)

- Self-awareness: How do you feel about yourself and the world around you? When you look in the mirror, does it ever appear to you that you are not connected to the person you see (depersonalisation). Or do you ever feel that you are detached from the world around you (derealisation)?

QUESTION B:

What factors do you need to consider when devising a management plan for patients with mental health disorders?

RESPONSE B:

- At this stage I should have some indication of a differential diagnosis which can be broadly divided in to a functional or organic mental illness or a personality disorder or clinical medical disorder. Some overlap may exist.

- I would need to address any acute medical issues, including dealing with high-risk suicidal intent. The patient will also need a psychological assessment.

- An important component of their management is to identify if the patient has insight into their condition, so I would ask 'Miss Willetts, can I ask whether you think you have a problem? Would it be OK to start you on some medication if this was found to be appropriate?'

- Social circumstances which are contributing to the patient's symptoms will need to be identified as well as methods to help deal with them.

- Define appropriate places of consultation and treatment: patients may need to be seen on an outpatient basis, others may require a short inpatient stay, while others may need to be referred to specialist psychiatry hospitals.

- Define the key members of the MDT who can help to play a role in the patient's care. These will include psychiatrists, psychiatric nurses, clinical psychologists, psychotherapists, counsellors, social workers, occupational therapists, mental health liaison nurses and community psychiatric nurses (CPNs).

Key points

- Divide a psychiatric assessment of a patient into a few individual sections: history taking, performing a mental state examination, assessing a patient's clinical risk of suicide and devising a management plan.

- Identify if a patient has insight into their condition.

- Be able to define some of the more common terms used in a psychiatric assessment, namely phobia, obsession, delusion and hallucination.

- The assessment and care of a psychiatric patient requires a multidisciplinary approach with several key members, so be able to list some of those involved.

Chapter 2

Examination skills

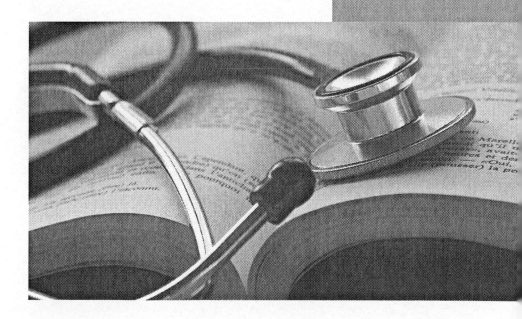

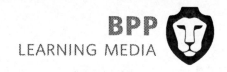
BPP
LEARNING MEDIA

Examination skills 1:

Examination of the knee

Level: * *

Mr Smith has come to your clinic complaining of a problem with his right knee.

Please examine his knees.

RESPONSE:

I would initially introduce myself to the patient and seek his consent to perform a knee examination. I would begin my examination with an inspection of both knees whilst he is standing, with his lower limbs exposed and undergarments on.

INSPECTION

I would inspect the patient from the front and side on.

- Is there any muscle wasting – particularly over the quadriceps?

- Are there any swellings – is it generalised, maybe indicating recent trauma; or is it localised, which could be suggestive of a bursa – or possibly a Baker's cyst if over the popliteal fossa.

- Are there any scars? Look for arthroscopic portal scars – placed laterally. Long, midline scars could indicate anterior cruciate ligament reconstruction or a knee replacement.

- Are there any obvious deformities detected on stance, eg 'bow legs' (genu valgus) or 'knock knees' (genu varus).

PALPATION

I would ask the patient to lie down on the examination table; at the same time, I would ask if the knee was hurting.

This may not only provide a clue to the diagnosis but, equally importantly, the examiner will be looking to ensure you take the patient's comfort into consideration whilst performing the exam.

- Wasting: Initially assess for quadriceps wasting by taking a tape measure in my hand and measuring the thigh circumference at a set distance (eg 10cm) above the patella, comparing both sides.

- Temperature: With the back of my hand, I would feel for warmth, sliding my hands over the anterior surface of both legs, proximal to distal.

- Tenderness: Note if this is localised or generalised.

- Effusion: This will be obvious if a large effusion is present. However some tests can be performed to help ascertain the presence of an effusion:

  - Patellar tap (for a moderate quantity of fluid): With my left hand on the thigh, just above the patella, I would push distally towards the foot; then, with the index finger of my right hand, I would push the patella proximally against the femoral condyles. In this way I am 'tapping' the patella against the proximal femur and feeling it bounce off.

  - Bulge test (for a small quantity of fluid): I would stroke the medial aspect of the joint to empty it. Then, keeping my eye on the medial side I would stroke the lateral aspect of the joint, the presence of excess fluid would produce a 'bulge' as fluid passes back into the medial side.

MOVEMENT

- I would ask the patient to press his thigh firmly against the table, noting if there is any hyperextension – if there is nil, then the limb is held at 0° extension. Similarly if the knee is flexed, I would estimate the angle of flexion and tell the examiner, eg 'the limb is held at 20° flexion.'

- I'd now assess the degree of flexion the patient can produce actively: 'Can you bend your knee? Slide your heel as far back as you are able.' (This is usually approximately 140°). Whilst the patient is performing this movement, I would place my hand over the knee and note any crepitus.

- I'd passively move the joint through its complete range of flexion and extension, without causing any pain or distress.

Special tests

- Cruciate ligaments

  - Anterior drawer test: The patient should have his knee flexed to 90° with quadriceps and hamstrings relaxed; you can sit on the foot to stabilise it – however, make sure the patient has no foot pain beforehand! Now using both hands, grasp the upper aspect of the shin just below the patella and with thumbs lying over the anterior surface. Pull the upper end of the tibia towards you. A positive 'anterior drawer' occurs when the tibia moves forward: this indicates an injury to the anterior cruciate ligament.

- Posterior sag: Whilst the knees are flexed to 90° with the feet firmly flat on the couch, examine the joints from a side view. If there is a 'sag' or drop of the upper end of the tibia, when compared with the opposite 'normal' side, this would indicate an injury to the posterior cruciate ligament.

- Collateral ligaments

  - Flex the knee to approximately 20° to 30°; grasp the knee with the left hand, with the fingers under the knee. With the other hand, grasp the lower tibia. Gently push in opposite directions. If there is an abnormal range of movement, this would suggest a lateral (or collateral) ligament injury.

The examination of the knee and hip are very commonly associated with patients who have osteoarthritis – hence you should be able to comment on symptoms and signs of this condition.

You may find that the joint appears swollen; this could be due to an effusion, haemarthrosis (less likely in the examination setting as this usually implies a recent trauma), or possibly a space-occupying lesion (eg excess bone formation, which restricts movement). In osteoarthritis, you may also find that the patient has a fixed flexion deformity (an inability to completely straighten the limb), the movements often being very painful. Be gentle and use the patient's verbal and non-verbal cues to identify how much active movement is possible.

At the end of your examination

Say that you would like to:

- Ask the patient questions relating to how his restriction in movement and pain is affecting his activities of daily living, with respect to his work, social life, night pain and ability to sleep etc.

- Assess the neurovascular status of the limb.

- Examine the hip and ankle joint. *With any joint examination it is imperative to get into the habit of always examining the joint above and below the joint of interest – pathology can be found at other closely related sites.*

Another common question is to be asked to state the radiographic findings in a patient with osteoarthritis.

Note the mnemonic **SCOL** *to remember the radiological features of osteoarthritis:*

Subchondral sclerosis at the joint margins
Cysts (bone cysts) close to the joint margins
Osteophyte formation
Loss of joint space

Key points

- Divide the examination of the knee into inspection, palpation, movement and special tests.

- To identify an effusion, carry out a patellar tap or bulge test.

- At the end of the examination get into the habit of stating you would examine the joint above (hip, in this case) and joint below (ankle, in this case).

Examination skills 2:   Level: * * *

Examination of a patient with a neck lump

Mr Jones has come to your clinic complaining of a lump in his neck, he has noticed this gradually getting larger over the previous 3 to 4 months.

Please examine his neck with a view to identifying the nature of this lump.

RESPONSE:

I would commence the examination by asking him to undo the top buttons of his shirt, so as to expose the neck adequately. I can now ask Mr Jones to sit on a chair and inspect his neck.

INSPECTION

I would inspect the patient by looking at the neck lump directly from the front and also from the side. I would state what I saw.

- 'There is a moderately sized lump measuring between 4 to 5cm in diameter on the anterior aspect of the neck in the midline'.

- I would comment on the presence (or absence) of scars, which would indicate previous surgery.

- I'd give him a glass of water, asking him to swallow. 'I notice that as he drinks, the lump rises on swallowing.'

- I'd ask him to open his mouth and stick his tongue out as far as possible, and observe the lump to see if it moves.

At this stage I should be able to make a comment about my findings. 'It is likely that from the position of the lump it is related to the thyroid gland. The most likely pathology is either a goitre or a thyroglossal cyst, as these are the only structures which would rise on swallowing. This is due to their attachment to the larynx.'

Note that if the lump moves on protrusion of the tongue, it is likely to be a thyroglossal cyst; this is due to the cyst being connected to the base of the tongue via a fibrous track which runs through the central portion of the hyoid bone.

PALPATION

I would ask the patient if the lump is tender; most likely they will say 'no', allowing me to proceed to palpation. Should the patient say it is painful, then it would be appropriate to make a comment like, 'Please let me know if I cause you any pain as I palpate the lump; I will try to be as gentle as possible'. I would then approach the patient from behind.

- Standing behind the patient, palpate the thyroid gland using fingers of both hands. Palpate both lobes as well as the isthmus (the central connecting structure) in a systematic fashion.

- Give the patient the glass of water and repeat the assessment as he swallows.

- Palpate the triangles of the neck and supraclavicular fossae to look for cervical lymphadenopathy, which could indicate metastatic disease.

On palpation I should be able to comment on certain features of the lump identified, namely:

- **Size**: Its estimated diameter, also noting the position of its lower border; a goitre may show retrosternal extension.

- **Shape**: Is it uniform and smooth, or does it show irregular or nodular enlargement?

- **Mobility**: A fixed, non-mobile gland would suggest a metastatic lesion.

- **Consistency**: A stony hard nodule is a further indication of carcinoma. A goitre, however, often appears firm but not hard.

- **Tenderness**: A tender nodule is often indicative of an inflammatory process, thyroiditis.

PERCUSSION

Following palpation, I would percuss the manubrium, to identify retrosternal goitre extension.

AUSCULTATION

Using my stethoscope, I would auscultate the lump to listen for any audible bruits. This may be heard in hyperthyroid states and is a sign suggesting an increased blood supply to this region.

Key points

- Ensure you have adequate exposure of the neck, allowing you to comment on the lump, and describing its appearance.

- Remember to ask the patient to open their mouth and stick the tongue out as far as possible.

- Comment on the movement of the lump as the patient swallows some water.

- Whilst standing behind the patient, palpate the lump in a systematic manner, commenting on your findings.

- Palpation also involves examining for any lymphadenopathy.

- Percuss to identify retrosternal extension and auscultate for bruits.

Further reading

This station should be read in conjunction with History taking 9: Thyroid disease in Chapter 1.

Ludman, H and Bradley, P (2012) *ABC of Ear, Nose and Throat (ABC series)*. 6th edition. Oxford: Wiley-Blackwell.

Examination skills 3: Clinical examination
Level: * *

Neurological: Motor examination of the lower limbs

 Mr Grant has come to your clinic complaining of pain in his legs on walking.

QUESTION A:

Please perform a motor system examination of his lower limbs.

RESPONSE A:

I would like to begin by carrying out a general inspection of his lower limbs, whilst he is standing with his lower limbs exposed and undergarments on.

INSPECTION/POSITION

I would inspect the patient standing (if they are physically capable) from the front and side on. I would look for:

- Muscle wasting/atrophy proximally or distally
- Muscle hypertrophy
- Asymmetry/deformity
- Fasciculation, this may be normal in the calf
- Evidence of foot deformity, for example, pes cavus, suggesting a Friedreich's ataxia
- Abnormal positioning of the legs or feet, for example, the presence of foot plantar flexion, indicating a foot drop.

Tone

Ask the patient to relax. Flex and extend each leg at the knee joint, noting any resistance.

Alternately roll each leg from side to side at the thigh. Now, suddenly lift the thigh from below; observe the response in the lower leg. The presence of increased tone causes the leg to raise upwards from the bed.

Assess for clonus: Apply a sudden and sustained dorsiflexion to the foot at the ankle joint (bend the foot upwards towards the head); the presence of a few oscillations may occur in a normal patient, however, when this is prolonged it is further indicative of increased tone.

Power

As you assess each movement in turn you must be aware of the main muscles and myotomes moving these joints.

For each lower limb movement, the main myotomes involved in each movement are highlighted in bold.

MOVEMENT	MUSCLES	MYOTOMES	NERVE
Hip flexion	Iliopsoas	**L1, L2,** L3	Femoral
Hip extension	Gluteus maximus	**L5, S1,** S2	Inferior gluteal
Hip abduction	Gluteus medius, Gluteus minimus, tensor fasciae latae	**L4, L5,** S1	Superior gluteal
Hip adduction	Adductors	**L2, L3,** L4	Obturator
Knee flexion	Hamstrings	L5, **S1,** S2	Sciatic
Knee extension	Quadriceps	L2, **L3, L4**	Femoral
Dorsiflexion of foot	Tibialis anterior	**L4,** L5	Deep peroneal
Dorsiflexion of big toe	Extensor hallucis longus	**L5,** S1	Deep peroneal
Plantarflexion of foot	Gastrocnemius, soleus	**S1, S2**	Tibial
Inversion	Tibialis posterior	**L4, L5**	Tibial
Eversion	Peroneus longus & brevis	**L5, S1**	Superficial peroneal

Table 2.1: Lower limb muscles, nerve supply and myotomes.

Reflexes

Knee jerk: L3,L4 roots

With the patient's leg relaxed, by hanging it over the edge of the bed or by resting it over your arm, tap the patellar tendon just below the patella with the hammer. Observe for quadriceps contraction; note any exaggerated response.

Ankle jerk: L5,S1 roots

Externally rotate the patient's leg; flex the knee and hold the foot in slight dorsiflexion. With the hammer, tap the Achilles tendon; look for calf muscle contraction and plantarflexion.

Plantar response:

Ensure the big toe is relaxed. Tell the patient you are going to 'scrape' the sole of his foot. With the sharp end of a tendon hammer, stroke the lateral aspect of the sole from the heel towards the fifth toe, and then across the forefoot towards the big toe. Watch the first movement of the big toe.

- The normal response is for the big toe and the others to show plantarflexion (bend downwards towards the bed)

- The abnormal response is to see big toe extension (dorsiflexion) and the other toes to fan. Extension occurs due to contraction of the extensor hallucis longus muscle. This is known as a 'Babinski' reflex and indicates an upper motor neuron lesion.

QUESTION B:

Do you know of any methods to enhance the knee or ankle reflexes, should you be unable to elicit them easily?

RESPONSE B:

Yes, they may be enhanced by asking the patient to clench the teeth, or to try to pull clasped hands apart when you are about to strike the hammer onto the tendon. This is known as reinforcement and has also been described as Jendrassik's manoeuvre.

Co-ordination

Heel shin: Ask the patient to put the heel of his right leg onto the knee of the left leg and run it down the shin to the big toe and back up again. Now ask him to do the same on the opposite side. Look for any inco-ordination of movement, also known as ataxia.

At the end of your examination

Say that you would like to:

- Perform Romberg's test to assess for sensory ataxia. Ask the patient to stand up, arms by his side and with heels together. Stand behind him and ask him to keep his eyes open, then to maintain his position with his eyes closed.

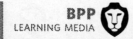

At each stage look for an exaggerated postural swaying or imbalance of movement. If this occurs only whilst the eyes are open, this would indicate a cerebellar deficit (cerebellar ataxia). However, if this was to occur only when the eyes are closed, it can be described as a 'positive' Romberg's test, indicating a proprioceptive deficit, or posterior column deficit (sensory ataxia).

- Assess his gait by asking him to walk in a straight line, as he would do normally. Abnormal gaits can include:

  - A wide-based posture, with evidence of swaying with the eyes open; he may need to hold on to things as he is walking. This would indicate cerebellar disease.

  - A high-stepping gait; on walking, the patient lifts the affected leg so that the toes clear the ground as he brings the leg through. This would indicate a foot drop, implying possible injury to the common (or deep) peroneal nerve on that side.

If he adopts a flexed posture, with loss of arm swing, and has small, shuffling steps, initiates walking by leaning forward and then speeds up (festinates) in an effort to 'catch up' on himself, this would suggest Parkinson's disease, the patient having a Parkinsonian (festinating) gait.

Key points

- The examination of the motor system in the legs requires good understanding of the anatomy of the lower limb to be interpreted adequately.

- Have your own systematic method and order to perform the examination. We suggest:

  1. Inspection

  2. Tone, including clonus

  3. Power, assess by performing the whole range of movements described

  4. Reflexes

  5. Co-ordination

  6. Gait

- Note the method of reinforcement when reflexes are not easily produced.

Examination skills 4:   Level: * *

Neurological: Motor examination of the upper limbs

Mr James is a 57-year-old male who has come to your clinic with some arm weakness.

Please perform a motor system examination of his upper limbs.

RESPONSE:

I would commence my examination by carrying out a general inspection of his upper limbs, with his hands, arms and shoulders exposed.

INSPECTION

I would look for the presence of:

- Muscle wasting/atrophy proximally or distally. Look for wasting over the shoulders and upper arms. Also observe the hands, palmar and dorsal surfaces.

- Muscle hypertrophy

- Asymmetry/deformity

- Abnormal movements such as tremor; is it occurring at rest or could it be an intentional tremor as often occurs in individuals with multiple sclerosis? Observe for chorea, the presence of random jerky movements. Is the patient using only one hand?

- Fasciculation, which are irregular, non-rhythmical contraction of groups of muscle fibres; they tend to increase on exercise and on tapping the muscle surface, for example, over the deltoid muscle. It is often a sign of subacute denervation, as in motor neurone disease. Fasciculation should be distinguished from 'fibrillation', which is excessive activity over a single motor unit; this tends to be visible only with electromyography studies.

- Abnormal posture affecting the upper or lower limbs, or both

Tone

Ensure the patient is relaxed. Tone can be assessed by alternately flexing and extending the elbow and wrist in a random manner. Tone can be described as normal, low or increased. Compare both sides; it is not easy to assess low tone.

Where there is an increase in tone, consider:

- Clasp-knife: The initial resistance to the movement is suddenly overcome; it is best brought about by rapid movements (upper motor neurone lesion).

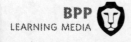

- Lead-pipe (cog-wheel): refers to a steady increase in resistance throughout the movement; it is best brought about by a slow movement (extrapyramidal lesion).

Power

For each upper limb movement, the main myotomes covering each movement are highlighted in bold.

MOVEMENT	MUSCLES	MYOTOMES	NERVE
Shoulder protraction, elevation & lateral rotation	Serratus anterior	**C5, C6, C7**	Long thoracic
Shoulder abduction	Deltoid	**C5**, C6	Axillary
Elbow flexion	Biceps	**C5,C6**	Musculocutaneous
Elbow extension	Triceps	C6, **C7**, C8	Radial
Finger extension	Extensor digitorum	**C7**, C8	Posterior interosseous
Thumb extension	Extensor pollicis longus and brevis	C7, **C8**	Posterior interosseous
Finger flexion	Flexor digitorum profundus I and II	C7, **C8**	Median
Finger flexion	Flexor digitorum profundus III and IV	C7, **C8**	Ulnar
Thumb opposition	Opponens pollicis	C8, **T1**	Median

Table 2.2: Upper limb muscles, nerve supply and myotomes

The extent of weakness can be graded using the MRC (Medical Research Council) scale:

Score 0: No muscle contraction or movement

Score 1: Flicker of muscle movement

Score 2: Active movement with gravity eliminated

Score 3: Active movement against gravity, but not against resistance

Score 4: Active movement against gravity and resistance but not normal

Score 5: Normal power

The way to eliminate gravity is by testing movement in a horizontal plane against a firm surface, for example a table. Make sure to examine both left and right sides, to determine the extent of any weakness.

Reflexes

- Biceps jerk: C5 root: With the patient's arm relaxed and in slight flexion, palpate the biceps tendon with your thumb and strike with the tendon hammer; observe for elbow flexion.

- Supinator jerk: C6 root: Strike the lower end of the radius over the supinator tendon with the hammer; watch for elbow and finger flexion.

- Triceps jerk: C7 root: Strike the triceps tendon just above the elbow; watch for elbow extension and triceps contraction.

Co-ordination

Finger-nose testing: The patient should be standing opposite you, about 50cm away. Point your index finger, away from you and at face level with the patient; ask him to, alternately, touch his nose with his index finger and then touch your index finger as quickly as he can. As the physician, you should move your own hand a little to make it harder for the patient. Now ask the patient to repeat the test with the other hand.

Here you are looking for signs of cerebellar disease; you may notice that the patient has *past pointing* or an *intention tremor*, as the patient's finger approaches your own, it does not home in on its target but shows a jerky tremor movement and overshoots its target (past pointing).

At the end of your examination

Say that you would like to:

- Complete your assessment on co-ordination by also testing for dysdiadochokinesia. This is an impaired ability to perform rapid, alternating movements. This can be demonstrated by asking your patient to rapidly supinate and pronate the forearms, or to perform rapid and repeated tapping movements on one hand on to another.

- Provide the examiner with a summary of your clinical findings.

Key points

Note the key steps in performing this examination:

1. Inspection
2. Tone
3. Reflexes
4. Power
5. Co-ordination

Examination skills 5:   Level: *

Examining the level of consciousness: Glasgow Coma Score (GCS)

Mr Chen has been brought to A&E by ambulance after being evacuated from his vehicle in a road traffic collision. He appears a little drowsy. As the A&E doctor, you have been asked to assess his Glasgow Coma Score (GCS).

QUESTION A:

How would you go about assessing the patient's GCS?

RESPONSE A:

I would start by introducing myself to the patient and asking his permission to examine him. The GCS is a scoring system which will give me an indication of his level of consciousness, by adding the sum of three responses.

Best eyes response: *score*

-    Open eyes   4
-    Open eyes in response to voice   3
-    Open eyes in response to painful stimuli   2
-    Does not open eyes   1

Best verbal response:

-    Orientated, converses normally   5
-    Confused, disorientated   4
-    Inappropriate words   3
-    Incomprehensible sounds   2
-    Makes no sound   1

Best motor response:

-    Obeys commands   6
-    Localises to painful stimuli   5
-    Withdraws from painful stimuli   4
-    Abnormal flexion to painful stimuli   3
  (decorticate response)
-    Extension to painful stimuli   2
  (decerebrate response)
-    Makes no response   1

BPP
LEARNING MEDIA

QUESTION B:

How do you interpret the result?

RESPONSE B:

- Individual elements, as well as the sum of the scores, are important. It is also good practice to state the time the GCS is recorded so that an accurate assessment of changes in conscious level over a period of time can be made. Hence, the score is expressed in the form, 'GCS E4V4M3 = 11, at 08:30 on 20.02.2013.'

- Like other scoring systems, the value of the GCS is that it allows clinicians to monitor changes in consciousness over time and in response to interventions.

- Brain injury is often classified as:

    - Minor: GCS ≥ 13
    - Moderate: GCS 9 – 12
    - Severe: GCS ≤ 8

- The possible scores range from 3 (worst) to 15 (best & normal).

QUESTION C:

The GCS is usually quoted in conjunction with pupil size, pupil reaction to light and limb movements; how are these parameters assessed?

RESPONSE C:

The pupil size is documented for each eye, between 1 and 8mm in size. The reaction to light is also stated for each eye; this can be:

- - : no reaction to light
- + : reacts to light
- C : eyes closed, ie patient is unable to open their eyes, usually due to localised ocular trauma

The patient's observation charts will also contain notes of his upper and lower limb movements for each side of his body. Hence for each arm and leg, document:

- Normal power
- Mild weakness
- Severe weakness
- Spastic flexion
- Extension
- No response

Key points

- The GCS gives an indication of a patient's level of consciousness by adding the sum of three responses (best eyes response, best verbal response and best motor response). Note and document the time and date each time the GCS is assessed.

- The lowest score is 3 out of 15, a normal score is 15 out of 15.

- Other parameters that should be assessed, along with the GCS, are a patient's pupil size, pupil reaction to light and limb movements.

Examination skills 6:   Level: *

Mini-mental state examination

Mr Jones is an 80-year-old male who has recently had several falls. His wife mentions that his memory has not been what it used to be, over the past few months and appears to be getting worse.

You have been asked to perform a mini-mental state examination to assess the severity of his intellectual impairment.

The mini-mental state examination (MMSE) is the most commonly used instrument for screening cognitive function. The examination is not suitable for making a diagnosis but can be used to indicate the presence of confusion and other cognitive impairment, as occurs in a patient following a head injury or someone with dementia. It has mainly been validated in the elderly.

Maximum score	Patient's score	Questions
5		What is the time? Day? Date? Month? Year?
		Score 1 mark for each correct response; note that the time should be given to the nearest hour
5		Where are we currently, and what is the name of hospital? Floor? Town/city? County? Country?
		Score 1 mark for each correct response
5		Can you subtract 7 from 100 (93); subtract a further 7 (86), and continue to subtract serial 7s for five answers in total (79, 72, 65).
		Score the total number of correct answers
3		Can you repeat the following address: '42 West Street'. I will ask you to repeat this later in the test.
		Score 1 mark for each correctly stated component

2	Show the patient two basic objects such as a pen and a wristwatch, ask the patient to name them.
	Score 1 mark for each correctly stated component
3	Show the patient a piece of A4 paper, ask him to 'Take this paper in your right hand, fold it in half, and put it on the table.'
	Score 1 mark for each component of the task performed correctly
1	Repeat after me, 'No ifs, ands, or buts'.
	Allow one chance only, score 0 or 1
1	Read what it states on this piece of paper and please follow the instruction.
	The written instruction being 'Close your eyes'.
1	Take this piece of paper and write a sentence about anything of your choice.
	The sentence must contain a noun and a verb to score 1 mark
3	Earlier I told you an address, can you repeat it for me.
	Score 1 mark for each correctly remembered component of the address
1	Take this piece of paper and pencil and please copy the picture below.

All 10 angles must be present and two must intersect to score 1 mark

Table 2.3: An example of questions used and scoring for the mini-mental state examination

Interpretation of MMSE

Score	Interpretation
24 – 30	No cognitive impairment
18 – 23	Mild cognitive impairment
0 – 17	Severe cognitive impairment

Sometimes time restrictions mean that it is not possible to do a complete mini-mental test. In this situation an abbreviated ten-point mental test can be performed, for example, by the bedside during a ward round. This gives a quick and effective assessment of the patient's cognitive function and you should also be able to use it in an OSCE station.

Score 1 for each correct response

1. What is your age?
2. What is your date of birth? (day and month sufficient)
3. What is the time, to the nearest hour?
4. Address for recall at end of test. "Can you repeat this address, '42 West Street'. I will ask you to recall this address at the end of the test." The patient is asked to repeat the address *at this stage* to make sure it has been heard correctly, and requested at the end of the test to repeat once more (score of 1 *only* if whole address is said correctly at the end of the test).
5. What year is it?
6. What is the name of the hospital or number of the residence we are in now?
7. Can you repeat after me, 'No ifs, ands or buts'?
8. What is the name of the current Prime Minister?
9. Count backwards from 20 to 1 (score of zero for any uncorrected error).
10. What are the years of the Second World War?

In this abbreviated test, a patient with no impairment should score 9 or 10 out of 10.

Table 2.4: Abbreviated ten-point mental test score

There are many different tests of memory impairment. A common feature of dementias is a loss of recent memory whilst having a relative preservation of distant memory.

Key points

- The MMSE is a useful tool to assess a patient's cognitive function including the presence of confusion.

- The test comprises a series of questions given to the patient; a score of less than 24 out of 30 indicates the presence of some cognitive impairment.

- It may not be feasible to do the complete test, in which case an abbreviated version can be performed: the "Abbreviated ten-point mental test score". A score of 9 or 10 out of 10 should be found in patients with no impairment.

- You could be asked to perform either of the two versions in your OSCE examination.

Further reading

Davies, T and Craig, T (2009) *ABC of Mental Health (ABC series)*. 2nd edition. Oxford: Wiley-Blackwell.

BPP LEARNING MEDIA

Examination skills 7:   Level: * *

Examination of the cardiovascular system

 Mr Hargreaves has come to the medical outpatient clinic complaining of a recent history of shortness of breath on minimal exertion.

QUESTION A:

Please examine his cardiovascular system.

RESPONSE A:

I would commence the examination by introducing myself to the patient, and eliciting his name and age. Then I would explain the examination to the patient and obtain his consent. Before proceeding I would also ask him to take his shirt off, exposing his chest and to lie on the couch so he is positioned at a 45° angle.

INSPECTION/POSITION

I would carry out an initial inspection by looking at the chest and other parts of the body that will give an indication of the patient's cardiovascular status. I would state what I saw.

- General: Whilst standing and observing the patient from the edge of the bed, look for any difficulty in breathing/shortness of breath, pallor, peripheral cyanosis, ankle swelling, scars suggestive of previous surgery and hear for any added audible sounds.

- Hands: Feel the hands for any obvious temperature changes. Also look out for features suggestive of endocarditis (such as Osler nodes, splinter haemorrhages, clubbing); cyanotic congenital heart disease (clubbing); peripheral vascular disease (nicotine stains).

- Pulse: Palpate the radial pulse with three fingers, assess for rate, rhythm, volume and character of the pulse:

    – Rate: Count the pulse for 15 seconds and multiply by 4

        - **Normal**   60-100 beats per minute
        - **Bradycardia**   <60 beats per minute
        - **Tachycardia**   >100 beats per minute

BPP
LEARNING MEDIA

- Rhythm: This may be divided into:

Regular	Sinus Rhythm
Regularly irregular	Second degree heart block or sinus arrhythmia
Irregularly irregular	Atrial fibrillation or atrial and ventricular ectopics

- Volume: Examine to identify the volume of the pulse:

  - **Low volume**   eg cardiac shock, tachycardia, left ventricular dysfunction, aortic and mitral stenosis

  - **High volume**   eg sinus bradycardia, thyrotoxicosis, aortic regurgitation

- Character: This, along with the volume, can be more accurately assessed by also palpating the carotid pulse in the neck.

- Arms: Inform the examiner I will move on to measure the patient's blood pressure in their arms using a sphygmomanometer.

- Face: Examine the patient's face:

  - Look at the skin, looking for a malar flush.

  - Look in and around the eyes, looking for features consistent with hyperlipidaemia, eg corneal arcus, xanthelesmata.

  - Inspect the tongue and mouth (central cyanosis).

- Neck: Here an assessment of the carotids and jugular venous pulse (JVP) should be performed. Palpate the carotid pulse with my thumb to assess its volume and character. ***Never palpate or compress both carotids simultaneously.*** Auscultate over the carotids to listen for bruits.

Assess the JVP, with the patient lying at 45° and with their head turned to one side. The internal jugular vein lies between the two heads (sternal and clavicular) of the sternocleidomastoid muscle; observe this to measure the JVP. The JVP is measured from the sternal angle. A normal value is less than, or equal to, 4cm from the sternal angle.

Mnemonic: EC PQRST

Pulmonary Embolism/Pericardial Effusion

Cannon waves

Constrictive Pericarditis

Quantity of fluid increased (resulting in a fluid overload)

Right heart failure

Superior vena caval obstruction

Tricuspid stenosis/Tricuspid regurgitation/Cardiac tamponade

Table 2.5: Causes of a raised jugular venous pulse

With the JVP, also assess the hepatojugular reflex. Apply firm pressure over the liver (right hypochondrium) for approximately 15 seconds and look for a rise in the JVP. A rise in the JVP in excess of 3cm, from the resting state after over 15 seconds of compression, is a positive 'hepatojugular reflux'. This occurs in conditions such as right ventricular failure, constrictive pericarditis and inferior vena cava obstruction. On the other hand, normal subjects will have a decrease in JVP with this manoeuvre, as there will be a reduced venous return to the heart.

Precordium: Inspect the precordium for the presence of scars, suggestive of previous surgery and pulsations.

PALPATION

Apex beat: Palpate the apex beat. This is usually located in the left fifth intercostal space at the level of the mid-clavicular line. Identify the character of the apex beat, and also whether it is displaced laterally, as would occur in left ventricular hypertrophy.

As you palpate also assess for the presence of any heaves or thrills.

AUSCULTATION

Using a stethoscope auscultate over the four areas of the heart; listen for heart sounds as well as additional sounds (such as clicks and snaps) and murmurs.

• Mitral area check: left fifth intercostal space, mid-clavicular line; roll the patient to the left side.

Listen for presence of mitral stenosis, best heard using the bell to identify a low-pitched murmur. Now ask the patient to breathe in and out, holding their breath in expiration. Using the diaphragm of the stethoscope, listen for mitral regurgitation at the apex. Auscultate the axilla to check for radiation of the murmur.

- Pulmonary area: left second intercostal space, left sternal edge, with the patient sitting up.

   Auscultate for pulmonary stenosis using the diaphragm of the stethoscope.

- Aortic area: right second intercostal space, right sternal edge, the patient remains sitting up.

   Auscultate for aortic stenosis; also check if there is radiation of the murmur to the carotids.

- Tricuspid area: left fifth intercostal space, left sternal edge, with the patient sitting up.

   Ask him to take a deep breath in and out, and once more hold the breath in expiration. Listen for aortic regurgitation.

   With the patient sitting up, also auscultate the back of the chest, including the lung bases, listening for wheezes and crackles.

OEDEMA

Examine for sacral oedema: look at the lower back and apply firm pressure with a finger.

Repeat for the patient's ankles to look for pedal oedema.

Pitting oedema is present if your finger leaves an indentation that persists for some time after pressure has been applied. Ensure you ask the patient if they feel pain as you press.

Oedema can be divided into pitting and non-pitting oedema, as shown in Table 2.6:

Pitting oedema: Heart failure, kidney disease (eg nephrotic syndrome), liver disease (eg cirrhosis, poor diet and malnutrition).

Non-pitting oedema: Lymphoedema, pre-tibial myxoedema (occurs in some patients with hyperthyroidism), deep vein thrombosis.

Table 2.6: Causes of oedema

QUESTION B:

What further tests or investigations would you do to complete your examination of the patient's cardiovascular system?

RESPONSE B:

- Examine the pulses in the patient's lower limbs.

- Measure the patient's BP.

- Perform an ECG.

- Perform a chest X-ray.

- Dipstick a urine sample and perform fundoscopy (both to look for signs of hypertension).

- Look at the patient's charts to note their oxygen saturation levels and temperature.

Key points

- Inspection of the patient includes an observation of their hands, face, neck and chest. It does not have to be in this order – however, develop your own system and adhere to it.

- Note the four areas of the heart that must be auscultated: mitral, pulmonary, aortic and tricuspid. This should be followed by listening to the back of the patient's chest.

- Look and feel for the presence of sacral and pedal oedema; note the possible causes of pitting and non-pitting oedema.

- At the end, remember to state that your examination of the cardiovascular system will be incomplete without the further investigations stated above.

Examination skills 8: Level: * *

Examination of the respiratory system

 Mr Fowler is a 63-year-old man who has been admitted to the medical assessment unit direct from the emergency department with a recent history of breathlessness.

QUESTION A:

Please show how you would examine his respiratory system.

RESPONSE A:

I would commence the examination by introducing myself to the patient, eliciting his name and age. Then I would explain the examination to him and obtain his consent. Before proceeding I would also ask him to take his shirt off, thus exposing his chest, and to lie on the couch so he is positioned at a 45° angle.

INSPECTION

An initial inspection should be performed by standing at the edge of the patient's bed, looking around for clues about the patient's respiratory status; look for nebulisers, oxygen masks, sputum pots and antibiotic drips.

- General: Is he comfortable, does he look ill?

- Colour: Pale or cyanotic, or does he have a good healthy colour and appear well-perfused?

- Breathing at rest: is there any obvious shortness of breath or dyspnoea?

- Is he using any accessory muscles of respiration?

- Can any audible added sounds be heard from the edge of the bed, eg stridor, wheeze or coughing?

- Look at the chest for any scars suggestive of previous surgery.

- Observe the chest shape: is there any asymmetry between the left and right sides; barrel shaped, pectus carinatum, pectus excavatum?

- Hands and arms:

    - Temperature: Feel his hands and note any obvious temperature change. Do they look warm and well-perfused?

- Peripheral cyanosis: Look for blue nail beds.

- Nicotine stains, on the fingernails, shows evidence of smoking.

- Clubbing of the nails: Occurring in a variety of respiratory conditions such as, asbestosis, bronchiectasis, bronchial carcinoma, cystic fibrosis and fibrosing alveolitis.

- Resting tremor: Ask the patient to straighten his arms, and observe the hands for a resting tremor. This can occur secondary to the use of a beta agonist (eg salbutamol).

- Retention flap: with the arms outstretched, ask him to cock his wrists backwards in extension. Look for an irregular jerking or flapping of the hands – identified with carbon dioxide (CO_2) retention.

- Pulse: Feel the radial pulse, assess the rate, rhythm and character. Also note the presence of a bounding pulse, a further indication of CO_2 retention.

- Respiration: Count the patient's respiratory rate over one minute.

- Face & Neck:

  - Look at the eyes for pale conjunctiva, a sign of anaemia.

  - Ask the patient to stick out their tongue, a pale blue appearance would indicate central cyanosis.

  - JVP, Assess the JVP, a raised and pulsatile JVP could indicate cor pulmonale which occurs in right heart failure.

PALPATION

- Neck

  Trachea: Check if the trachea is central or deviated to one side by placing the index and middle finger of one hand on either side of the trachea. Noting beforehand the patient has no areas of pain in this area and warn them it may feel temporarily uncomfortable. In most people the trachea is slightly deviated to the right side.

  Lymph nodes: With the patient sat forward palpate for enlarged lymph nodes in the cervical or supra-clavicular fossa. Lymphadenopathy here could indicate lung malignancy or TB.

- Chest

   Apex beat: Identify the apex beat, by palpating the furthest pulsating point of the heart; it is normally located at the level of the 5th intercostal space in the mid-clavicular line. If it is displaced, this could indicate a pneumothorax or pleural effusion.

   Chest expansion: Determine if the chest expands equally on both sides by placing your hands on his chest, with thumbs just touching each other in the midline and fingers spread out on the ribcage. Now ask the patient to take deep breaths in and out. As he breathes in and the chest expands, measure the distance between your thumbs. Normally you would see a chest expansion of >5cm, also note, if there is a reduction, whether it is unilateral or bilateral.

- Tactile Fremitus

   Assess by placing your hand over the patient's chest wall, over the right second intercostal space; ask the patient to say the number 'Ninety-nine'. A positive result will be a vibration felt over the patient's chest when they say the number. Tactile fremitus is pathologically increased (more pronounced vibration) over areas of consolidation, and decreased or absent over areas of pleural effusion or pneumothorax.

PERCUSSION

- Percussion is performed by placing the middle finger of your non-dominant hand (left hand in right-handed individuals) on to the chest wall of the patient. Now strike the centre of the middle phalynx of this hand with the middle finger of the other. Percuss each area of the chest in turn; this can be divided into an upper, middle and lower zone. Remember to extend the percussion to include the axilla, and compare the percussion sound heard on one side with the other.

- Percussion sounds are usually described as normal, dull, stony dull, resonant and hyper-resonant.

Dull	Fluid overload, consolidation, pulmonary fibrosis, lung collapse
Stony dull	Pleural effusion
Resonant	Normal individuals
Hyper-resonant	Pneumothorax

Table 2.7: Character of percussion sound

AUSCULTATION

- Ask the patient to sit up and take deep breaths in and out of his mouth. Now auscultate using a stethoscope to listen for breath sounds (vesicular, bronchial, or absent), noting the presence of added sounds (wheezes, crepitations and crackles) begin at the clavicles, before progressing downwards. Compare left and right sides, and remember to listen to the axilla on each side.

Crepitations (crackles)	
fine:	pulmonary fibrosis, congestive heart failure
coarse:	bronchiectasis, pneumonia
Wheeze (rhonchi)	asthma, COPD (chronic bronchitis & emphysema) Pleural rub pneumonia, pulmonary embolism

Table 2.8: Additional chest sounds heard on auscultation

At the end of the physical examination look for oedema. Examine for sacral and pedal oedema by applying firm pressure with your finger over the lower back and ankle respectively. Ensure to ask the patient if they feel pain as you press. Observe for the presence of pitting.

QUESTION B:

What further tests or investigations would you do to complete your examination of the patient's respiratory system?

RESPONSE B:

- Request a chest X-ray
- Peak flow and spirometry
- Sputum analysis
- Arterial blood gas
- Look at the patient's charts to note oxygen saturation levels, pulse, blood pressure and temperature

Key points

- On inspection, remember to look around a patient's bed, if appropriate, to identify clues regarding his or her respiratory status.

- Practise distinguishing different percussion sounds and the pathologies they represent.

- In the same manner, practise distinguishing different sounds heard on auscultation, along with the pathologies they represent.

- As with the cardiovascular system examination, remember to feel for sacral and pedal oedema.

- At the end of your examination, inform the examiner of the additional tests and investigations you would perform to complete the assessment of the patient's respiratory status, if not asked.

BPP
LEARNING MEDIA

Examination skills 9:   Level: * *

Examination of the gastrointestinal system

Mr Choo is a 56-year-old male who has been admitted to the medical assessment unit from the emergency department with a recent history of generalised abdominal pain.

QUESTION A:

Please show how you would examine his gastrointestinal system.

RESPONSE A:

I would commence the examination by introducing myself to the patient, eliciting his name and age. Then I would explain the examination to the patient and obtain his consent. Before proceeding I would also ask him to lie flat on the couch, arms by his side; he should be exposed from 'nipples to the knees'. In the first instance, his external genitalia should be covered.

INSPECTION

An initial inspection should be performed by standing at the edge of the patient's bed, if this is practical:

- General: Is the patient comfortable or in pain?

- Colour: Does the skin colour appear normal, are they pale or jaundiced?

- Look at the surrounding environment, look for sickness bowls, IV fluid drips or even an IV antibiotic drip running. This will help to give an indication of the current state of the patient.

- Hands and arms: Look at, and feel, the patient's hands and inspect his nails. The state of the skin may give important clues: turgor (dehydration), scratch marks, jaundice, purpura (clotting abnormalities).

Clubbing	Liver cirrhosis, coeliac disease, Inflammatory bowel disease
Koilonychia (spoon-shaped nails)	Iron deficient anaemia
Leukonychia (whitening of the nails)	Liver cirrhosis, ulcerative colitis, hypoalbuminemia
Palmar erythema	Chronic liver disease
Dupuytren's contracture	Liver cirrhosis

Table 2.9: Hand signs seen on abdominal examination

- Examine for a retention flap: with the arms outstretched, ask the patient to cock their wrists backwards in extension. Look for an irregular jerking or flapping of the hands which is indicative of liver failure. This is also known as asterixis. The same test is performed when carrying out a respiratory examination and here can indicate CO_2 retention.

- Face: look at the face for the following features:

    - Eyes: for pale conjunctiva (anaemia), yellowing of the sclera (jaundice)

    - Lips: for presence of pigmented brown freckles (seen in Peutz-Jeghers syndrome)

    - Mouth

Blue tongue	Central cyanosis
Atrophic glossitis or angular stomatitis	Iron, folate, Vitamin B_{12} deficiency
Macroglossis	Hypothyroidism or acromegaly
Ulcers	Crohn's disease, coeliac disease
Dry tongue	Dehydration
Breath	Hepatic foetor, ketosis, alcohol excess

Table 2.10: Signs to look for in the mouth during a gastrointestinal examination

- Chest: look at the patient's chest for the presence of spider naevi, telangiectasia, gynaecomastia in males and scratch marks and axillary hair loss. Their presence may indicate chronic liver disease.

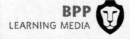

- Abdomen: look at the patient's abdomen. Look for scars suggestive of previous surgery, distended abdominal veins, distension, swellings, visible peristalsis and pulsations (query abdominal aneurysm), stoma sites (ileostomy, colostomy), hernias, presence of indwelling catheters, eg suprapubic.

PALPATION

Neck: Palpate the left supraclavicular fossa to identify Virchow's node, also known as Troisier's sign and seen in patients with gastric carcinoma.

Abdomen: Before palpating the abdomen, ask the patient if he has any areas of tenderness. Ensure your hands are warm, and kneel down at the side of the bed, so you are at the same level. Palpate non-tender areas first, being systematic in your approach. Continue to look at the patient's face as you palpate, to look for signs of pain.

- Light palpation: Palpate all nine quadrants (non-tender sites first). Look for the presence of rebound tenderness (increased pain felt on releasing pressure), guarding (a reflex contraction of the abdominal muscles) and rigidity.

- Deep palpation: Subsequently palpate all quadrants more deeply; feel for masses and the presence of tenderness. If a mass is felt, this should be described in relation to its location, size, shape, consistency, edge, sound heard on percussion, as well as presence or absence of bowel sounds or bruits on auscultation.

- Note and describe any organomegaly.

Liver: Palpate from the right iliac fossa (RIF), towards the right hypochondrium, ask the patient to take deep breaths in and out.

Spleen: Palpate from the RIF, towards the left hypochondrium, use the same technique as with the liver.

Kidney: Ballot the kidneys on inspiration.

AAA: Feel for an abdominal aortic aneurysm by placing two fingers in the epigastric area, above the umbilicus. Feel for an expansile, not a transmitted pulsation.

PERCUSSION

- Liver: Percuss from the right nipple down to the RIF.

- Spleen: Percuss from the left nipple down to the left iliac fossa (LIF).

- Bladder: Percuss suprapubically listening for dullness suggestive of bladder distension.

- Kidney: Percuss both flanks.

ASCITES: To test for ascites, two tests should be performed:

- Shifting dullness: first percuss from the umbilicus laterally towards the flanks. Ascertain that the percussion note is resonant at the umbilicus (gas), and dull in the flanks (fluid). If this is not the case, then the patient does not have ascites. Note the point of dullness.

    Next, ask the patient to roll over towards you (on his right side), whilst keeping your finger over the same point where dullness appeared (on his left flank). Wait for approximately 30 seconds before percussing again. The fluid should drain towards the patient's right flank, with bowel gas remaining in the left flank; the percussion note should now be resonant (in the left flank).

    Finally, return the patient to the supine position; wait for a further 30 seconds and percuss again. The note over the left flank should now be dull again.

- Fluid thrill: This can be detected by asking the patient to place his hand along the midline of his abdomen. Then place your 'detecting' hand on the patient's flank. Flick the opposite flank area with your index finger; the presence of a fluid thrill transmitted to your detecting hand is suggestive of severe ascites.

AUSCULTATION

- Auscultate close to the umbilicus for peristaltic bowel sounds.

    Over a 30-second period, at least two or three sounds should be heard: identify if the sounds are increased (tinkling quality, in obstruction), reduced or absent (paralytic ileus or generalised peritonitis).

- Abdominal aorta: auscultate to listen for bruits, which could indicate an aneurysm or arteriosclerosis.

- Renal artery: auscultate approximately 3 to 4cm supero-lateral to the umbilicus. A bruit here could suggest renal artery stenosis.

QUESTION B:

If the abdomen is distended what could be the possible causes?

BPP
LEARNING MEDIA

RESPONSE B:

Remember the mnemonic – the 5Fs of abdominal distension:

- Fat
- Fluid
- Foetus
- Flatus
- Faeces

QUESTION C:

What further tests or investigations would you do to complete your examination of the patient's gastrointestinal system?

RESPONSE C:

- Hernias: To examine for the presence of hernias, I would ask the patient to cough as I feel for a cough impulse over the hernial orifices.

- I'd examine for inguinal lymphadenopathy.

- I would request a urine dipstick and send for culture.

- I would also perform an examination of the groin and external genitalia.

- I would perform a rectal examination.

- I would look at the patient's charts, to note their oxygen saturation levels, pulse, blood pressure and temperature.

Key points

- On inspection, remember to look around the patient's bed, if practical, to look for clues regarding his GI status.

- When commencing palpation of the patient's abdomen, divide your approach systematically into nine quadrants; start at non-tender areas.

- Have your own system to palpate and percuss to look for various organomegaly.

- Look for ascites using both techniques of shifting dullness and fluid thrill.

- Remember the causes of abdominal distension: the 5Fs.

- At the end of your examination, inform the examiner of the additional tests and investigations you would perform to complete the assessment of the patient's gastrointestinal status, if not asked.

Examination skills 10:   Level: * *

Examination of the groin and external genitalia

Mr Poules is a 38-year-old male who has noticed a lump in his groin; as the surgical FY2 doctor in the clinic, you have been asked by your consultant to assess him.

QUESTION A:

Please examine his groin with a view to identifying the nature of this lump.

RESPONSE A:

- I would commence by introducing myself to the patient and eliciting his name and age. I would explain what the examination involves and seek his consent. I'd ensure we were in a quiet, private area with a chaperone present.

- I'd ask the patient to undress to expose the groin and external genitalia, and ask the patient to be standing if possible.

INSPECTION

- Look for any scars or swellings over the groin and scrotum; compare left with right side.

- Where a lump is noted, identify its position relative to the pubic tubercle:

    - Inguinal hernias lie above and medial to this point.
    - Femoral hernias are located below and lateral to it.

PALPATION

I would make sure my hands are warm before beginning palpation. I would ask the patient if he has any areas of pain or tenderness in the groin and scrotum.

- Hernia examination:

    If you suspect a lump is a hernia, place one hand on the pubic tubercle, and ask the patient to cough. An inguinal hernia lies above and medial to the pubic tubercle, a femoral hernia being below and lateral to this point.

    Now state your knowledge of this region to the examiner by mentioning that the inguinal ligament is a band which lies between the anterior superior iliac spine (ASIS) and the pubic tubercle. The deep inguinal ring is a point half-way along this line, known as the mid-point of the inguinal ligament. The superficial inguinal ring is a structure which lies 1cm above and medial to the pubic tubercle.

With this in mind, ask the patient whether they can reduce the swelling by manually pushing the lump in with his fingers. If so, then identify the deep inguinal ring and apply direct pressure over this point. When the hernia is controlled and reduced at the deep inguinal ring, ask the patient to cough and feel for a cough impulse. If a cough impulse occurs in the deep inguinal ring, in the absence of a swelling or lump in the superficial inguinal ring, this would indicate the presence of an indirect inguinal hernia.

In contrast, if there is no cough impulse over the deep ring, but a lump appears in the superficial ring, this would indicate a direct inguinal hernia.

- Indirect inguinal hernia: a hernia that passes through the deep inguinal ring, running obliquely along the inguinal canal and out through the superficial inguinal ring. It can pass into the scrotum. Indirect hernias are more common in younger males and comprise 85% of all hernias.

- Direct inguinal hernia: This type of hernia arises from a defect in the posterior wall of the inguinal canal and then passes through the superficial inguinal ring. They tend to be more common in elderly patients.

- Testis: Hold and then roll each testis between your thumb and index finger. Note the absence of a testis – this could suggest a previous orchidectomy, or even an undescended testis. Where an enlarged and tender testis is palpable in the acute setting, testicular torsion is the primary concern.

- Epididymis: The epididymi (plural) can be identified above and posterior to the testis. Presence of a swelling here would suggest an epididymitis.

- Spermatic cord: These structures are located above the epididymis; a swelling on palpation here could indicate an epididymal cyst.

- Each time a lump is identified, you should be able to identify certain features.

Site	Testicular/separate (scrotal). Can you get above it? If so, it will be a scrotal swelling. If not, it could be an inguinal scrotal hernia
Size	Use a ruler to measure its length and width
Shape	Irregular or spherical
Consistency	Is it soft, firm, hard or spongy?
Trans-illuminate	If so, it could be a hydrocele or cystic in nature. If not, it will likely be a solid structure
Edge	Are you able to palpate the upper border? If not, it could be an inguino-scrotal hernia
Temperature	Does it appear warm/cold?
Pulsatile	Can you feel a pulsatile lump?
Bruit	Auscultate to identify any bruit
Structures	Note its relation to surrounding structures, such as nerves, vessels and lymph nodes

Table 2.11: Salient features of a scrotal lump

- Lymph node: Palpate for presence of surrounding lymphadenopathy, para-aortic nodes would indicate possibility of a testicular tumour.

PERCUSSION
Percuss the lump and listen for increased resonance, suggesting the presence of bowel contents in the lump itself.

AUSCULTATION
Auscultate for bruits and the presence of bowel sounds.

QUESTION B:

What further tests or investigations would you do to complete your examination of the patient's groin and external genitalia?

RESPONSE B:

- I would examine and compare external genitalia and the groin on both sides.
- I would palpate the femoral arteries on both sides and auscultate for the presence of bruits.
- I would perform an abdominal examination.
- I would perform a rectal examination.

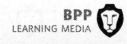

Key points

- With a groin lump, note its position relative to the pubic tubercle. If it is a hernia, inguinal hernias lie above and medial to this point and femoral hernias are below and lateral to this point.

- The deep inguinal ring lies half way along the inguinal ligament, also known as the midpoint of the inguinal ligament. The superficial inguinal ring lies 1cm above and medial to the pubic tubercle.

- Be able to describe the salient features of a scrotal lump.

- At the end of your examination, remember to tell the examiner you would also examine the groin on both sides, as well as perform an abdominal examination and a rectal exam.

Examination skills 11:   Level: * * *

Examination of gait

Mrs Adderton is a 53-year-old female who has come to the neurology clinic today after being referred by her GP with a recent history of falls and unsteadiness on walking. As the FY2 trainee in the clinic, you have been asked to see her.

QUESTION A:

How would you proceed?

RESPONSE A:

I would commence by introducing myself to the patient, eliciting her name and age.

INSPECTION

I would initially look at the soles of the patient's footwear for any pattern of wear and tear. If visiting the patient's home, I would also look around the room for walking sticks or any other walking aids.

I would ask the patient to sit down on a chair. As she sits, I would look for any instability or postural abnormality.

Then I would ask her to stand up from the chair. I would look for any difficulty in standing from the sitting position, also known as 'truncal ataxia'. I would make sure, as the person performing the examination, I am in a position to aid her in case she falls.

I would ask her to walk to a specific point in the room, eg the door, then turn round and return to the starting position. I would allow her to use a walking aid, if that is what she normally uses. At this point I would observe each stage of the gait, including the initiation of movement, rate, type of gait, how she turns around, and the presence or absence of arm swinging.

Parkinsonian	Slow and hesitant to initiate movement; small steps, shuffling gait, there is often little or no arm swing.
Cerebellar	Broad-based, ataxic gait with patient often falling to one side.
Hemiparesis	One leg is in extension, is spastic and stiff. On walking, this leg is circumducted (namely the leg swings in a semicircle fashion from a medial to lateral direction) as the patient walks, the toe hits the ground before the heel does. Often the arm on the paretic side does not swing well and is flexed at the elbow.
High-stepping	Patient has a foot drop, here the patient flexes the hip, in an effort to clear the foot from the floor. This often occurs with a peroneal nerve palsy, causing weakness of foot dorsiflexors.
Waddling	Occurs due to weakness of the proximal muscles of the pelvic girdle. The patient circumducts to compensate for gluteal weakness.

Table 2.12: Types and descriptions of common gait disturbances

QUESTION B:

How and why would you perform a Trendelenburg's test?

RESPONSE B:

A Trendelenburg's test is used to assess for hip abductor weakness. It can be performed by facing the patient and asking her to stand on her good leg, and the foot on the contralateral side is elevated from the floor by bending at the knee. I would ask the patient to rest the palms of her hands on your hands. The test should be repeated on the other leg.

In normal function, the hip is held stable by the gluteus medius muscle acting as an abductor in the supporting leg. If the pelvis drops on the unsupported side, this is a positive Trendelenburg's test. This implies the hip on which the patient is standing is painful or has a weak gluteus medius muscle.

QUESTION C:

What other tests are required to complete the examination?

RESPONSE C:

- I would do a full neurological examination of the lower limbs.

- Examine the patient's hips and spine.

- Assess for leg length discrepancies, which could also cause problems with gait.

Key points

- Inspection of gait should commence with a careful observation of the patient's environment including footwear and the presence of walking aids.

- Observe every stage of a patient's gait, including the initiation of movement, rate, type of gait, how they turn around and the presence or absence of arm swinging.

- Remember there are both neurological (eg Parkinson's disease, cerebellar dysfunction) and mechanical causes for gait instability (eg abductor weakness).

Examination skills 12:   Level: *

Examination of ear, nose and throat

Mr Gates is a 58-year-old male who has come to your clinic with a recent history of flu-like symptoms, now complaining of a sore throat with hearing difficulty in both ears. You have been asked to examine his ear, nose and throat.

How would you proceed and what equipment do you require?

RESPONSE:

I would start by introducing myself to the patient and obtaining his consent to perform the examination.

POSITION

The patient should be asked to sit on a comfortable stool or chair.

I would need the following equipment in order to perform the examination: otoscope, light source, syringe for wax removal, a direct endoscopy mirror, tongue depressor with local anaesthetic spray and a nasal speculum.

INSPECTION

Ears:

*   Inspect each ear in turn; look at the pinna and external auditory meatus, comment on any abnormality of shape and asymmetry between the two sides; in addition, look for discharge from the ears.

*   Inform the patient that you need to look inside his ears '...using this instrument, it's called an otoscope, it basically contains a magnifying glass and has a built-in light source. It should not cause you any pain, but it may feel uncomfortable for a couple of minutes.'

*   Begin by examining the good ear (if applicable) first.

*   Pinna: Look at the pinna for scars, sinuses, abscesses, and/or discolouration. Remember to look behind the pinna.

*   Canal: Now examine the external ear canal and look for any discharge. A clue may be the presence of any foul smell: eg a purulent smell may indicate an otitis media; if 'cheesy', this is often indicative of a cholesteatoma.

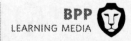

- Hold the otoscope like a pen-torch, using your thumb and index finger. Rest the medial border of your hand against the patient's cheek. Ensure the size of the speculum is appropriate for the patient's ear canal. Pull the pinna upwards and backwards and insert the otoscope into the ear canal. Look inside the ear canal for foreign bodies, discharge or inflammation.

- Tympanic membrane: Look at the tympanic membrane (eardrum) with the otoscope; observe to see if it is intact or perforated and look at its colour and shape. Establish the presence of a light reflex.

- To verify the patency of the eustachian tube, ask the patient to gently perform a valsalva manoeuvre by pinching their own nose, keeping their mouth closed and exhaling. Patency of the eustachian tube can be demonstrated by movement of the tympanic membrane.

- Inform the examiner you would also assess the integrity of the VIII (8th) cranial nerve (vestibulocochlear nerve). This includes performing Weber's and Rinne's tests (see Examination skills 19: Examination of the cranial nerves).

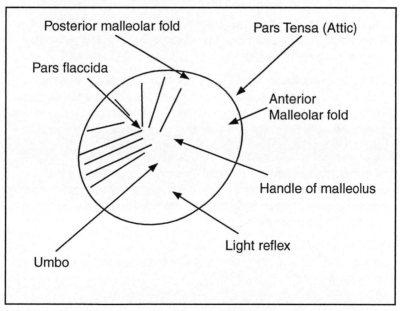

Figure 2.1: Diagrammatic representation of the tympanic membrane

Nose and throat:

- Inspect the nose from the front, from above (as the patient is sitting) and from the side. Look for any obvious deviation, scars, swellings, or discharge. Now raise the tip of the nose gently and examine the vestibule of the nose. Note the presence of cartilaginous collapse, noted to occur with cocaine use and previous surgeries.

- Apply some local anaesthetic spray into the patient's mouth and throat. Use a tongue depressor to observe the oropharynx and note general dental hygiene, tonsils and pharynx. Continue to look for bleeding, discharge or the presence of abscesses.

- Use a nasal speculum or an otoscope with a wide speculum attachment; observe the internal aspect of the nose. Examine the post-nasal space; look at the nasal septum, middle and inferior turbinates and the nasal mucosa. Look for bleeding, perforation presence of ulcers or nasal polyps and note any asymmetry or deviation.

- Inform the examiner 'I can also test the sense of smell using specific scented odour bottles.'

- Assess the patient's swallowing function, along with tongue movements, by testing cranial nerves glossopharyngeal (IX), vagus (X) and hypoglossal (XII).

- Offer to examine for lymphadenopathy, palpating the lymph nodes in the cervical, submandibular, sublingual and parotid regions.

Key points

- As this station involves physically inserting objects into the patient, remember to inform them *at the start of any examination* that there may be some discomfort during the assessment but that it should not be painful.

- Practise using an otoscope on your colleagues, learning to identify 'normal' structures – particularly in relation to the tympanic membrane.

- Remember that, when performing the examination of the ear, nose and throat, you should be able to state, and perform examination of, the relevant cranial nerves which are involved in the functioning of these structures.

Examination skills 13:   Level: *

Examination of the spine

Mr Kendall is a 67-year-old male who has been referred by his GP with a complaint of worsening lower back pain. You have been asked by your consultant to assess him when he arrives at the outpatient clinic.

QUESTION A:

How would you proceed with the examination?

RESPONSE A:

I would start by introducing myself to the patient and obtaining his consent to perform the examination.

POSITION

I would ask him to take his shirt off, so his back is adequately exposed and to stand in front of me.

INSPECTION

- Observation from behind: look for scoliosis (lateral curvature of the spine), presence of scars or swellings.

- Observation from the side: look for an exaggerated kyphosis – a bowing or rounding of the back, which leads to a hunchback or slouching posture; also look for scars and a lumbar lordosis.

- Other general features to look for include sinuses, pigmentation, abnormal skin creases and/or an abnormal hair distribution.

PALPATION

Palpate the full length of the spine, including over the spinous processes, paraspinal muscles and interspinous ligaments. As you palpate, feel for a raised temperature along with the presence of tenderness, where tenderness occurs make a note of the site of the pain.

MOVEMENT

I would actively and passively assess the following movements:

- Forward flexion: ask the patient to keep his knees straight and touch his toes.

- Extension: stand behind the patient and ask him to lean backwards as far as he comfortably can.

- Lateral flexion: ask him to slide his right hand as far down his right leg as possible, then repeat this on the left side. Lateral flexion is often restricted in the early stages of ankylosing spondylitis.

- Rotation: ask him to sit on a stool (or alternatively fix his pelvis from behind whilst he is standing). Now ask him to rotate his body, head, shoulders and chest to either side as far as he can.

- Expansion: measure the chest circumference of the patient, both in full expiration and then in full inspiration. In most individuals, chest expansion of around 7cm is expected. When chest expansion of less than 5cm occurs, this is further suggestive of ankylosing spondylitis.

QUESTION B:

Are there any additional tests you would perform?

RESPONSE B:

Yes, I would assess the patient's ability to carry out a straight leg raise (the leg is kept straight as it is flexed at the hip) and then perform passive dorsiflexion of the foot – Bragard's test. If the pain is increased when the foot is dorsiflexed, nerve aetiology is likely at L4, L5 or S1 levels. If there is no increase in pain, muscle aetiology is likely.

I would also perform another variant of the straight leg raise, namely passively extend the patient's knee once the leg has been flexed at the hip – Lasègue's test. Both of these tests are useful in determining the presence of sciatic nerve irritation, usually from a prolapsed disc.

QUESTION C:

How would you complete your examination?

RESPONSE C:

I would:

- Perform a neurological examination of both upper and lower limbs.

- Assess urinary and bowel sphincter integrity.

- Examine other upper limb joints, namely the shoulders, elbows and wrists.

- Perform radiographs (plain X-rays) of the spine, with AP and lateral views.

Key points

- Observe the patient both from the side and the back.

- As you palpate the patient's back, try to identify any raised temperature along with the presence of tenderness.

- Assess the movements of the spine both passively and actively.

- The examination of the spine is not complete unless further tests, including a neurological examination of the upper and lower limbs, have been performed.

Examination skills 14:   Level: *

Examination of the shoulder

Mr Beard is a 45-year-old male presenting to the orthopaedic outpatient clinic with a recent history of stiffness affecting his left shoulder. As the FY2 doctor covering the firm, you have been asked to assess him.

QUESTION A:

How would you proceed with the examination?

RESPONSE A:

I would start by introducing myself to him, eliciting his name, date of birth, hospital number and obtaining his consent to perform the examination.

POSITION

I would ask him to remove his shirt and adequately expose his shoulders, neck and chest. The patient should be examined standing.

INSPECTION

I'd inspect the patient from the front, behind and side on, looking for:

- Asymmetry of the shoulders
- Winging of the scapula (seen from behind), suggesting injury to the long thoracic nerve and weakness of serratus anterior muscle
- Muscle wasting; the deltoid, in particular, shows wasting with a proximal myopathy
- Scars suggestive of previous surgery, sinuses and discolouration (bruising)
- Large effusions (smaller effusions in the shoulder are usually not visible)

PALPATION

I'd palpate the shoulder joint and state the areas I was feeling: sternoclavicular joint, clavicle, acromioclavicular joint, glenohumeral joint as well as the axilla.

While doing so, I'd feel for any areas of tenderness or pain, or any areas of increased warmth or swelling (bogginess) of the joint. On gentle movement I'd comment on the presence of crepitus if this was apparent.

MOVEMENT

I'd assess active and passive movements of the shoulder.

- Examine passive movements whilst standing behind the patient. The starting position should have the patient with arms hanging by his sides with palms semi-pronated, facing inwards. When examining the left shoulder, use your right hand to hold the scapula and superior aspect of the shoulder, over the deltoid muscle. This method will allow you to fix the scapula and identify whether apparent shoulder movements are arising as a result of the scapula sliding on the chest wall. Use your left hand to move the patient's left arm as described below. During the movements remember to comment on restriction or limitation of movement, along with any tenderness or pain. Also look out for joint crepitus. Remember to compare each side and begin your examination with the 'good' shoulder.

- Abduction: Hold the elbow and abduct the arm. The initial movement is at the glenohumeral joint, up to 90°. Now ask the patient to rotate the palm anteriorly so it is facing upwards; further abduction should now be possible to around 180°, the normal range of motion.

- Adduction: Move the arm across the front of the chest to the midline, across their body so that the hands are now on the opposite shoulders. Shoulder adduction can occur to around 50° normal range of motion.

- Forwards flexion: Move the arm forwards as far as possible, normal range of motion being 180°.

- Backwards extension: Move the arm backwards as far as possible, normal range of motion is 65°.

- External rotation: Ask the patient to flex his elbow to 90°, firmly placed against the side. Now rotate the arm laterally as far as possible, normal range is 60°.

- Internal rotation: Ask the patient to place his hands behind his back and try to touch the opposite scapula; the normal range of motion is 90°.

QUESTION B:

Are there any additional tests you would perform?

RESPONSE B:

Yes, I would check sensation in the regimental badge area over the lateral aspect of the shoulder over the deltoid muscle. This tests for axillary nerve damage, which supplies the deltoid muscle.

QUESTION C:

How would you complete your examination?

RESPONSE C:

- Perform a neurological examination of the upper limbs.
- Perform an examination of the cervical spine.
- Perform an examination of the elbow.
- Obtain an X-ray of the shoulder, anteroposterior (AP) and lateral views.

Key points

- As with other joint examinations, have your own sequence for examining the shoulder. A common method, as described, is:
  - Position the patient
  - Inspection
  - Palpation
  - Movement
  - Then any additional relevant special tests.

- Winging of the scapula, on inspection, indicates damage to the long thoracic nerve; this results in weakness of the serratus anterior muscle.

- Remember to compare left with right sides. During palpation look for tenderness, pain, swellings, warmth and crepitus.

- Assess for loss of sensation over the regimental badge area, indicating axillary nerve damage, causing weakness in the deltoid muscle.

Examination skills 15:　　　　　Level: * *

Examination of the hip

Mr Harcourt is a 53-year-old male presenting to the orthopaedic outpatient clinic with a recent history of pain in his right hip. You have been asked to assess him by your consultant.

QUESTION A:

How would you proceed with the examination?

RESPONSE A:

I would start by introducing myself to the patient, eliciting his name, date of birth, hospital number and obtaining his consent to perform the examination.

POSITION

I would ask him to undress to his undergarments. The patient should initially be examined standing.

INSPECTION

I'd inspect the patient from the front, behind and side on, and look at or for:

- Alignment of the shoulder, hips and patella. I'd also check to see that the anterior superior iliac spines (ASIS) are aligned at the same level as each other.

- Scars suggestive of previous surgery.

- Muscle wasting or pelvic tilting.

- I'd look from behind for a scoliosis and, from the side, a lumbar lordosis (fixed flexion deformity).

PALPATION

I'd palpate the hip, with the patient lying on a couch. As I do so, I'd examine bony landmarks, such as the head of the femur along with the greater and lesser trochanters on each side, and feel if there are any areas of warmth or the presence of effusions. I'd compare each side.

MOVEMENT

I'd identify any limited range of movements, or complaints of pain on movement. I would also test movements actively and passively, and ask him to lie flat on his back on the couch during the examination.

- Flexion: Flex the knee so that you are not doing a straight leg raise test; now stabilise the iliac crest with one hand (so that the pelvis does not rise from the bed) then, with the other hand, move the thigh towards the patient's chest. The normal range of movement is 130°.

- Thomas' test (to assess for a fixed flexion deformity). Place one hand under the patient's lumbar spine to identify a lumbar lordosis. Now fully flex the 'normal' hip, so that the thigh just touches the abdomen; the lumbar spine should be noted to flatten to obliterate the lumbar lordosis and the opposite (tested) leg should remain in contact with the couch. However, if this tested leg rises off the couch and is unable to flatten or straighten fully, this implies a fixed flexion deformity of the hip on this side. The angle of fixed flexion is the angle through which the thigh rises. Repeat these steps to test the other hip.

- Rotation: Flex the knee and hip to 90°. With one hand, hold the knee; with the other, hold the patient's ankle. Move the foot medially, to test external rotation (the normal range is 45°). Move the foot laterally, to test internal rotation, the normal range also being 45°.

- Abduction: With one hand, hold the heel of the leg to be tested; use your other hand to fix the pelvis on the other side, by pressing over the ASIS. Now move the leg as far outwards as possible. The normal range is 50°.

- Adduction: With both legs on the couch, adduct one by moving it medially to cross the other as far as it will go; the normal range is 45°.

- Extension: Ask the patient to turn over, so he is lying flat on his stomach. Now, placing one hand over the sacroiliac joint, use the other hand to elevate the leg. The normal range is 30°.

Carry out the above movements on both sides to compare the range of motion.

QUESTION B:

Are there any additional tests you would perform?

RESPONSE B:

Yes, I would like to assess for limb shortening by testing the true and apparent leg lengths; I would also perform a Trendelenburg's test.

- Leg length measurement: Apparent leg length is measured from the xiphisternum to the medial malleolus on each side. True length is measured from the ASIS to the medial malleolus on each side. Compare the values obtained on each side.

  If the apparent limb lengths are unequal, but the true limb lengths appear the same, this could be due to a fixed adduction deformity of the hip as occurs in arthritis.

  When the true limb length measurements are unequal, this is true limb shortening. True limb shortening occurs in conditions such as Perthes' disease, hip dislocation, arthritis, avascular necrosis and slipped femoral epiphysis.

- A Trendelenburg's test is used to assess for hip stability and, more specifically, abductor weakness. It can be performed by facing the patient and asking him to stand on his good leg; the foot on the contralateral side is elevated from the floor by bending at the knee. Ask the patient to rest the palms of his hands on your hands. The test should be repeated on the other leg. In normal function, the hip is held stable by the gluteus medius muscle acting as an abductor in the supporting leg.

  If the pelvis drops on the unsupported side, this is a positive Trendelenburg's test. This implies the hip on which the patient is standing is painful or has a weak gluteus medius muscle. Other conditions where you may find a positive Trendelenburg's test include hip dislocation and shortening of the femoral neck, as occurs when there is a fracture of the neck of the femur.

QUESTION C:

How would you complete your examination?

RESPONSE C:

- Obtain an X-ray of the hip, anteroposterior (AP) and lateral views.
- Perform an assessment of the patient's gait.
- Perform a neurological examination of the lower limbs.
- Perform an examination of the patient's knee.

Key points

- When testing movements, Thomas' test is used to test for a fixed flexion deformity of the hip; note that you are testing the leg which should be lying flat in contact with the couch, while the opposite hip is flexed.

- When apparent limb lengths are unequal, but true leg lengths are the same, this could be due to a fixed adduction deformity of the hip. However, when there is a difference in true limb lengths, this implies true limb shortening, which occurs in Perthes' disease, hip dislocation arthritis, avascular necrosis and slipped femoral epiphysis.

- A Trendelenburg's test helps to assess for hip stability, in particular abductor muscle (gluteus medius) weakness.

- State that you would perform an X-ray of the hip (AP and lateral views) to complete the examination.

Examination skills 16:   Level: *

Examination of the breast

Mrs Sharma, a 34-year-old female, has been referred by her GP after noticing a lump on her right breast. You have been asked to assess her by your consultant in the outpatient clinic.

QUESTION A:
How would you proceed?

RESPONSE A:
I would start by introducing myself to the patient and obtaining her consent to perform the examination. I would inform the patient that I will require a chaperone, and obtain one, for example this could be a nurse.

POSITION
I would ask the patient to undress to her waist, adequately exposing her chest.

INSPECTION
I would begin the inspection with the patient's arms by her sides (not elevated). I would repeat the inspection, asking her to sit on the edge of the couch with her hands pressing against her hips and ask her to squeeze inwards. This has the effect of tensing the pectoralis major muscles, making it easier to identify any masses tethered to the underlying muscle. I'd look out for, and comment on as appropriate:

- Breast symmetry – I'd look at both breasts and observe for symmetry with respect to size and shape.

- Skin changes.

- Scars suggestive of previous surgery.

- Ulceration.

- Erythema/redness.

- Peau d'orange, where there is dimpling of the skin as occurs in breast carcinoma.

- Nipples and areolae. Here, I'd look for any discharge, and also assess if they look inverted: nipple inversion can occur congenitally, but it is also a feature of breast cancer. Eczema around the nipples can be seen in Paget's disease.

I would repeat the inspection, after asking the patient to elevate her arms above her head. Also I would examine the axillae and arms for muscle wasting and swellings, which may indicate lymphadenopathy (enlarged lymph nodes).

PALPATION

I would ask the patient to lie on the couch at a 45° angle, with hands behind her head. Before beginning palpation, I would ask the patient if she has any areas of pain or tenderness or if she has noticed any breast lumps. Begin your examination by palpating the 'normal' side first.

- Perform a systematic examination of all four quadrants; use your other hand to steady the breast as you use the palmar surface of the fingers of the examining hand to palpate.

- Use a rotatory action of your fingers whilst palpating. Gently press the breast tissue against the chest wall, to identify any swellings. Palpate the whole breast in a concentric ring fashion commencing at the nipple and working your way to the borders of the breast, before moving on to the axilla.

- Axilla: palpate all four walls of the axilla, identifying the presence of any lymphadenopathy.

- Neck, palpate for the presence of supra and infra-clavicular lymphadenopathy.

QUESTION B:

If during your examination you identified a breast lump, how would you describe it?

RESPONSE B:

I would describe the salient features of the lump in relation to its location (site), size, shape, consistency, mobility and temperature.

Site	In relation to the quadrant, describe it as upper outer, upper inner, lower outer, lower inner
Size	Use a ruler to measure the height and diameter
Shape	Regular or irregular
Consistency	Firm, soft, stony hard, rubbery
Mobility	Mobile, fixed or tethered
Temperature	Warm or cold

Table 2.13: Describing the characteristics of a breast lump

QUESTION C:

How would you complete the examination, if a breast lump is identified?

RESPONSE C:

The patient should be referred for triple assessment, this comprises:

- A full history and examination
- Appropriate imaging in the form of ultrasound or mammography
- Histological/cytological diagnosis via Trucut biopsy or fine needle aspiration

Key points

- Inspection of the breasts should be performed with the patient sitting up facing you and with her hands pressing against the hips. It should be repeated with the patient having their arms elevated above her head.

- Have a systematic method to palpate all four breast quadrants along with the axillae.

- Where a breast lump is identified, it should be described in relation to its size, shape, consistency, mobility and temperature.

- Patients with a breast lump should be referred to a clinician for triple assessment.

Examination skills 17: Level: *

Examination of the skin (dermatology)

Miss Kay has presented to the medical outpatient department with a skin lesion on her right leg. As the medical FY2 doctor in the clinic today, you have been asked to review her and present your findings.

How would you proceed?

RESPONSE:

I would start by introducing myself to the patient and obtaining her consent to perform the examination. I would inform her that I will require a chaperone, and obtain one – for example, a nurse.

I would ask the patient to expose the lesion, ideally to be undressed to her undergarments.

POSITION

I would begin the inspection by asking the patient to stand up in front of me.

INSPECTION

I would describe the lesion to the examiner in relation to its location (site), size, shape, colour, fluid type, surface features and edge.

Site	Which body part or parts are affected
Size	Use a ruler to measure the height and diameter
Shape	*Macule*: a flat discoloured spot <0.5cm in diameter, eg lentigo
	Plaque: raised lesion with a flat top, eg psoriasis
	Papule: <0.5cm of raised elevated skin, eg lichen
	Nodule: >0.5cm raised palpable mass, eg basal cell carcinoma
Colour	Pink, red or purple: caused by blood:
	Erythema – blood within blood vessels
	Purpura – blood leakage outside blood vessels
	Brown: due to pigment deposition:
	Melanin – melanin in the dermis, resulting in varying shades of brown or black
	Haemosiderin – follows purpura
	Yellow: due to bilirubin or lipids, eg jaundice, corneal arcus
	White: indicating a lack of pigment
Fluid type	*Vesicle*: <0.5cm, clear/serous fluid, eg chickenpox
	Bulla: > 0.5cm, eg impetigo
	Pustule: contains pus, usually <0.5cm eg folliculitis; a larger lesion implies an abscess
Surface features	Normal: pathology must be in the dermis, eg a haemangioma
	Abnormal: depends on the layer(s) involved:
	Crust: dried exudates and overlies an ulcer or erosion; can be picked off, eg impetigo
	Erosion: superficial, involving the epidermis only, eg pemphigus
	Ulcer: extends into the dermis, eg a venous leg ulcer
	Fissure: A small, deep but narrow ulcer, eg anal fissure
Edge	Smooth
	Uneven, eg scaly
	Rough, eg keratin or crust
Consistency	Firm, soft, stony hard, rubbery
Mobility	Mobile, fixed or tethered
Temperature	Warm or cold

Table 2.14: Features to describe a skin lesion

PALPATION

Before palpation, I would ask the patient if she is in any pain – and if so, is it directly centred over and around the lesion and/or does it radiate to other parts of the body?

- Palpate the skin lesion or rash, identify its surface characteristics, texture, sweating differences and temperature.

- Observe the rest of the body to see any associated distribution; areas commonly missed that should be inspected include the soles of the feet, extensor surfaces of the upper limbs, particularly the elbows.

- Look for features of psoriasis, by inspecting the nails (onycholysis, pitting) and hair. You will find scaly, erythematous lesions with a well-defined edge, mostly prominent over extensor surfaces.

- Also observe for features that could suggest an eczema. The commonest form is an atopic eczema, usually found in skin flexures, with associated erythema and scaling.

- Palpate the lymph nodes to assess for lymphadenopathy, which could suggest an underlying malignancy.

Key points

- Ideally the patient should be exposed to their undergarments; it is not just the lesion you are examining, but also its associated distribution.

- Describe the lesion in relation to its location, size, shape, colour, fluid type, surface features and edge.

- Before palpating, remember to ask the patient if he or she is in any pain.

- Commonly encountered pathologies are psoriasis and eczema, hence be able to recognise their features.

Examination skills 18:   Level: *

Examination of the retina (ophthalmoscopy)

Mr Watkins is a 43-year-old male, known to be a diabetic. He has been complaining of blurred vision over the past few weeks. You have been asked to examine his retina.

QUESTION A:

How would you proceed and what equipment do you require?

RESPONSE A:

I would start by introducing myself to the patient and obtaining his consent to perform the examination.

POSITION

I would ask him to sit on a comfortable stool or chair, and I would sit on a chair directly opposite him. I would need a fundoscope, also known as an ophthalmoscope, to proceed.

INSPECTION

I would inspect around each eye for scars suggestive of previous surgery, periorbital swelling, redness or foreign bodies. I would concentrate on specific components of each eye:

- Eyelid: look for ptosis (drooping of the eyelid), presence of styes, eyelids turned in (entropion), eyelids turned out (ectropion).

- Conjunctiva: presence of chemosis (swelling or oedema), conjunctivitis (inflammation of the conjunctivae), pallor (indicating possibility of anaemia).

- Sclera: this may appear yellow in jaundice, blue in osteogenesis imperfecta.

- Cornea: corneal arcus – a yellow ring of fat around the iris which is indicative of hypercholesterolemia; or Kayser-Fleischer rings – dark rings that encircle the iris (due to copper deposition as a result of particular liver diseases such as Wilson's disease).

- Iris: look for inflammation (iritis).

- Pupils: check for the presence of dilated or constricted pupils.

- Also test for pupillary reflexes, direct, consensual and accommodation.
- Test eye movements in all directions, and look for any asymmetry between left and right eyes.

QUESTION B:

Please show how you would use the fundoscope/ophthalmoscope.

RESPONSE B:

The procedure should be performed in a dimly-lit room. I have already obtained the patient's consent to proceed. The examination can be performed easier with certain eye drops to help dilate the eyes, such as tropicamide.

- Ask the patient to fixate on a distant object as you switch the ophthalmoscope on.

- When examining the right eye, hold the ophthalmoscope in your right hand; when examining the left eye, the ophthalmoscope should be held in your left hand. With your free hand, steady the patient's head, hand above the eyebrow.

- Look for the presence of a red reflex, and focus on the patient's pupil approximately a foot away from their eyes. An absent red reflex occurs in conditions such as cataract, retinoblastoma or a detached retina.

- Move closer to the patient, initially focus on structures in the anterior segment of the eye (namely the cornea and iris) then move on to the fundus. You should be very close to the patient at this point, almost touching him.

- Focus on the optic disc. Follow the blood vessels passing centrally from the disc to the periphery.

- Now examine each of the four quadrants of the retina: superior temporal, inferior temporal, superior nasal, inferior nasal.

- Now ask the patient to look directly into the light source as you examine the macula. Note its colour: pink is normal; a pigmented macula indicates senile macular degeneration.

Inform the examiner that you would examine the other eye in the same fashion and do so unless you are stopped.

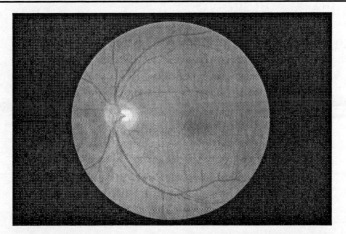

Note the optic disc to the left of the image; vessels can be seen converging on the disc.

Centrally, the darkened structure is the macula.

Figure 2.2: Fundus in a normal eye

Key points

- Perform a general inspection, and comment on any areas of abnormality to the relevant structures: eyelids, conjunctiva, sclera, cornea, iris and pupils.

- When performing fundoscopy, hold the instrument in your right hand to examine the patient's right eye and in your left hand to examine their left eye. Use your other hand to steady the patient's head, hand above their eyebrow.

- With the fundoscope, start by looking for the red reflex at a distance of approximately a foot from the patient. This is absent in conditions such as cataract, retinoblastoma and a detached retina.

- Move closer to the patient to assess the fundus; this should be examined systematically. Look at the optic disc, the vessels passing from it, the four quadrants of the retina, along with the macula.

Examination skills 19:   Level: * * *

Examination of the cranial nerves

Miss Kyle is a 38-year-old female presenting to the neurology outpatient clinic with a recent history of numbness affecting her face. You have been asked to examine her cranial nerves. Fundoscopy is normal.

How would you proceed?

RESPONSE:

I would start by introducing myself to the patient and obtaining her consent to perform the examination.

POSITION

I would ask the patient to sit up on a chair or bed.

INSPECTION

As I speak with the patient, I would try to identify any dysphasia; if present, I would note if it is expressive or receptive.

I would look for any involuntary movements, fasciculation, tremor, choreiform; I'd also look for facial asymmetry/facial weakness, ptosis or craniotomy scars suggestive of previous surgery. I'd work through the cranial nerves in a definite sequence:

-   I   Olfactory
-   II   Optic
-   III, IV & VI   Oculomotor, Trochlear & Abducens
-   V   Trigeminal
-   VII   Facial
-   VIII   Vestibulocochlear
-   IX, X   Glossopharyngeal & Vagus
-   XI   Accessory
-   XII   Hypoglossal

I   Olfactory nerve

Test the sense of smell, both perception and identification using aromatic non-irritant materials (to avoid stimulation of trigeminal nerve fibres in the nasal mucosa) such as peppermint or tobacco, with the patient's eyes shut. Also ensure that they can breathe through each nostril.

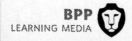

II   Optic nerve

A complete assessment of the optic nerve would comprise testing the visual acuity, visual fields and fundoscopic examination of each eye. You have already been informed in this case that fundoscopy is normal.

*   Visual acuity: Test acuity by asking the patient to read letters and numbers on a Snellen chart. Test at a distance of 6m or 3m. Each eye should be tested separately, the patient keeping her glasses on if she wears them.

*   Visual fields: Gross testing by confrontation. Sit on a chair directly opposite the patient, at the same level. Ask her to cover her right eye whilst you cover or shut your left eye. The patient's open eye should look straight into your open eye directly opposite. Now compare the field of vision by advancing a moving finger, or more precisely, a red 5mm pin from the extreme periphery towards the fixation point. Test each of the four field quadrants in this way.

*   Blind spot: Identify the blind spot, using a 2mm pin. Start with it held laterally in the periphery, then bring it slowly towards the centre along the horizontal, until it disappears and reappears. Ensure that both the patient and you continue to look straight ahead.

*   Visual inattention: Test for visual inattention using bilateral stimulation. Wiggle two fingers simultaneously on either side of the patient's head, and ask whether she is able to see one or both fingers move. In a parietal lobe lesion, only the ipsilateral finger to the lesion is seen.

*   Pupillary reflexes: Ask the patient to fixate on an object in the distance. Inspect each pupil's size (constriction/dilatation) and shape (regularity). Use a pen torch to assess the direct and consensual reflex: shine the light directly in one eye, look for a pupillary response, observe for pupillary constriction. As you illuminate one eye, observe for pupillary constriction in the adjacent eye. Repeat this test and illuminate the other eye.

*   Test the accommodation reflex by asking the patient to remain fixated on an object in the distance – and then, very quickly, to look at your finger, which you would rapidly move close to the patient's nose (20–30cm away).

III, IV & VI Oculomotor, trochlear and abducens nerves

Test the cranial nerves involved in eye movements (III, IV and VI) in unison.

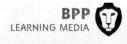

Initially inspect for ptosis (a drooping of the upper or lower eyelid, seen in a 3rd nerve palsy); also look for strabismus (squint). If present, note if this is divergent or convergent.

Ask the patient to keep her head straight and assist her by steadying her head (hold the patient at arm's length with my hand on her chin). Now ask the patient to follow your finger with her eyes. Move your finger vertically and horizontally, in an 'H' sign. As you move your finger, ask if she has any double vision or pain. Look for any nystagmus. Cranial nerve IV supplies the superior oblique muscle which moves the eye down and out. Cranial nerve IV supplies the lateral rectus muscle which abducts the eye (away from the nose). The remaining extra-ocular muscles which control eye movement are supplied by Cranial nerve III.

- Diplopia, commonly known as double vision:

  - Is maximal when looking in the direction of the impaired muscle.

  - The false image appears less defined/distinct than the true image.

  - The false image is displaced furthest in the direction of action of the impaired muscle.

- Nystagmus:

  - This is an impairment in the normal balance of eye control. A slow drift in one direction is followed by a fast corrective movement. 'Physiological' nystagmus (ie nystagmus is normal) when the eyes deviate to the endpoint/extreme of gaze. Nystagmus is named according to the direction of fast movement, and may be horizontal or vertical. Nystagmus is maximal when looking in the direction of fast movement.

  - Peripheral lesions eg damage to the vestibular apparatus causes nystagmus (fast movement away from the side of the lesion).

  - Central lesions eg unilateral cerebellar damage causes nystagmus (fast movement towards the side of the lesion.)

V   Trigeminal nerve

- Sensation: Test each of the divisions of the trigeminal nerve, use the sternum to demonstrate the normal sensory stimuli. Use a piece of cotton wool to assess light touch in the ophthalmic, maxillary and mandibular regions on left and right sides of the face. Ask the patient if sensations are the same on each side. Repeat the assessment using a pin-prick to check pain sensation.

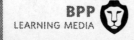

- Corneal reflex: This is the most important sign to examine if there is any suspicion of trigeminal nerve damage. As with all other reflexes, the corneal reflex has an afferent and an efferent arc, ie sensory – ophthalmic (CN V), motor – facial (CN VII).

    - Ask the patient to keep her head straight and to look up to the ceiling, ie by rolling her eyes upwards, hence exposing the lower cornea.

    - Approach from the side of the patient (to avoid an aversion response) with a small wisp of cotton wool, lightly touch the lower cornea. If this reflex is impaired, the patient will not blink.

- Motor: The trigeminal nerve gives motor supply to the muscles of mastication (the masseters, temporalis and pterygoids). Observe for wasting and thinning of the temporalis muscle – 'hollowing out' of the temporalis fossa. Test the strength of the muscles (on both sides) by asking her to perform the following commands:

    - 'Clench your teeth together': See the temporalis and masseter muscles, palpate them to check their bulk.

    - 'Open your mouth against resistance': Pterygoids.

    - 'Open your jaw slightly and move it from side to side': Masseters.

- Jaw jerk: Ask the patient to open her mouth slightly. Place your index finger on her chin. Now use a tendon hammer to gently strike your finger. A normal response will show a slight jerk whereby the muscles contract and the mouth will close. An increased jerk is a sign of a bilateral upper motor neuron lesion above the level of the pons.

VII   Facial nerve

This is predominantly a motor nerve to the muscles of facial expression. On inspection, look at the patient's face to look for facial asymmetry or asymmetrical elevation of one corner of the mouth. Mild facial weakness is best seen through flattening of the nasolabial fold.

- Test the muscles of facial expression by asking the patient to perform the following commands:

    - Wrinkle the forehead by raising the eyebrows (frontalis).

    - Close eyes while you attempt to open them (orbicularis oculi).

    - Purse the lips and blow out the cheeks while you press against the cheeks (buccinators).

    - Show teeth (orbicularis oris).

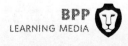

- Taste: Test taste to the anterior two-thirds of the tongue using sugar, salt, or tartaric acid; state that you would place a small quantity of each substance anteriorly on the appropriate side of the protruded tongue.

Make sure you are able to distinguish between an upper motor neurone lesion and a lower motor neurone lesion of the facial nerve.

Upper motor neurone lesion:	eg tumour or CVA (stroke).
	Here, there is sparing of the forehead due to the bilateral innervation of the upper part of the face. There is weakness in the contralateral (opposite) lower quadrant of the face. The mouth deviates to the normal side.
Lower motor neurone lesion:	eg Bell's palsy, tumour or herpes zoster.
	Affects all muscles on the same side as the lesion. On that side there is loss of wrinkling of the forehead, impaired blinking and eye closure. On attempting to close the eye on the affected side, the eye does not close, and the eyeball rotates upwards and outwards – Bell's phenomenon (normal eyeball movement on eye closure). On the affected side there is lower facial muscle weakness. The mouth deviates to the normal side. There is also loss of taste in the anterior two thirds of the tongue.

Table 2.15: Distinguishing the types of facial nerve weakness

VIII   Vestibulocochlear nerve:

- To assess hearing, stand behind the patient and quietly whisper a set of numbers and letters in each ear and ask the patient to repeat what you have said. Mask hearing in the other (non-examined) ear by rubbing your fingers and thumb together in front of the external auditory meatus. If the patient makes a mistake repeat the assessment up to three times.

- State that if the hearing was impaired, you would examine the external meatus and the tympanic membrane, using an otoscope to exclude ear wax or infection.

- Now state that you would like a 512Hz tuning fork to perform Weber's and Rinne's tests to differentiate conductive (middle ear) deafness from perceptive (nerve) deafness:

  - **Weber's**: strike the tuning fork on your knee then hold the base of the instrument against the patient's vertex. Ask the patient where the sound is heard loudest, ie in the centre or does it lateralise to one side. Normally, the sound is heard equally in both ears.

    - Conductive deafness: here the sound is louder in the affected ear, since distraction from external sounds is reduced in that ear.

    - Nerve deafness: Sound is louder in the normal ear.

  - **Rinne's**: Strike the tuning fork on your knee, place the base on the patient's mastoid bone. Ask the patient if she can hear the vibrations, then tell her to indicate (perhaps by raising her hand) when she can no longer hear the note. When the note can no longer be heard, hold the prongs of the tuning fork 1 to 2cm from the external auditory canal (without touching the ear). Ask the patient if she can hear the note again, if so, also ask whether the note was loudest when the base of the tuning fork was against the mastoid, or when the prongs were placed next to the ear.

    Normally air conduction is more sensitive (ie better) than bone conduction; this means that the sound should be heard when the tuning fork prongs are placed next to the ear after they can no longer hear it when held against the mastoid.

    - Conductive deafness: If the patient is unable to hear the tuning fork after the mastoid test, this indicates that her bone conduction is greater than her air conduction.

    - Sensorineural deafness: Here the ability to detect the tuning fork by both bone and air conduction is equally impaired.

    State you would repeat the test on the other side.

IX, X Glossopharyngeal & vagus nerves:

These nerves are examined together since their actions are rarely individually impaired.

- Gag reflex: Ask the patient to open her mouth and depress her tongue with a suitable tongue depressor. Use an orange stick to touch the palate, pharynx or tonsil on one side until the patient gags. Compare sensitivity on each side and observe symmetry of palatal contraction. Afferent route – CN IX, efferent route CN X.

  An absent gag reflex indicates a loss of sensation and/or loss of motor power. CN IX supplies taste in the posterior one third of the tongue which is impractical to test.

- Uvula deviation: Ask the patient to open their mouth and say 'Ahh'. Depress the tongue and use a pen torch to look for uvula deviation. The uvula swings to the opposite side of any lesion.

XI Accessory nerve:

- Stand behind the patient as they are sitting on a chair. Look for wasting of the sternomastoid and trapezius muscles.

- Ask the patient to rotate her head against resistance, compare power and muscle bulk on each side (sternomastoid). Note that the left sternomastoid turns the head to the right side, and vice versa.

- Now ask the patient to shrug her shoulders (trapezius) and to hold them in this position against resistance. Once more compare the power on each side.

XII Hypoglossal nerve:

- Ask the patient to open her mouth and use a pen torch to inspect the tongue and look for atrophy (wasting, increased folds) and fibrillations (small wriggling movements) – a lower motor neurone sign.

- Then ask the patient to protrude her tongue, and note any difficulty or deviation. A protruded tongue will deviate to the side of the weakness, due to the unopposed action of the normal muscles on the other side.

Key points

- A complete assessment of the optic nerve would consist of testing the visual acuity, visual fields and fundoscopic examination of each eye.

- The trigeminal nerve (CN V) gives motor supply to the muscles of mastication. The corneal reflex is the most important sign to examine if there is a suspicion of trigeminal nerve damage.

- The facial nerve (CN VII) is predominantly a motor nerve to the muscle of facial expression. Mild facial weakness is best seen through flattening of the nasolabial fold.

- Be able to distinguish an upper motor neurone lesion and a lower motor neurone lesion of the facial nerve.

- Glossopharyngeal (CN IX) and vagus (CN X) nerves are examined together since their actions are rarely individually impaired.

Examination skills 20: Level: * *

Examination of the peripheral vascular system, upper and lower limbs

Mr Richards is a 74-year-old male, a lifelong smoker who has been referred by his GP with a recent history of pain in his legs on walking short distances. You have been asked by your consultant to perform an examination of his peripheral vascular system, upper and lower limbs.

QUESTION A:

How would you proceed?

RESPONSE A:

I would start by introducing myself to the patient, eliciting his name, date of birth and obtaining his consent to perform the examination.

POSITION

I would ask the patient to undress so that he is adequately exposed; a pair of shorts and vest will suffice. The patient should be sitting down on a chair or bed for the upper limb component of the examination and should lie down on a bed for the lower limb examination.

INSPECTION

I would begin the inspection by commenting on any signs of cardiovascular disease at rest, namely if he appears short of breath or cyanotic. I would check to see:

- If he appears obese, suggesting he may have a raised BMI.

- If there any obvious signs of (pre-) gangrene, such as black, dark or missing toes, or any evidence of nail infection.

- If there are any scars suggestive of previous surgery; look at the groin and the medial aspect of the thigh.

- If there is any ulceration. If so, describe this in relation to its size, shape, edge, presence of slough and the surrounding skin. Be able to comment on whether it is likely to be venous (varicose veins, varicose eczema, these are usually painless) or arterial (punched out in appearance and painful).

- If there are varicose veins. These are best identified with the patient standing.

- If there are any clues in the surrounding environment, if practical: is the patient taking oxygen, can I see a GTN spray by his bedside, for example.

Upper limb & neck

PALPATION

- Hands: Look for further clues about the patient's cardiovascular status, by checking:

    - Temperature changes

    - Palms: pallor

    - Nails: splinter haemorrhages, clubbing, nicotine staining

    - Examine the capillary refill time: This is done by pressing the tip of the nails on both hands for 5 seconds. The nail bed should blanch, on releasing the pressure measure the time taken for the nail bed to turn pink. A normal capillary refill time is less than 2 seconds.

- Radial Pulses: identify the rate and rhythm. Examine for the presence of a radial-radial or radial-femoral delay. Also test for a collapsing pulse, which is a sign of aortic regurgitation.

- Assess the blood supply to the hand by performing Allen's test:

    - Ask the patient to elevate his hand and make a fist. After around 30 seconds, occlude both the ulnar and radial arteries.

    - Still elevated, the hand is opened; it should appear blanched (whitish). Now release the pressure on the ulnar artery. The hand should re-perfuse and the colour return in 7 to 10 seconds. If, however, the colour does not return in this time period, the test is considered positive and the ulnar artery supply to the hand is not sufficient. The clinical significance is that the radial artery cannot be safely cannulated or used for radial arterial blood sampling.

    - Repeat the test, steps as above, but this time release the pressure on the radial artery. In this way Allen's test is a useful method to demonstrate an adequate collateral circulation.

- Brachial pulses: Use these to assess the blood pressure bilaterally. The axillary artery originates at the lateral border of the 1st rib as a continuation of the subclavian artery. Auscultate for the presence of bruits.

  Palpate to feel for presence of a cervical rib.

- Carotid pulses: Assess the rate, rhythm and character; auscultate for presence of carotid bruits.

Lower limb

Complete your inspection as stated above.

PALPATION

I would assess the temperature, by running the back of my hands along both limbs and the soles of both feet. I would identify any points where the temperature changes from warm to cool on both sides.

> **Pain**
> **Paraesthesia** (numbness)
> **Pallor** (pale)
> **Pulseless**
> **Paralysis**
> **Perishing cold**

Table 2.16: The 6Ps – Signs and symptoms of acute ischaemia

Capillary refill time: Normal value should be less than two seconds, as with the upper limb.

Pulses: Examine the peripheral pulses on both legs; compare and note any differences.

Femoral:	Located midway between the pubic symphysis & ASIS.
Popliteal:	Ask the patient to flex his knee, foot resting on the bed. Now place your thumbs on the tibial tuberosity, and feel the pulse with both sets of fingers (all eight) in the popliteal fossa.
Posterior tibial:	Behind the medial malleolus.
Dorsalis pedis:	On the dorsum of the foot, feel with three fingers in the cleft between the 1st and 2nd metatarsal.

Table 2.17: The location of the lower limb peripheral pulses

QUESTION B:

What is Buerger's test and how would you perform it?

RESPONSE B:

Buerger's test is also known as Buerger's angle; it is the angle to which the leg has to be raised before it becomes pale. It is used to assess the adequacy of the arterial supply to the leg. In a limb with normal circulation, the toes remain pink and well-perfused, even when the limb is raised by 90°. In a patient with an ischaemic leg, elevation to 15° or 30° for 30 to 60 seconds may cause pallor. An angle of less than 25° indicates critical ischaemia.

The test is performed by supporting the patient's heel and gently elevating the leg. I would note the angle when the leg blanches (in relation to the leg and bed, Buerger's angle). Then I would ask the patient to sit up and place the leg over the side of the bed (dependent at 90°). If cyanosis occurs – the leg becomes engorged and purple in appearance, this implies a positive Buerger's test.

QUESTION C:

How would you complete the examination?

RESPONSE C:

- Examine the rest of the cardiovascular system.

- Listen over the femoral artery and abdominal aorta for bruits.

- Perform arterial doppler ultrasound assessment of the lower limbs.

- Measure the ankle brachial pressure index, ABPI.

- If indicated, organise an angiogram to assess the lower limb vasculature.

Key points

- The patient should be sitting down on a chair or bed for the upper limb component of the examination and should lie down on a bed for the lower limb examination.

- Allen's test is performed to demonstrate an adequate collateral circulation to the hand. It is of particular clinical significance when considering cannulating the radial artery or performing a radial artery stab (for a blood gas measurement).

- Remember the **6Ps**, a useful mnemonic for the signs and symptoms of acute ischaemia: Pain, Paraesthesia, Pallor, Pulseless, Paralysis, Perishing cold.

- Buerger's test (Buerger's angle), is used to assess the adequacy of the arterial supply to the leg.

Examination skills 21:   Level: * *

Examination of a patient with an ulcer

Mr Price has come to your general surgical clinic with a complaint of having several ulcers.

QUESTION A:

Please examine him and present your findings.

RESPONSE A:

I would commence by eliciting the patient's name and date of birth, and obtaining the patient's consent to perform the examination.

POSITION

I would proceed by asking him to remove any clothes and shoes, as appropriate, so as to expose the area adequately. I would ask him to lie on the couch with the legs lying flat.

INSPECTION

I would perform an initial inspection by observing the patient at rest; does he look comfortable or is he in any obvious distress or pain?

- Comment on the presence (or absence) of scars, particularly in the groin or limbs which would indicate previous surgery.

- From the end of the couch, note the presence of any ulcers; comment on their site, size and shape:

    - Site:

        - Venous ulcers, usually located in the medial gaiter region

        - Arterial ulcers, located on pressure sites and at the periphery of limbs.

        - Neuropathic ulcers, often found at the sole of the foot or heel.

    - Size: Use a ruler to measure the width and length of the ulcer.

    - Shape: This can be described as round, oval or irregular.

- Comment on the edge:
  - Flat, sloping: Often venous ulcers. The skin surrounding the ulcer has a reddish-blue appearance as a consequence of haemosiderin.
  - Punched-out or squared: Arterial or neuropathic ulcers. As a result of pressure applied to areas associated with an inadequate circulation, such as the feet in a diabetic patient.
  - Rolled: Classically seen with a rodent ulcer (basal cell carcinoma). Here there is a necrotic centre with a build-up of tissue at the periphery.
  - Everted: Seen in squamous cell carcinoma and ulcerated adenocarcinoma. Due to the rapid proliferation of tissues at the ulcer periphery, it passes out of the ulcer site and overlaps the normal skin.

- Comment on what you see at the base of the ulcer:
  - Tissue: look for granulation or necrotic tissue, or the presence of abnormal neoplastic features (as seen in squamous cell carcinoma).
  - Colour: White, yellow, green, blue, pink, grey, black or brown. The base of a venous ulcer is usually red. It may also be covered with yellow fibrous tissue, or there may be a green or yellow discharge if the ulcer is infected. The base of an arterial ischaemic ulcer usually does not bleed. It has a yellow, brown, grey or black colour.
  - Penetrating features: Does it appear to invade surrounding tissue such as muscle, tendons or bone?

- Look at any surrounding discharge, which could indicate an infection. Discharge can be described as either serous, sanguineous, serosanguineous or purulent. Mention that you would take a bacterial swab of the ulcer and any surrounding discharge for microbiological analysis.

- Examine for tenderness and temperature.
  - Tenderness: Before touching the patient, ask whether they have any pain in and around the region of the ulcer. Pain may indicate an arterial ulcer.
  - Temperature: Examination can be performed by running the back of your hand over the affected limb and compare with the opposite normal side. Note the point where the temperature changes.

- Examine the neurovascular status of the surrounding tissue.

  - Neurological status: On both sides, assess light touch, such as by using a cotton wool ball. To assess pain, you should say that you would use the pin prick test. However, it is unlikely that you will be asked to physically perform this modality assessment. Also assess proprioception and vibration sense – this requires a tuning fork (128Hz).

  - Vascular status: Assess the capillary refill time (CRT), by applying pressure to the tips of the nails on both feet for five seconds, which would give a whitish appearance over the nail bed, and then let go. A normal CRT is when the colour of the nails returns pink in less than two seconds.

Palpate the lower limb pulses: On both lower limbs, compare pulses for the posterior tibial artery, dorsalis pedis artery, popliteal artery and femoral artery. Tell the examiner that, if you can't palpate any of the pulses, you would perform an ABPI using a doppler ultrasound.

- Lymph nodes: Examine for regional lymphadenopathy; note any lymph node enlargement or tenderness, which could indicate an infection or be suggestive of malignancy.

QUESTION B:

How would you complete your examination?

RESPONSE B:

- I would want to assess if the patient is diabetic, by checking their BMs and performing a urinalysis. If it was known that the patient is already a diabetic, I would want to check their diabetic control, by testing their HbA1c levels.

- If there was suspicion of a poor circulation on vascular assessment, I would arrange for an angiogram.

- I would also arrange for an ABPI measurement.

- At the end, I would thank the patient and cover his exposed limbs.

Key points

- On inspecting a patient from the edge of the bed, ensure they are adequately exposed and appear comfortable before assessing for ulcers.

- Comment on the site, size and shape of the ulcer, along with its associated edge.

- Before palpating to check the skin temperature, remember to ask the patient if there is any tenderness.

- Assess the neurovascular status of the surrounding tissue.

- Examine for regional lymphadenopathy.

Examination skills 22:   Level: *

Examination of a newborn

Mrs Thomas is a mother who has just had a child, delivered by the midwife.

QUESTION A:

Examine the neonate to identify any abnormalities using the APGAR scoring system.

RESPONSE A:

I would commence by seeking the mother's consent to examine her child, in so doing perform and mark the examination as follows using the APGAR scoring system:

The general condition of a newborn should be assessed at one and five minutes after birth. It may be repeated later if the score is, and remains, low.

> **A**PPEARANCE
> 2: Completely pink, body and extremities
> 1: Body pink, blue at extremities
> 0: Blue or pale all over
>
> **P**ULSE RATE
> 2: ≥100 beats/minute
> 1: <100 beats/minute
> 0: Absent
>
> **G**RIMACE/reflex irritability to stimulation
> 2: Cough, sneeze, vigorous cry or pull away when stimulated
> 1: Grimace or feeble cry when stimulated
> 0: No response to stimulation
>
> **A**CTIVITY/muscle tone
> 2: Flexed arms and legs that resist extension
> 1: Some flexion
> 0: Limp, no movement
>
> **R**ESPIRATORY EFFORT
> 2: Strong, good cry
> 1: Weak, irregular crying
> 0: Crying absent

QUESTION B:

How would you interpret the score obtained?

RESPONSE B:

The total score is the sum of all five assessments, it ranges from zero (0), the poorest, to ten (10), the best grade.

- Score ≥7; generally normal

- Score 4 - 6; fairly low, neonate requiring assistance

- Score ≤3; critically low: resuscitation required

A low score at the one-minute test may well indicate that the neonate requires medical attention, but this does not necessarily mean there will be problems long term, particularly if the five-minute test shows an improvement. If the APGAR score remains 3 or below, if and when performed subsequently (such as at 15 or 30 minutes) there is a risk that the child may suffer some form of long-term neurological damage. There is also a small, but significant increase in the risk of developing cerebral palsy.

Note, however, that the purpose of the APGAR score is to determine quickly whether a neonate needs immediate medical care. It is not designed to make long-term predictions on a child's future health.

Key points

- As a useful guide, neonates with an APGAR score ≤6 need a review; resuscitation is likely to be required if the score is ≤3.

- The APGAR scoring system is useful to identify if a neonate needs immediate medical care: it should not be used to make long-term predictions on a child's health.

BPP
LEARNING MEDIA

Examination skills 23:   Level: *

Examination of paediatric developmental milestones

Please record the milestones a child should develop as their development progresses into the first few years of life.

RESPONSE:

AGE	Development

2 months

speech:	makes cooing sounds; eg says 'ooh' or 'aah'
motor:	arms extend forward when prone
social:	smiles

4 months

speech:	responds to voice of others
motor:	reaches out, pulling objects towards mouth
social:	squeals with pleasure appropriately

6 months

speech:	responds to name; starts imitating heard sounds
motor:	applies weight on hands when lying prone
social:	appearing anxious in the presence of strangers

9 months

speech:	'mamma, dadda'
motor:	pulls to stand; grasps objects between finger and thumb
social:	separation anxiety

12 months

speech:	two words beyond just 'mamma, dadda'
motor:	walks with support; plays 'pat a cake'; waves goodbye
social:	drinks from a cup

15 months

speech:	speaks jargon; four to five words
motor:	walks without support; draws lines with pen and paper
social:	points to needed items

18 months

speech:	says own name; speaks seven to ten words
motor:	walks up steps with support; builds a two-cube tower
social:	uses spoon and fork

2 years

speech: speaks two-word sentences; names six body parts

motor: walks steps without support; undresses; builds a four-cube tower

social: mimics play activities of others

3 years

speech: sentences includes prepositions: 'of, to, for, in, but, like', etc.

motor: rides a tricycle; washes and dries hands; builds an eight-cube tower

social: able to dress and undress, except use buttons

4 years

speech: understandable; tells stories

motor: copies a circle/cross; hops

social: toilet-trained; plays co-operatively; buttons clothes

Key points

- When asked about developmental milestones, try to divide your response into a few categories, as in the example outlined above, ie speech, motor functions, and social development.

- Developmental stages stated above relate to an 'average' child. If a child falls short in one particular category at that age group, it is not necessarily a cause for concern.

Examination skills 24: **Level: * ***

Examination of visual fields

 Mr Craig is a 53-year-old male who has been complaining of problems with his vision. He states that he has been bumping into objects recently and does not realise how close he is to items of furniture. You have been asked to assess his visual fields.

QUESTION A:

How would you proceed and is there any equipment you would like?

RESPONSE A:

I would start by introducing myself to the patient, eliciting his name and date of birth, and obtaining his consent to perform the examination.

POSITION

The patient should be asked to sit on a comfortable stool or chair, I will sit on a chair directly opposite and facing him.

INSPECTION

I would perform the examination in a darkened, private area.

To test the visual fields, this requires an assessment of the function of the peripheral and central retina, along with the optic pathways and the cortex.

Visual fields can be tested manually by a method of confrontation, where perimeters are mapped out. A crude test of visual fields can be performed by moving my hand quickly towards the patient's face. A normal response would be for the patient to blink.

Normal fields extend 130° vertically, and 160° horizontally; the blind spot is 15° from fixation in the temporal field.

To perform the examination I would request a couple of red hat pins, 5mm and 2mm sizes.

QUESTION B:

How would you perform the examination to assess visual fields by direct confrontation testing?

RESPONSE B:

- I would examine each eye separately.

- Whilst sitting opposite the patient, I would ask him to cover one eye with his hand. I would close my own eye which is directly facing the patient's closed eye.

- Ask the patient to look with his open eye directly straight at my (opposite) open eye.

- Using the 5mm red hat pin (or my index finger) I would examine the outer extent of the patient's visual fields. I'd have the red hat pin half-way between myself and the patient, then extend my arm so that the red hat pin lies beyond my own peripheral vision. Now, slowly move my finger towards the midline (fixation point) into the field of vision in a curve, until it is visible in my own visual field, I would ask the patient to let me know when he can also see the red colour of the pin. If both the patient and I have normal fields, we will both see the red hat pin at the same time.

- I would carry out the same exercise, but approach from the periphery at several points in the circumference of the upper and lower nasal and temporal quadrants of the fields. This maps out 'cone' vision.

- The physiological blind spot may be identified in the temporal portion of the visual field.

- It should be possible to map out central field defects by moving a 2mm red hat pin across the visual field. Central field defects may only manifest as a loss of colour perception.

- Once one eye is tested, I would repeat the above steps with the patient's other eye.

- To test for visual attention, I would ask the patient to inform me when my index finger is moved on one or both sides simultaneously whilst looking straight at me. If there is inattention, the patient will identify single targets but will ignore targets when the two fields are stimulated simultaneously.

QUESTION C:

What other methods of detecting visual field defects are you aware of?

RESPONSE C:

- Peripheral visual field defects are more sensitive to a moving target, so they can be tested with a Goldmann Perimeter. Here, the patient is asked to fix his or her vision on a central point. A target beam of light is then slowly moved towards the centre from the extreme of the periphery. The position at which the patient identifies the target is marked on a chart. By repeating the testing from multiple directions, it is possible to provide an accurate record of the visual fields. Each eye is tested separately.

- Central fields can also be charted with a Goldmann Perimeter using a small light source of lesser intensity. An alternative and rather sensitive method (for testing central fields) is the use of the Humphrey Field Analyser; this can record the threshold at which the patient observes a static light source of increasing intensity.

Key points

- Visual fields can be assessed manually by a method of confrontation, where perimeters can be mapped out.

- More accurate methods for testing visual fields are the use of the Goldmann Perimeter and the Humphrey Field Analyser.

- Normal fields extend 130° vertically and 160° horizontally; the blind spot is 15° from fixation in the temporal field.

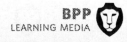

Examination skills 25:

Level: * *

Male genital examination

Mr Thornton is a 27-year-old male with a recent history of scrotal swelling. He has presented as a GP-referral to the surgical outpatient clinic. You have been asked to perform an examination of his genitalia.

QUESTION A:

How would you proceed? Use the mannequin provided as necessary.

RESPONSE A:

To start with I would introduce myself to the patient, elicit his name and date of birth. I would then explain the need to perform the examination, and obtain his verbal consent 'I need to examine your genitalia to identify whether there are any problems that could explain the scrotal swelling you have noticed recently. Is that OK?'

It is good practice to have a chaperone present (this could be a nurse) when performing genitalia examination for any patient, but mandatory when examining patients of the opposite gender.

POSITION

I would ask the patient to stand, with his undergarments off.

QUESTION B:

Please talk me through the procedure, using the mannequin provided.

RESPONSE B:

I would wash my hands and put on a pair of gloves. Once the patient is in the correct position, I would proceed.

INSPECTION

I would examine for:

–   Ulcers or lesions around the scrotum and penis.

–   Mucosal ulceration around the glans penis (first ask the patient if he has any pain; if not, gently retract the foreskin).

–   Urethral discharge. If any is seen, indicate that you would send it for microbiological examination, culture and sensitivity.

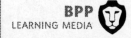

I would observe the scrotum, usually the left side testis hangs slightly lower than the right.

PALPATION

I would palpate each testis, epididymis and vas deferens, using the index finger and thumb of my hand. The testes should be equal in size; the consistency should be smooth and firm.

- An absent testis could be secondary to a failure of descent, or there may have been a surgical removal (eg due to tumour or torsion).
- Palpate for an undescended testis in the inguinal canal.
- The presence of small testes (hypogonadism) suggests that an endocrine disorder may be the cause.

- If a mass in the scrotum is felt:

  - See if you can get above it; if not, consider if there is a hernia.
  - If the mass is confined to the scrotum, is it separate or part of the testis? Can you trans-illuminate it (use a pen-torch).

  Note that a solid testicular mass is likely to be a tumour (eg teratoma or a seminoma).

  A hydrocele is a cystic mass and the testes lie within it.

  Consider if a varicocele could be present; this will feel like a mass of soft cord-like structures posterior to the testes, extending up to the epididymis.

Key points

- Talk to the model or examiner as you perform this examination.
- Look for ulcers and lesions around the penis and scrotum and for mucosal ulceration and urethral discharge.
- Remember to state you would swab any discharge and send it for microbiological analysis.
- Palpate each testis, epididymis and vas deferens, and comment on presence of these structures: their size, shape and consistency.
- Identify any masses; if present trans-illuminate them.

Examination skills 26:

Level: * *

Digital rectal examination

Mr Elwell is a 72-year-old male with a recent history of rectal bleeding. He has presented as a GP-referral to the surgical outpatient clinic. You have been asked to perform a digital rectal examination (DRE).

QUESTION A:

How would you proceed? Use the mannequin provided as appropriate.

RESPONSE A:

To start with I would introduce myself to the patient, elicit his name and date of birth; I would then explain the need to perform the procedure, and obtain his verbal consent: 'I need to examine your back passage, using my finger to identify whether there are any problems there to explain the bleeding you have had. Is that OK?'

He should be told of any complications that can occur, namely intestinal bleeding or (rarely) perforation.

It is good practice to have a chaperone present (this could be a nurse) when performing the procedure for any patient, but mandatory when examining patients of the opposite gender.

POSITION

I would ask the patient to lie down, turn onto his left side (also known as a left lateral decubitus position), and with his knees drawn up towards the chest. The chaperone, if present, should be on the left side of the bed facing the patient so that he or she can also provide reassurance, and assist in positioning.

QUESTION B:

What items of equipment do you need to prepare for the procedure?

RESPONSE B:

- KY Jelly
- Gauze swabs
- Occult blood test kit

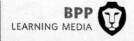

QUESTION C:

Please talk me through the procedure, using the mannequin provided as required.

RESPONSE C:

I would wash my hands and put on a pair of gloves.

Once the patient is in the correct position, I would gently part the buttocks and inspect the anus and perianal region for:

- Skin tags
- Ulcers
- Warts
- Prolapsed piles (haemorrhoids)
- Fistulas
- Fissures

I'd note that, if the patient has a fissure, a rectal examination may be too painful.

- Apply lubricant (KY Jelly) to the gloved index finger of your right hand, and tell the patient he may feel some discomfort and pressure; he should try to take 'easy breaths'.

- Insert your finger into the anus. Run the finger along the midline to the anus. Exert pressure on the anus towards the back and gently push the finger into the rectum.

- As the finger is inserted, assess for pain, eg secondary to anal fissure.

- Examine the rectum in a systematic manner. Rotate your hand clockwise and anticlockwise.

PALPATION

As I palpate the rectum, I'd ask myself the following questions:

- Is there any obvious mass, or intrinsic lesion of the rectum, eg hard, non-smooth edge of a carcinoma?

- Is there faecal loading (the rectum should normally be empty).

- Where faeces are felt, note if they are hard or soft; this will affect your treatment for constipation.

- In males, assess if the prostate feels normal. If not, is it enlarged or irregular? Is there a palpable nodule?

- I'd remove my finger and look at the glove:

  - I would look for any blood or mucus.

  - If there is faeces, is this dark/black in colour? If so, this could indicate malaena or somebody on iron therapy.

- I'd wipe the anus and perianal region with gauze; I'd then dispose of the gloves and wash my hands.

QUESTION D:

What would you do and tell the patient once the examination has been performed?

RESPONSE D:

- I would document I have performed the procedure in the patient's notes along with any findings.

- I would tell the patient that further tests may be required. I would inform him of my findings, but also let him know of the next steps in management. He may, for example, require a biopsy (if a lump is found) or other further investigation.

- The patient should also be told that they may experience bleeding and mild cramps per rectum over the next few weeks.

Key points

- Ask for a chaperone.

- Obtain the patient's verbal consent; remember to inform him of complications, namely bleeding and perforation (rare).

- During each step, give clear instructions to the mannequin.

- Inspect the anus and perianal region, informing the examiner what you are looking for.

- Apply lubricant to your gloved finger.

- Palpate the rectum in a systematic manner; in males, remember to comment on the prostate.

- On taking your finger out, comment on the presence or absence of blood or faeces on your gloved finger.

- At the end of the examination, wipe the anus, dispose of equipment correctly and wash your hands.

Examination skills 27:   Level: * * *

Examination of the hands (patient with rheumatoid arthritis)

 Mrs Sharma is a 55-year-old female presenting to the clinic as a referral from her GP, with a several-month history of stiffness affecting her hands. She denies any history of trauma. As the FY2 doctor covering the firm, you have been asked to assess her.

QUESTION A:

How would you proceed with the examination?

RESPONSE A:

I would start by introducing myself to the patient, eliciting her name, date of birth and hospital number, and obtaining her consent to perform the examination.

POSITION

I would ask her to rest her hands on a pillow with her sleeves rolled up.

INSPECTION

I'd inspect the ventral (palm) and dorsal aspects of the patient's hands for:

- Swelling
- Skin changes
- Muscle wasting of the intrinsic muscles
- Symmetrical deformities (polyarthropathy of joints)
- Ulnar deviation at the metacarpophalangeal (MCP) joint
- Radial deviation at the wrist
- Swan-neck or boutonnière's deformities in the fingers
- A Z-thumb deformity
- Sparing of the distal interphalangeal (DIP) joints
- Any vasculitic changes, pale beds or pitting in the nails
- Palmar erythema as well as pale palmar creases

I would also:

- Examine the elbows for nodules.

- Look for, and comment on, any evidence of previous surgery suggesting tendon repair or joint replacement.

PALPATION

Before feeling the hands, I would ask the patient if she has any areas of pain or tenderness.

- Feel the temperature of the hands: are they warm?

- Palpate the joints in turn: wrist, metacarpals, PIPs and DIPS. At each set of joints, also comment on synovitis and deformity.

- Heberden's nodes at the DIPs.

- Bouchard's nodes at the PIPS.

- In rheumatoid disease, you would normally identify a symmetry in the polyarthropathy and sparing of the DIPs. There may be tenderness over the ulnar styloid.

MOVEMENT

- Assess the range of active and passive movements of each set of joints.

- Assess flexion, extension, radial and ulnar deviation.

- Examine (and comment on) the function of the hand, it is not uncommon for patients to still be able to use hands that are very deformed. Test the hand and pinch grip strength. Ask her to hold a pen, write an address, undo/redo a shirt button.

Joint stability:

- Comment on any subluxation of the joints and arthritis mutulans (more often seen in psoriatic arthropathy).

Sensation:

- Examine sensation in the territories of the median, radial and ulnar nerves.

QUESTION B:

Are there any additional examinations or tests you would perform?

RESPONSE B:

To complete the hands examination, I would:

- Perform a neurological examination of the upper limbs.

- Perform a systems examination, to look for extra-articular manifestations of rheumatoid disease. This may affect the neurological, cardiovascular, respiratory, abdominal systems, along with the eyes and skin.

- Request radiographs of the hands.

Key points

- Inspect the ventral (palm) and dorsal aspects of the patient's hands, and comment on any obvious deformities, swellings or other abnormalities.

- Remember to ask whether the patient's hands are tender or painful before touching them.

- Examine and comment on the function of the hand; assess hand and pinch grip strength.

Examination skills 28:

Level: *

Examination of the sensory system in the upper limbs

Mr Arkwright is a 49-year-old male who has come to the neurology clinic today after being referred by his GP with a recent history of numbness affecting his arms.

How would you test sensation in this patient's upper limbs?

RESPONSE:

I would start by introducing myself to the patient, eliciting his name and date of birth and obtaining his verbal consent to proceed. The main sensory modalities I need to assess are:

- Pinprick – ie superficial pain
- Vibration
- Joint position sense – proprioception
- Light touch

POSITION

I would ask the patient to stand upright with his upper limbs adequately exposed in the anatomical position, with the hands supinated (palms facing uppermost).

Pinprick

- I would perform this assessment using disposable neurological pins. To start with I would demonstrate the pinprick sensation over the sternum: 'This is sharp, now this is blunt. Can you please shut your eyes and say sharp or blunt when you feel the pin.'

- I would test the patient's ability to feel pinprick sensation throughout the upper limb and upper thoracic dermatomes, C4 (shoulder) to T2 (chest wall). While assessing these along with the nerves of the hand, if any abnormality is detected, I would delineate the loss by moving from the centre of the area of loss/ abnormal sensation to the normal area.

Vibration

- This should be tested using a vibrating (128Hz) tuning fork, applied over a bony prominence.

- To ensure that the patient is feeling the actual vibration and not

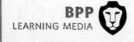

the cold metal of the tuning fork, I would ask him to close his eyes and apply the vibrating fork over the nail beds, wrists, elbows and sternum. I would ask him to tell me or indicate when he can feel the vibration, and also when he can no longer feel the vibration. (This can be stopped by touching the tines of the tuning fork.)

Joint position sense

To perform this accurately:

- Initially I would ask the patient to keep his eyes open and demonstrate what I want to show him. 'I am now moving your finger up, now moving it down; please say *up* or *down* when you detect any movement.' Now carry out the assessment with the patient's eyes closed.

- Ensure I grasp the finger at the sides, so that the patient does not have an indication of movement through pressure.

- Commence with the most distal joint (DIP); move proximally until sensation is detected.

- Use fine and not gross movements as I move the finger up and down.

Light touch

This should be the last modality to be tested as it is the most difficult to do well and interpret correctly; patients often find it difficult to identify, consistently, any differences or abnormalities in sensation.

- Use a cotton wool ball with a fine touch, not a stroking movement.

- I would ask the patient to close his eyes and say: 'As I touch your skin with this cotton wool, can you say yes when you feel something.'

When testing sensation, pinprick or light touch, always test in the middle of each dermatome. For example, if the patient has a sensory loss over the medial border of the arms (T1/T2 distribution), then subsequently test the torso to identify if a lower sensory level is present.

C5:	Lateral side of the antecubital fossa, just proximal to the elbow
C6:	Proximal phalynx of the thumb
C7:	Proximal phalynx of the middle finger
C8:	Proximal phalynx of the little finger
T1:	Medial side of the antecubital fossa, just proximal to the medial epicondyle of the humerus
T2:	At the apex of the axilla
T5:	At the nipple
T10:	At umbilicus
T12:	At midpoint of the inguinal ligament

Table 2.18: Thoracic and upper limb dermatomes: levels to remember

Key points

- Give clear and concise instructions to the patient as you perform the examination.

- Be able to show how to test sensation in a dermatomal/nerve distribution.

- Test pinprick sensation.

- Test vibration sensation.

- Test joint position sense.

- Test light touch last.

Examination skills 29:   Level: *

Examination of the sensory system in the lower limbs

Mr Witchell is a 57-year-old male who has come to the GP clinic today stating that, over the past few months, he has been having an odd sensation when he walks. He says, 'It feels like I'm walking on cotton wool.'

QUESTION A:

How would you test sensation in this patient's lower limbs?

RESPONSE A:

I would start by introducing myself to the patient, eliciting his name and date of birth and obtaining his verbal consent to proceed. The main sensory modalities I need to assess are:

- Pinprick – ie superficial pain
- Vibration
- Joint position sense – proprioception
- Light touch

POSITION

I would ask the patient to stand upright, with his upper limbs adequately exposed in the anatomical position.

INSPECTION

- **Pinprick**

    I would perform this assessment using disposable neurological pins. To start with, I would demonstrate the pinprick sensation over the sternum, and say: 'This is sharp, now this is blunt. Can you please shut your eyes and say sharp or blunt when you feel the pin'.

    I would test his ability to feel pinprick sensation throughout the lower limb dermatomes, L1 to S1 (in practice I would not routinely assess the peri-anal sensation, lower sacral dermatomes unless clinically indicated).

- **Vibration**

    This should be tested using a vibrating (128Hz) tuning fork, applied over a bony prominence. I would start at the malleolus; if there is a sensory deficit here, then move up to the head of the fibula, then anterior superior iliac spine.

To ensure that the patient is feeling the actual vibration and not the cold metal of the tuning fork, I would ask him to close his eyes and then apply the vibrating fork over these bony prominences. I would ask him to tell me or indicate when he can feel the vibration and also when he can no longer feel the vibration. (This can be stopped by touching the tines of the tuning fork.)

- **Joint position sense**

  To perform this accurately, I would initially ask him to keep his eyes open and demonstrate what I want to show him: 'I am now moving your big toe up; now moving it down. Please say *up* or *down* when you detect any movement.' Then I would carry out the assessment with the patient's eyes closed. If there is any abnormality, test ankle joint position sense in the same way. I'd use fine and not gross movements as I moved the big toe up and down.

- **Light touch**

  This should be the last modality to be tested as it is the most difficult to do well and interpret correctly. Patients often find it difficult to identify, consistently, any differences or abnormalities in sensation. I'd use a cotton wool ball with a fine touch, not a stroking movement, and would ask the patient to close his eyes. 'As I touch your skin with this cotton wool, can you say yes when you feel something'.

When testing sensation, pinprick or light touch, I would always test in the middle of each dermatome.

- **Mobilise**

  If the patient is physically able, ask him to stand up, then ask him to walk (see Examination skills 11: Examination of gait)

- **Romberg's test**

  Stand behind the patient and ask him to stand with his heels together, at first with eyes open, then with the eyes closed.

  Look for any excessive postural swaying or loss of balance. If this is present when the eyes are either open or closed this is a sign of cerebellar deficit (cerebellar ataxia). If, however, this swaying or loss of balance is only present when the eyes are closed, this is called a positive Romberg's test and indicates posterior column disease, proprioceptive deficit (sensory ataxia).

QUESTION B:

What do you think is the problem in this patient?

RESPONSE B:

Well, as he is complaining of 'walking on cotton wool', this is very often suggestive of a peripheral neuropathy; this is often secondary to diabetes mellitus. Such a peripheral neuropathy causes a stocking loss, which is usually more common on the left side, but does not have to be perfectly symmetrical.

L1:	Upper anterior thigh
L2:	At the antero-medial thigh (mid-thigh level)
L3:	At the medial epicondyle of the femur
L4:	Over the medial malleolus
L5:	On the dorsum of the foot, namely at the third metatarsophalangeal joint
S1:	At the lateral aspect of the calcaneus
S2:	Popliteal fossa
S3:	Over the ischial tuberosity
S4:	Outer perianal area
S5:	Inner perianal area

Table 2.19: Lower limb dermatomes, levels to remember

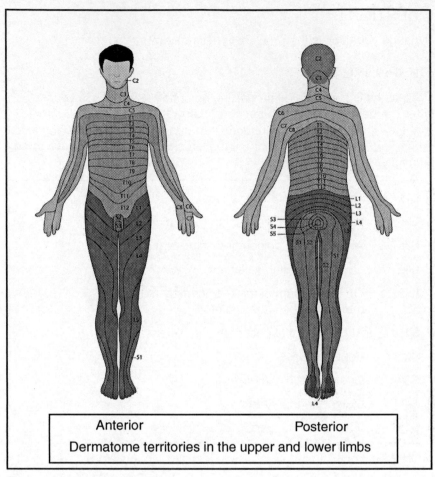

Anterior   Posterior

Dermatome territories in the upper and lower limbs

Figure 2.3: Dermatomal patterns

Key points

- Give clear and concise instructions to the patient as you perform the examination.

- Be able to show how to test sensation in a dermatomal/nerve distribution.

- Test pinprick sensation.

- Test vibration sensation.

- Test joint position sense.

- Test light touch, as the final item.

- Ask the patient to stand up and then walk (if physically able).

- Perform Romberg's test to look for signs of posterior column disease.

Further reading

Useful texts for examination skills:

Cox, N and Roper, T eds. (2005) *Clinical skills: Oxford Core Text*. Oxford: OUP.

Douglas, G et al (2009) *Macleod's Clinical Examination*. 12th edition. Oxford: Churchill Livingstone.

Gleadle, J (2012) *History and Clinical Examination at a Glance*. 3rd edition. Oxford: Wiley-Blackwell.

Glynn, M and Drake, W eds. (2012) *Hutchison's Clinical Methods*. 21st edition. Oxford: Saunders Ltd.

Thomas, J and Monaghan, T (2007) *Oxford Handbook of Clinical Examination and Practical Skills*. Oxford: OUP.

Chapter 3

Clinical procedure

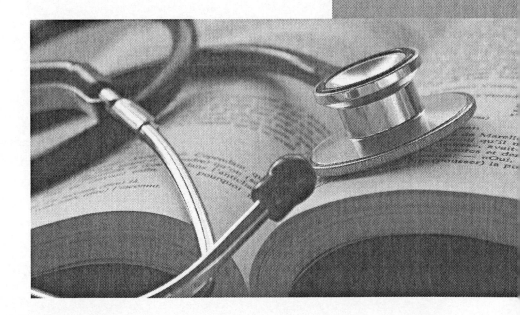

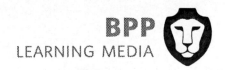

Clinical procedure 1:

Level * *

Arterial blood gas sampling

Mr Turner is a 53-year-old male, admitted to the medical admissions unit with an infective exacerbation of COPD. As the FY1 doctor on call you have been informed by the nurse that his saturations have dropped on room air and he appears to be having some difficulty in breathing.

QUESTION A:

Please use the mannequin provided to show how you would proceed to take an arterial blood gas sample.

RESPONSE A:

*   INTRODUCTION: To begin with I would introduce myself. I would check I am speaking to the right patient by eliciting his name and date of birth. At this stage I would try to establish a rapport and make him feel at ease.

*   EXPLANATION: I would explain the reasons for taking the blood gas: 'Hello Mr Turner, my name is James Peters. I'm the doctor on call today. I understand you have been having some difficulty in breathing. To help keep an eye on your progress, I need to take a blood test from your wrist. It may cause you some temporary pain, but it shouldn't last long; it's usually a reasonably quick procedure.'

*   CONSENT: Ask the patient if that is OK. Also check with them if they have any questions or concerns.

*   POSITION: The patient should be sitting or lying comfortably. Select an arm and place a pillow underneath the arm to support it.

QUESTION B:

What equipment do you need to perform the arterial blood gas sampling?

RESPONSE B:

I would have the following equipment to perform the procedure:

*   A pre-heparinised syringe
*   Alcohol steret
*   Cotton wool or gauze
*   A pair of gloves
*   An arterial blood gas syringe, 23G (blue) needles
*   A sharps container

 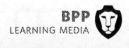

QUESTION C:

Can you describe the procedure to me?

RESPONSE C:

- I would wash my hands with an appropriate disinfectant, then dry them.

- Put on a pair of gloves.

- Clean the area of radial pulsation with an alcohol steret; to do this, I use a circular motion, moving from the centre to the periphery. Allow to air dry.

- With the patient positioned comfortably, and having their wrist and elbow extended, palm facing upwards, I would locate their radial pulse with the index and middle finger of my non-dominant hand. Use my fingers to palpate the size, depth and direction of the artery.

- Inform the patient he will feel a 'sharp scratch'.

- Insert the needle (attached to the blood gas syringe) at an angle of 30° to the skin at the point of maximal pulsation.

- Advance the needle until arterial blood passes back into the syringe.

- Allow the blood to fill the syringe under arterial pressure, aspirate gently if required.

- If the artery has been missed, slowly withdraw the tip of the needle and insert at a slightly different angle.

- Aim to aspirate approximately 2ml of blood into the syringe, then withdraw the needle.

- Apply a piece of cotton wool or gauze over the puncture site and apply firm pressure for 5 minutes. I can ask the patient to press, using his other hand.

- Remove the needle and put it in the sharps container.

- Expel any air from the syringe and cap it.

- I would now label it with patient's name, date of birth, hospital number, date and time the sample is taken. Then I would take the sample quickly to the blood gas analyser.

QUESTION D:

How do you go about interpreting the results of the arterial blood gas (ABG)?

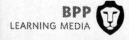

RESPONSE D:

- First, I would identify the inspired oxygen concentration, or note if the patient was breathing room air.

- Next, look at the pCO_2 and pO_2 concentration, to see if there is any evidence of respiratory failure.

  Where there is hypoxia (low pO_2) and low CO_2, this would indicate a ventilation perfusion mismatch, or type 1 respiratory failure.

  Hypoxia (low pO_2) with a raised pCO_2, indicates a type 2 respiratory failure.

- I look at the pH to see if there is an acidosis or an alkalosis.

  If pH > 7.45 this indicates alkalosis
  pH < 7.45 indicates acidosis

- I identify the metabolic and respiratory components:

  Acidosis and a high pCO_2 (>6.0 kpa): respiratory acidosis
  Acidosis and a low HCO_3 (<22mmol/l): metabolic acidosis
  Alkalosis and a low pCO_2 (<4.5 kpa): respiratory alkalosis
  Alkalosis and a high HCO_3 (>30mmol/l): metabolic alkalosis

	pH	pCO_2	HCO_3	Examples
Metabolic alkalosis	↑	↑*	↑	Diarrhoea and vomiting, use of diuretics
Metabolic acidosis	↓	↓*	↓	Renal failure, lactic acidosis, ketoacidotic states, such as diabetes and alcoholism
Respiratory alkalosis	↑	↓	↓*	Pulmonary embolism, pneumonia, asthma attack, anxiety
Respiratory acidosis	↓	↑	↑*	COPD, asthma, neuromuscular disease eg Guillain-Barré syndrome, opiate overdose

Table 3.1: Examples of the different types of acid/base disorders

- pH ↑ implies pH greater than 7.45
- pH ↓ implies pH less than 7.35

For pCO_2 and HCO_3:

  ↑ implies a primary increase
  ↓ implies a primary decrease
  ↑* implies a compensatory increase
  ↓* implies a compensatory decrease

QUESTION E:

What is the anion gap?

RESPONSE E:

The anion gap, the difference in the measured cations (positively charged ions) and the measured anions (negatively charged ions), is a useful test to determine the cause of a metabolic acidosis. Once you know the serum electrolytes including the chloride value, the anion gap can be calculated:

Anion gap $= [(Na^+ + K^+)] - [(Cl^- + HCO3^-)]$

The usefulness of calculating the anion gap is in distinguishing a metabolic acidosis resulting from an accumulation of lactic acid (lactic acidosis), ketoacids (as occurs in diabetic ketoacidosis) or that occurring secondary to poisoning with drugs such as salicylate. In this setting (salicylate poisoning), there is no compensatory rise in chloride and the anion gap exceeds 10mmol/l.

If, for example, the patient has renal failure, this can result in an impairment of hydrogen ion excretion causing an acidosis. As pH and bicarbonate falls, the serum chloride value rises to maintain electrical neutrality so that the anion gap is less than 10mmol/l. A normal anion gap is often defined as being within the prediction interval of 3–11 mEq/L, however this will vary slightly from one laboratory reference range to another.

Key points

- Inform the patient why you need to perform the ABG, making them aware it may cause some pain, and obtain their consent.

- Palpate the radial artery using the index finger and middle finger of your non-dominant hand; avoid using your thumb, as this has its own pulse, which can be confused with that of the patient.

- At least approximately 2ml of arterial blood will be required to obtain an accurate analysis.

- Cap the syringe as soon as the sample is taken, noting the concentration of inspired oxygen the patient is on.

- Taking the pH into account, methodically work out the acid/base disturbance.

Clinical procedure 2:   Level * *

Aspirate a knee joint

An anatomical model of a knee joint is available at this station. You are given a trolley containing various items, including a pair of gloves, povidone-iodine solution (Betadine), dressing pack, a couple of syringes and needles, alcohol sterets, cotton gauze, specimen pots for fluid collection and a glucose tube.

Please regard this model as the knee of a 60-year-old man who has presented to the emergency department with a swollen, tender and painful right knee. You have performed an examination and note that he has a large effusion present.

QUESTION A:

Describe the indications for performing a diagnostic knee aspiration.

RESPONSE A:

There are several reasons for performing a knee joint aspiration:
- To drain off a haemarthrosis (blood in the joint cavity) following trauma.

- To establish a diagnosis from the fluid obtained; depending on a patient's background, they may have a crystal arthritis, an inflammatory or non-inflammatory process, a septic arthritis or even a haemarthrosis.

- Aspiration of a joint can also be therapeutic to provide symptomatic relief of a large effusion; it can be performed to administer a steroid injection or drain infection.

QUESTION B:

Are you aware of any contraindications to needle aspiration of a joint in general – not necessarily to aspiration of the knee only?

RESPONSE B:

I would be hesitant to perform a joint aspiration in the following circumstances:
- If there is overlying infection in the joint soft tissues
- In the presence of a severe coagulopathy
- If the patient has a joint prosthesis or the joint is inaccessible

- If there is a bacteraemia
- If the patient is uncooperative

QUESTION C:

Using the model provided, demonstrate the technique of knee joint aspiration.

RESPONSE C:

- I would begin by introducing myself to the patient, verifying his name, date of birth, hospital number and obtaining his consent.

- I would ask the patient to sit on a couch; I would position his knee slightly flexed and support it using a pillow.

- Ensure all the equipment required (as stated above) is available and on a procedure trolley.

- Wash my hands and apply a pair of gloves.

- Clean the knee with betadine-soaked swabs, place the drapes (from the dressing pack) around the knee puncture site to create a sterile field. Once the betadine has dried, re-clean the puncture site with alcohol sterets as betadine can affect culture results.

- Attach a green (21G) needle to a 10ml syringe.

- Apply pressure on the medial aspect of the patella with my free hand to displace fluid laterally, in this way opening the space between the patella and femur.

- Insert the needle through the skin, entering from the supero-lateral aspect of the joint with the needle directed infero-medially. Aspirate as the needle is advanced. Stop advancing the needle when fluid is encountered.

- Withdraw as much of the fluid as possible, before taking the needle and syringe out. Apply firm pressure over the puncture site with a cotton swab until any bleeding has stopped. Apply a gauze dressing over the site.

- Inform the patient the procedure is over and advise that they should take some bed rest to take the weight off the joint and take analgesia as required.

- Fill the specimen pots and glucose tube with the fluid extracted and label the microbiology & biochemistry requests correctly.

- Ensure all sharps and waste are disposed of appropriately and wash my hands.

QUESTION D:

What would you document in the patient notes?

RESPONSE D:

- I would document the procedure: in this I would include the amount of fluid aspirated as well as its colour – for example, it could be clear (suggesting a non-inflammatory process), turbid (suggesting a possible inflammatory process), milky (which can be found in a crystal arthritis) or even bloodstained (as occurs with a haemarthrosis).

- I would also state that the sample has been sent for microscopy, culture and sensitivity along with biochemistry (glucose) analysis.

Key points

- The technique of joint aspiration can be both diagnostic as well as therapeutic.

- Infection of the knee or any other joint can have severe debilitating consequences, hence you should emphasise the need to take sterile precautions whilst performing the technique of joint aspiration.

- The volume and colour of the fluid obtained can provide an indication of the diagnosis.

Clinical procedure 3: Level *

Blood pressure measurement

Mr Wells is returning to the OPD for a follow-up following his recent inpatient admission with an acute coronary syndrome. As part of his clinical examination, you should take a blood pressure reading.

QUESTION A:

How would you proceed?

RESPONSE A:

- INTRODUCTION: To begin with I would introduce myself. I would check I am speaking to the right patient by eliciting his name, date of birth and hospital number. At this stage I would try to establish a rapport and make him feel at ease.

- EXPLANATION: I would explain the reasons for taking the blood pressure: 'Hello Mr Wells, my name is Paul Knight. I'm the doctor in the clinic today. In view of your recent admission I would like to measure your blood pressure as part of your routine assessment. Could I ask you to remove your jacket and sit up straight on the chair? Then I'll place the blood pressure cuff around your arm above the elbow.' I can then measure the blood pressure with my stethoscope, the end of which I will hold against the patient's arm.

- CONSENT: I would ask the patient if that is OK. Also check with him if he has any questions or concerns.

QUESTION B:

What equipment do you need to perform the blood pressure measurement?

RESPONSE B:

I would have the following equipment to perform the procedure:

- Cuff: Choosing the appropriate size cuff for the patient, from a choice of two. Large and obese patients will require a large cuff, children will need a small cuff.

- BP machine: Ensure that the cuff is deflated fully and correctly attached.

- Stethoscope.

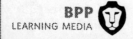

QUESTION C:

Please describe the procedure to me.

RESPONSE C:

- Apply the appropriate-sized cuff to the patient's arm, ensure it is completely deflated and attached to the BP machine correctly.

- Have the patient with the arm fully extended and horizontal. Place the BP machine in line with the level of the heart.

- Palpate the brachial or radial artery as I inflate the cuff. Identify the systolic pressure by palpation, inflate the cuff above the systolic pressure (so that the brachial artery is compressed and the radial pulse is impalpable). When this point has been reached, inflate the cuff by a further 20 30mmHg; now let the pressure release slowly, until I feel the pulse return.

- Auscultate over the brachial artery (with the diaphragm of the stethoscope) to identify the systolic pressure using my stethoscope. Again inflate the cuff 20–30mmHg over the systolic pressure. Now I would release the pressure slowly (2mmHg/sec).

- Note when I can hear the first sound (called 1st Korotkoff sound); this is the systolic pressure. I would record this value to the nearest 2mmHg.

- Continue to deflate the cuff; the Korotkoff sound then gets louder before appearing muffled (4th Korotkoff sound), and then the sound disappears; on disappearing this is the diastolic pressure (5th Korotkoff sound).

- After the 5th Korotkoff sound, deflate and release the cuff.

- I would state that I would repeat the blood pressure measurement in the other arm and with the patient standing; this will allow me to observe for a postural drop.

- If I identify (on standing) a drop of 20mmHg systolic pressure that remains sustained at 2 minutes, the patient has a postural hypotension.

- State that I would take at least two blood pressure measurements, as features such as anxiety and recent exercise may cause falsely raised readings.

- Ask the patient if he has any concerns and document the results in the patient notes.

Key points

- Ensure the appropriate size cuff is chosen for each patient.
- Identify the systolic pressure both by palpation and auscultation.
- Remember to state that you would check for a postural drop in blood pressure.
- Also, state you would obtain at least two readings, lying and standing, to account for variable factors, such as exercise and anxiety.

Clinical procedure 4:   Level **

Blood transfusion

> Mrs Gulati is a 46-year-old female who is one day post-op. She has returned to the ward following a sigmoid colectomy for bowel cancer. Her haemoglobin level today is 7.1g/dl. You have been asked by your consultant to organise a two-unit blood transfusion. She already has an IV cannula in situ; the nurse tells you that the blood has been cross-matched and the porter has brought the first unit on to the ward.

QUESTION A:

Explain how you would proceed to organise the transfusion.

RESPONSE A:

- I would start by introducing myself to the patient. I would check that I am speaking to the right patient by eliciting her name, date of birth and hospital number, which should all be on the patient's ID label, usually on the patient's wrist.

- I would give her the explanation that she requires a blood transfusion, as she has lost a large volume of blood during her procedure.

- I would ask her if she has any questions or concerns, and obtain her verbal consent to go ahead with the transfusion.

- Check the prescription chart to confirm the blood has been prescribed, review the date, time, number of units required along with the infusion rate.

- Verify if the patient has any allergies, any past history of blood transfusion reactions. Also check if she has recently been pregnant, within the past three months or so.

- Ensure that she is seated or lying comfortably in bed. The arm through which the transfusion will be run can be rested on a pillow for added support.

- Have a note of the patient's vital signs, temperature, saturation, blood pressure and heart rate.

QUESTION B:

What equipment do you need to perform the transfusion?

RESPONSE B:

I would gather the following equipment:

- A unit of blood
- Blood transfusion giving set
- A syringe containing normal saline flush
- A pair of gloves

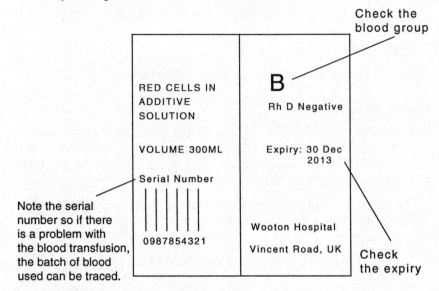

Check the blood group

RED CELLS IN ADDITIVE SOLUTION

B

Rh D Negative

VOLUME 300ML

Expiry: 30 Dec 2013

Serial Number

Note the serial number so if there is a problem with the blood transfusion, the batch of blood used can be traced.

0987854321

Wooton Hospital

Vincent Road, UK

Check the expiry

Figure 3.1: Showing the front label on a unit of blood

QUESTION C:

Describe how you would perform the procedure.

RESPONSE C:

- I would commence by washing my hands with an appropriate disinfectant, drying them thoroughly and putting on a pair of gloves.

- Flush the cannula, which is already in situ, with 5-10ml of normal saline to check its patency. A size 16G (grey) cannula would be ideal.

- Two people (one of whom is myself) should check the patient's identity. Confirm her full name, date of birth, hospital number against her identity band, blood compatibility report, blood unit label and the drug chart.

- With another colleague or nurse, check the serial number of the blood unit against that on the compatibility report. Also, make sure the blood unit has not expired and check the bag for any leaks, clots or discolouration.

- Flush the blood giving set with normal (0.9%) saline; this will help to remove any air (I should not use any solution containing dextrose).

- Connect the giving set to the blood bag for transfusion. Infusion should take place through a blood administration set with an integral filter (double-barrel set).

- Using the roller clamp, alter the drip rate as necessary.

- The patient should be advised to contact a nurse or member of staff if she develops breathing difficulties, a fever, joint pains, a rash or itchiness.

- Ensure that the nurse taking care of the patient routinely monitors her observations, and in so doing check for adverse reactions to the transfused blood – at 0 minutes (ie initially), 15 minutes, 30 minutes and at 1 hour. Check the hospital policy for frequency of observations.

- Document and sign in the drug chart and blood compatibility report the date and time of transfusion. The patient's notes should also contain the transfusion details, including the number of units given, patient's blood group, the rate of infusion and any adverse reactions.

- At the end of the transfusion, make sure the patient remains comfortable; check if she has any concerns.

- If there is a concern about fluid overload, then I would give the patient Furosemide 20mg (a diuretic) by mouth with alternate bags.

- Re-check the patient's haemoglobin level (FBC bottle) around 12 to 24 hours after the final unit has been transfused.

QUESTION D:

You are told Mrs Gulati develops an urticarial skin rash one hour into the transfusion. She becomes breathless, with a raised temperature (38.1°C), severe headache and abdominal pain. What do you think has happened and what would you do?

RESPONSE D:

It is likely from this history that our patient has developed a haemolytic transfusion reaction. This needs to be treated as a matter of urgency. I would:

- Immediately stop the blood transfusion. Replace the giving set, keeping the line patent with normal saline.

- Check the patient's identity against the blood bottle used for transfusion, to verify she has not received the wrong patient's blood.

- Perform venepuncture to take blood for analysis, FBC, urea and electrolytes, coagulation screen; repeat a cross-match and send off some blood cultures.

- Return the giving set along with the remaining blood to the laboratory.

- Contact the haematology registrar or consultant on call for senior help.

St. John's NHS Trust, Wiltshire, UK

PRESCRIPTION for Inpatient Blood Transfusion

Name _____	Patient Location _____
Address _____	Consultant _____
_____ Date of Birth ___ / ___ / ____	Date of transfusion(s) ____ / ____ / _____
Hospital No. _____	

Indications for Red Cell Transfusion

1. Acute blood loss (especially if > 1.5L in adult)
2. Symptomatic anaemia with no easily treatable cause (e.g. treat FE deficiency with Fe!),
   i.e. Hb <8g/dl (age <75yrs),   or   Hb <9g/dL (age >75yrs, or cardiac or respiratory disease)
3. Long-term transfusion-dependent anaemia
4. Radiotherapy patient (Hb < 10g/dL)
5. Chemotherapy patient (Hb <9g/dL)

- Indication for Transfusion (according to list above) _____
  (This must also be clearly documented in the patient's medical records)
- Patient's Blood Group _____   Pre-Transfusion Hb: _____ g/dL   (Date: _____)
- History of transfusion reaction/allergy? YES/NO.   If YES, Please specify _____
- Special Requirements (please circle):   Irradiated blood / CMV negative / Blood warmer

(ONCE ONLY MEDICATIONS)
Under NO circumstances should any drugs be added to blood or component transfusions

DRUG	DOSE	ROUTE	Doctor's Signature	Date	Time given	Signature
Hydrocortisone	100 mgs	IV bolus				
Chlorpheniramine	10 mgs	IV bolus				
0.9% N/Saline flush	5 ml	IV				

TRANSFUSION ROTA

Product	Duration	Diuretic (if required)	Doctor's Signature	Date

MILD Reactions	ACTION	SEVERE Reactions	ACTION
Rising pulse Rising temperature Flushing Shivering Tingling Headache Urticarial rash	Slow or stop transfusion Inform nurse in charge who will inform doctor	SHOCK. Fall in BP Rapid thready pulse Pain – Lumbar, Chest or abdomen Rigor Dyspnoea Vomiting Incontinence	Stop transfusion Inform nurse in charge who will immediately summon doctor

After use Please File in Patient's Medical Records with the Nursing Notes

Figure 3.2: Example of an inpatient blood transfusion prescription

Key points

- In general, consider a transfusion if the haemoglobin is <8g/dl or if the patient is symptomatic from their anaemia. Seek advice from your seniors.

- Blood transfusion usually occurs at a rate of one unit between 2- and 4-hourly.

- Always remember to check the patient's details – and that of the blood to be transfused – to make sure the right blood is being given to the right patient. It is prudent to do this with a colleague or nurse.

- During and after transfusion, observe for symptoms that could indicate an adverse transfusion reaction, such as fever, breathlessness, flushing, headache, abdominal pain, rash and itchiness. Act urgently if these are recognised.

Clinical procedure 5:   Level *

Hand washing

You are the surgical FY2 doctor on call, attending a ward round with your consultant. You have just finished reviewing a patient with an infected abdominal wound and are about to proceed to see the next patient.

QUESTION A:

Explain how you would approach and wash your hands before you examine the next patient.

RESPONSE A:

I would start by introducing myself. I would roll up my shirt so the sleeves are above the elbows. Then remove my wristwatch, along with any other jewellery. If I had a tie on I would tuck it into my shirt.

QUESTION B:

OK, now what steps would you take to ensure effective hand washing?

RESPONSE B:

*   I would turn on the hot and cold water taps ensuring a suitable, lukewarm temperature.

*   Then wet both my hands and apply about 5 to 10ml of liquid disinfectant, such as hibiscrub.

*   I then rub my hands to develop a lather, applying this between my fingers, under the nails, on the palm and back of the hand. This I would do for between 30 to 60 seconds.

*   I would then rinse my hands under the tap so that the water drips downwards to the elbows, not the other way round.

*   I then take paper towels from the dispenser to dry each hand thoroughly.

*   Finally I would switch off the taps using my elbows and discard the paper towels in the appropriate container.

QUESTION C:

In what other ways can you ensure effective hand hygiene between patients?

RESPONSE C:

Instead of washing hands with water, alcohol antiseptic from a dispenser can also be used, allowing the alcohol to air dry.

QUESTION D:

Apart from the wards, are there any other settings where you should be washing your hands in a hospital?

RESPONSE D:

- I would want to wash my hands in virtually every setting prior to patient contact. This would include seeing patients in clinics. In A&E, and especially in an ITU setting and in theatre when scrubbing up for a procedure.

- It is also good practice as a doctor to carry an alcohol-dispensing bottle whilst walking around the hospital seeing patients on the same and in different wards.

Key points

- Effective hand washing may seem a trivial task; however, when commencing work as a junior doctor, poor compliance and bad technique will be picked up on by seniors and nursing staff.

- Remember to rinse appropriately from hands to elbows, reducing the risk of re-contaminating your fingers and hands.

- It would look professional as a trainee (even someone doing their clinical examination) to attach an alcohol-dispensing bottle to your belt, or keep in a pocket. Show the examiner the act of taking it out and using it before touching a patient.

Clinical procedure 6:   Level *

Intravenous drug injection

Mrs Bailey is a 46-year-old female who has been admitted to the general surgical ward with abdominal obstruction. She has had a few episodes of vomiting whilst in A&E. As the FY1 doctor on the ward you have been asked by your registrar to administer 10mg of metoclopramide via an IV injection.

QUESTION A:

How would you proceed?

RESPONSE A:

- INTRODUCTION: To begin with I would introduce myself. I would check I am speaking to the right patient by eliciting her name, date of birth and hospital number. At this stage I would try to establish a rapport and make her feel at ease.

- EXPLANATION: I would explain the reasons for giving the anti-emetic (anti-sickness). 'I have been asked to give you an anti-sickness drug called metoclopramide. This should help the feelings of nausea you have been having recently and help to prevent sickness. The quickest way for it to act is through a vein in your arm as an injection; for this purpose we can use the cannula already in your arm. Do you have any questions?'

- CONSENT: I would obtain verbal consent from the patient and warn her of some of the more common side effects of the drug (metoclopramide) such as drowsiness, dizziness and fatigue.

- POSITION: The patient should be sitting or lying comfortably.

QUESTION B:

Explain how you would perform the procedure; prepare the equipment as you do so.

RESPONSE B:

- I would start by checking the patient's drug chart to verify the name of the drug, its dosage, dilutant and volume of dilutant (if required), the route of administration (intravenous in this case), date and time to be given and the signature of the requesting clinician – ie the validity of the prescription.

- Clarify if the patient has any drug allergies, and specifically to the drug to be administered.

- Check the British National Formulary (BNF) to see if the drug and dose are appropriate.

- Wash my hands using a disinfectant, dry thoroughly and put on a pair of gloves.

- Check the name, strength and expiry date of the drug in the ampoule with a nurse or colleague.

- Now prepare the correct volume of the drug, dilute as per the manufacturer's guidelines, draw into a syringe using a green (21G) needle.

- Expel any excess air from the syringe and needle by inverting the syringe and tapping.

- Draw up a 10ml normal saline flush.

- Remove the cap from the cannula port already in situ. Use an alcohol steret to clean the injection port, allow to air dry (for about 30 seconds). Flush the cannula port with 5ml normal saline to confirm its patency. Inject and administer the medication at the correct speed as stated in the BNF. Follow this with a further 5ml normal saline flush.

- Ensure that the patient is comfortable during the procedure and no localised swelling has occurred at the injection site.

- Remove the syringe, close the cap on the cannula port.

- Dispose of the syringe, my gloves and any soiled material.

- Document, in the drug chart, the time the drug was administered and sign.

BPP
LEARNING MEDIA

Key points

- Before administering any drug, it is paramount that some basic checks are performed: this includes the patient's identity, their allergies, the drug, its dosage, strength, dilution, expiry date and method of administration. Always mention that you would also check the drug with a nurse or colleague before administering it.

- Explain to the patient why they need the drug and seek their consent to administer it.

- Administer the IV injection at the correct rate, as stated in the BNF.

- Document in the drug chart that the drug has been administered, along with the dosage and route of administration. State the date and time, and sign.

Clinical procedure 7:   Level * *

Lumbar Puncture

Mrs Chen is a 29-year-old female who over the last 36 hours has been complaining of headaches, nausea with three episodes of vomiting, problems with looking at bright light and neck stiffness. Her GP has seen her and is concerned she may have meningitis; she has now been referred under your consultant's care. He has asked you to perform a lumbar puncture with cerebrospinal fluid (CSF) analysis to help verify the diagnosis.

QUESTION A:

Name some of the indications for performing a lumbar puncture.

RESPONSE A:

The cerebrospinal fluid (CSF) obtained from a lumbar puncture is required:

- If acute or chronic infection of the brain or meningitis is a possibility.

- If the diagnostic possibilities include neurological disorders such as multiple sclerosis, Guillain-Barré syndrome and sarcoidosis.

- In situations where subarachnoid haemorrhage is a likely diagnosis, when patients have a negative CT Head scan, or if CT imaging facilities are not available.

- When patients have an excessive amount of fluid in the ventricles of the brain, hydrocephalus – in this situation repeated lumbar punctures over a few days may be of benefit by draining the CSF.

QUESTION B:

In what situations is a lumbar puncture contraindicated?

RESPONSE B:

- Where there is an intracranial space occupying lesion – CSF withdrawal can result in a pressure gradient which may result in tentorial herniation.

- Papilloedema or other signs of raised intracranial pressure.

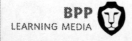

- A low platelet count – less than 40,000 or in the presence of any other clotting abnormality.

- A relative contraindication is if there is localised infection over the lumbar puncture-needle insertion site.

QUESTION C:

Can you explain the procedure to me?

RESPONSE C:

- I would inform the patient what the procedure involves, explaining the risks and benefits and obtain her informed consent before proceeding.

- I would ask the patient to lie on the edge of a couch in the left lateral position, with knees up to her chest. An assistant would stand in front of the patient to help keep her in position and talk to her to keep her calm during the procedure.

- I would identify my landmarks by palpating the iliac crests; the L4/5 interspace lies level with the iliac crests.

- I would then clean her back with antiseptic solution such as chlorhexidine.

- Once I have identified an appropriate level, I would inform the patient I am about to give the local anaesthetic.

- After allowing the anaesthetic a couple of minutes to act, I would then insert the spinal needle, until I feel a 'give' suggesting the dura has been punctured. I can then remove the stylet from the needle slowly to obtain and collect CSF.

- Once I have collected 3 to 5mls of CSF I will take out the needle, clean the wound site with a chlorhexidine soaked swab and then apply a mepore dressing.

- I would ask her to lie flat for at least a couple of hours after the procedure to reduce the risk of a post-lumbar puncture headache.

QUESTION D:

At what level does the spinal cord end?

RESPONSE D:

The spinal cord in adults ends at the L1/2 interspace; for that reason I would not insert the spinal needle above the L2/3 interspace.

QUESTION E:

Can you explain what Queckenstedt's test is?

RESPONSE E:

Yes, as part of the lumbar puncture I may have to have to perform this manoeuvre. It involves placing my hands round the patient's neck momentarily and compressing the internal jugular vein. A positive test is suggested by no rise in CSF pressure on compression of this vein. This would suggest that the flow of CSF is blocked in the spinal canal.

QUESTION F:

When you ask the patient for consent to perform the lumbar puncture, what should you make her aware of?

RESPONSE F:

Well, I would tell her that, during the procedure, she may experience a sudden sharp numbness or pain affecting one or both legs; I would tell her that this should not last more than a few minutes. She should also be told she may experience an ache in her lower back for some time after the procedure. Perhaps most importantly she should be warned of the risk of a headache following the lumbar puncture. For this reason I would request she lay flat on her back for some time. Both the headache and backache should respond to basic analgesia such as paracetamol and codeine phosphate.

Key points

- Ensure that you obtain informed consent for the lumbar puncture; this can be written or verbal. Where verbal consent is obtained, make sure you document the risks explained to the patient.

- Remember this scenario is a favourite for examiners, particularly to assess communication skills, hence talk to the patient in an approachable and empathetic manner.

- The examiner will want to see that you are technically safe in performing the procedure – it is especially important you know your landmarks, eg the point of termination of the spinal cord.

- Be able to state some of the indications and contraindications for this procedure. Note that determining the presence of meningitis is not the only reason for performing a lumbar puncture.

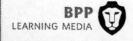

Clinical procedure 8:   Level *

Nasogastric intubation

> Mrs Joshi is a 56-year-old female who has been admitted to the
> surgical assessment unit with what appears to be intestinal
> obstruction. Over the past three days she has been complaining of
> abdominal pain, inability to open her bowels, a distended abdomen
> along with several episodes of vomiting and constant nausea. The
> nurse taking care of her has asked you to insert a nasogastric tube.

QUESTION A:

State the indications for inserting a nasogastric tube, also known as a
Ryle's tube.

RESPONSE A:

By inserting a wide-bore nasogastric tube, you are gaining access to
the stomach and its contents, allowing the application of suction. This is
indicated:

- When gastric emptying is required
    - When intestinal obstruction/ileus is suspected
    - At the time of gastro-intestinal surgery, pre and post-op
    - Situations where there is a risk of aspiration, as may occur
      in serious illness
    - To perform gastric lavage in drug overdose or poisoning
- When aspiration of stomach contents is required, for example, to
  assess the state of GI bleeding in trauma scenarios.

QUESTION B:

Are you aware of any contraindications to, or complications of, inserting
a nasogastric tube?

RESPONSE B:

- Inserting a nasogastric tube is contraindicated in the presence
  of severe facial trauma, and certain cranial fractures, cribriform
  plate or base-of-skull fractures. This is due to the possibility of the
  tube being misguided intra-cranially. In these circumstances an
  orogastric tube can be inserted instead.

- The main complications of nasogastric tube insertion are tissue trauma during insertion, along with initiating aspiration. The act of inserting the catheter (tube) can produce gagging or vomiting; for this reason it would be prudent to have suction available and at hand.

QUESTION C:

When would you use a fine-bore tube instead of a wide-bore one?

RESPONSE C:

- When a nasogastric tube is needed for feeding or giving medication enterally.

- When the tube is required to stay in situ for more than seven days.

These fine-bore tubes collapse on the application of suction; they are also too fine to allow air to be syringed through them rapidly. Hence the only way to ensure they are in the correct position is by X-raying – (the tube has a radio-opaque marker).

QUESTION D:

Please describe the procedure of nasogastric tube insertion.

RESPONSE D:

- I would begin by introducing myself to the patient, eliciting her name, date of birth and hospital number, and obtaining her consent.

- Arrange a signal so that the patient can communicate that she may want to stop, for example, 'raise your hand if you are in pain'.

- Assist to sit her in a supported upright position, with the neck slightly flexed, either in a bed or chair.

- I would wash my hands with soap and water, put on an apron and wear gloves. Then I would assemble all the equipment required.

- Next, I would select the appropriate length of tube required by measuring the distance from the patient's ear lobe to the tip of the nose to the xiphisternum, marking this distance with a piece of tape on the tube.

- The procedure can be very uncomfortable for the patient, so to help alleviate the discomfort I would squirt some xylocaine jelly into her nostril and spray some xylocaine to the back of the throat.

- Lubricate the distal (end) two to four inches of the tube with KY jelly, using gauze.

- Pass the tube into a nostril, sliding it backwards and inwards along the floor of the nose to the nasopharynx. If any obstruction is felt, remove the tube and try again in a slightly different direction; alternatively use the other nostril.

- As the tube passes down the nasopharynx and the patient becomes aware that the tube is in the back of the throat, ask her to swallow water via a straw. The action of swallowing closes the epiglottis, allowing the tube to pass into the oesophagus.

- Each time the patient swallows, advance the tube into the oesophagus by a few (two to three) centimetres. I would continue to do this until the predetermined mark has been reached.

- If the patient shows any signs of distress, such as coughing, gasping for air or cyanosis, I would remove the tube immediately.

- Check that the tube is in the correct position by asking an assistant to inject a small volume of air into it from a syringe and simultaneously I would listen with a stethoscope.

- Secure the tube to the nostril and cheek using appropriate tape or fixation device.

Key points

- Nasogastric (Ryle's) tube insertion is a skill which is usually performed by nursing staff on the wards. However, you will be called on to do this task when the nurses are unsuccessful, hence you would do well to become competent in performing this early in your training.

- Note that fine-bore tubes are able to stay in for a longer time (more than one week) compared with wide-bore tubes. They are used for feeding purposes and administering medication enterally.

- It is contraindicated and unsafe to insert a nasogastric tube in patients with severe facial trauma and certain cranial (cribriform plate and base-of-skull) fractures.

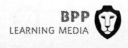

Clinical procedure 9:   Level *

Performing basic life support

The technique of performing basic life support (BLS) refers to the acute initial management of the airway, the support of breathing and circulatory support. Cardiac and cardio-pulmonary dysfunction are a leading cause of death in society; as a junior doctor you should be able to initiate treatment by following a basic algorithm when assessing and managing these patients. You are likely to be severely marked down, if not failed, if you cannot give a competent demonstration of how to perform well in this setting.

You and a friend are walking down a street when you witness an elderly man, who is walking towards you, suddenly collapse a few metres from you. Can you show me what you would do?

RESPONSE:

INITIAL ASSESSMENT

- Ensure that I, the patient and anyone else nearby are safe; I would indicate that I would move the person to an area of safety.

- Check if the person is responsive by gently shaking his shoulders and asking in a loud voice, 'Are you all right?'

  The examiner tells you there is no response!

- Shout for help.

AIRWAY MANAGEMENT

- Now I would turn the patient on to his back.

- Then open his airway by placing my hand on to the forehead and gently tilting the head back (head tilt), and put my fingertips under the patients chin and lift his chin (chin lift).

- I would look for any visible obstruction in the patient's mouth; if found, this should be removed using a finger sweep method. I may find items such as displaced dentures, vomit or a foreign body. Leave correctly fitting dentures in place.

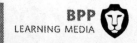

ASSESS BREATHING

- With the airway open, bring my ear adjacent to the patient's mouth and *Look, Listen* and *Feel* for breathing for 10 seconds:

- Look for chest movements.

- Listen for breath sounds.

- Feel for breathing against my cheek.

- If no breathing can be detected, I would send my friend to get some help. (If I was alone, I would leave the patient in a safe area and call for an ambulance. On returning, I would immediately move on to assessing the circulation.)

CIRCULATORY ASSESSMENT

- Check for signs of a circulation; I should take no more than 10 seconds to do this.

- Feel for a carotid pulse.

- Observe for any movement, including regular breathing or swallowing pattern.

  If signs of a circulation are evident, I would continue to give the patient rescue breaths, until he can manage to breathe independently. With every 10 breaths, or after one minute, I should re-check for the signs of a circulation, taking no more than 10 seconds to do this.

- If no signs of a circulation can be elicited, or I am in any doubt, chest compressions should be commenced.

- Identify the costal margin and the xiphisternum. I would have one hand on top of the other, the fingers interlocked, keeping my arms straight, in a position so that the shoulders are above the wrists. I place the heels of my hands two finger-breadths above the xiphisternum and commence chest compressions.

- I would use the following technique: Press down the sternum, depressing it by a depth of 4–5cm; the same duration of time should be taken for compression and release of pressure. Make sure I don't press on the ribs.

- Maintain a compression rate of 100 per minute.

- After every 30 compressions, the patient should receive 2 breaths, ie continue compressions and breaths in a ratio of 30 to 2.

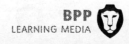

- If there is more than one rescuer, I would change over every 1–2 minutes, to avoid tiredness.

    I would only stop if:
    - Help arrives
    - I become exhausted
    - If the patient shows signs of life, for example, by making a movement or takes a spontaneous breath, I would re-check for signs of a circulation

As you approach the scene, observe for danger – look for anything that is dangerous to you, bystanders or the casualty.

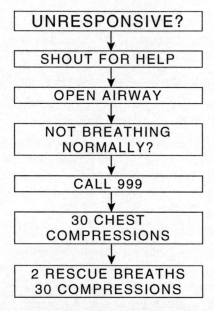

Figure 3.3: Algorithm for adult basic life support

Key points

- BLS is a well-defined clinical skill; you are very likely to be tested on this at some point during your final exams.

- Note the steps of the algorithm above and practise until it becomes second nature.

- Remember the chest compression rate is 100 per minute, the compression-to-ventilation rate being 30:2.

Clinical procedure 10:   Level *

Surgical scrubbing, gowning and gloving

As the orthopaedic FY1 doctor on call, you have been bleeped by your registrar who wants you to come to theatre to assist him in performing a hip hemiarthroplasty.

QUESTION A:

Before going into theatre, how would you prepare yourself to assist in the procedure?

RESPONSE A:

- I would introduce myself to the theatre staff.
- I would remove my wristwatch; if I had on any jewellery I would take this off too.
- Before walking into the operating room I would change into surgical scrubs (greens or blues), wear theatre shoes along with a disposable hat (non-sterile).
- In the operating theatre I would apply a face mask (non-sterile) before scrubbing, covering my mouth and nose.
- Now I would need to open up a sterile gown pack on a procedure trolley, thereby creating a sterile field. I would open a glove pack and drop the sterile inner gloves into this aseptic field.

QUESTION B:

How would you go on and scrub, gown and glove for the procedure?

RESPONSE B:

- Turn on the hot and cold water taps, and adjust the water temperature.
- Open a sterile sponge/brush pack, leaving this to the side.
- Wash and wet my forearms and hands. Keep my hands above my elbows, ensuring the water passes downwards from hands to elbows, not the other way around.

- Obtain the disinfectant by using my elbow to dispense either the betadine or hibiscrub disinfectant solutions onto my hands. Lather the detergent from my hands to 2cm above the elbows and perform a pre-scrub; then rinse, again making sure the water drips from my hands to my elbows. Scrub one arm (using the technique stated below) before moving to the other arm.

- Take the nail cleaner from the brush pack. Brush and file under the fingernails for approximately 1 minute. Using the scrub side of the scrub brush, scrub each of the four sides (anterior, posterior, medial and lateral) of each finger. Also scrub the palm of the hand, the dorsum as well as the heel of the hand, for a further minute per hand.

- Discard the sponge.

- Wash each arm in turn, starting from the hand to the elbow in the correct fashion, ensuring water runs away from the hand to the elbow. Do this for 1 minute per side.

- Now continue to hold my hands above the elbows and dry each hand and forearm in turn using the sterile towels provided in the gown pack. Starting from the hand, move proximally towards the elbows. Use opposite sides of the same towel for each hand and forearm. Use a different towel for each side.

- Pick up the gown from the reverse side, holding it away from me, and gently shake to unfold. Pass each hand into the gown sleeves and move them forwards up to, but not beyond, the cuffs. Ensure the gown does not touch the floor. Ask a colleague or theatre staff to tie the back of the gown.

- Pick up the internal part of the left glove through the gown cuffs without touching the outer surface. With the palm of the glove facing down, insert the hand into the glove. Use the sleeve-covered right hand to stretch the glove over the sleeve-covered left hand, by pulling it at the edge of the glove fold. Repeat with my right hand (this time, when I stretch the glove over the right hand, the left hand will already be gloved).

- Hold the paper belt tab found at the front of the gown and pass it to an assistant or scrub nurse. Whilst this is held by the assistant, swivel anticlockwise before grasping the belt (not the paper tab) and pull so that the paper is left behind in the assistant's hands. Now tie the belt at the front.

QUESTION C:

How long should you scrub for?

RESPONSE C:

The first scrub of the day should last for five minutes. Subsequent scrubs for procedures on the same day should last three minutes.

QUESTION D:

Can you explain why we don't use the brush on the skin; and how long is scrubbing thought to be effective in removing surface organisms?

RESPONSE D:

By not using the scrub brush on the skin we prevent exposing deeper organisms in the hair follicles to the surface of the skin. Scrubbing is thought to be effective for around two hours to remove surface skin organisms.

Key points

- The technique of surgical gowning requires meticulous attention to ensure sterility is maintained throughout.

- When washing and drying your hands and forearms always remember to work from distal (hands) proximally towards the elbows. In this way you reduce the risk of desterilising the fingers and hands.

- Note that during the technique there will be occasions when you require an assistant to gown up, namely when tying the gown from behind after scrubbing up, as well as when tying from the front; someone will need to hold the paper belt as you turn.

Clinical procedure 11:   Level *

Urethral catheterisation

Mr Patel is a 35-year-old male who has returned to the ward following elective abdominal surgery. He has not been able to pass urine since he arrived at the ward eight hours ago and is complaining of lower abdominal pain, with a feeling of needing to pass urine.

On examining him you note that he has a distended suprapubic region, which is also dull to percussion. You correctly diagnose that he has a distended bladder, and that he will need to be catheterised. You have been asked by your consultant to describe to him your understanding of the procedure before explaining how you would perform it.

QUESTION A:

State the indications for carrying out urethral catheterisation using a Foley catheter.

RESPONSE A:

Indications for urethral catheterisation include:

- Urinary retention
- Urinary incontinence
- Poor mobility
- Administration of intra-vesical drugs, particularly common in chemotherapy
- Monitoring of urine output, eg in a patient with suspected cardiac and/or renal failure
- Urodynamic investigations, such as micturating cystourethrography

QUESTION B:

State the contraindications and complications of this procedure.

RESPONSE B:

- An absolute contraindication is a suspicion of urethral trauma. I would look out for this by observing for blood at the meatus and/or the presence of perineal bruising. Also suspect this if the patient has a high riding or boggy prostate.

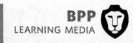

- A relative contraindication is a history of urethral strictures.
- Complications associated with urinary catheter insertion are:
    - Infection
    - Bleeding
    - Stricture formation, in long-dwelling rubber (less likely with silicone) catheters
    - Pain

QUESTION C:

Now please explain how you would perform the procedure.

RESPONSE C:

- I would first introduce myself to the patient, eliciting his name, date of birth, hospital number and then obtain consent to proceed.
- Ensure he is lying comfortably on his back with legs slightly separated.
- Choose a size 12 or 14FG catheter.
- Have the catheterisation pack open on the trolley, put on my sterile gloves.
- Clean and drape the penis and surrounding region, retracting the prepuce and clean with antiseptic around the meatus.
- As I am right-handed, I would hold the penis with my left hand using a gauze swab. With my right hand insert approximately 8 to 10ml of lubricant jelly or anaesthetic jelly into the urethral meatus.
- Now change my gloves to another sterile pair; whilst doing so give the jelly/anaesthetic three to four minutes to act.
- Hold the catheter over its sleeve, allowing myself to introduce the catheter tip into the urethra, ie use a 'non-touch' technique.
- Advance the catheter either with my hand (non-touch technique), or with a pair of sterile, non-toothed forceps. Advance the catheter until either I see urine passing out of it or the end arm of the catheter is up to the level of the meatus, whichever comes first.
- Check the balloon size, inflate the balloon with 10ml of saline.
- Attach the catheter to the drainage bag.

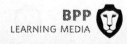

QUESTION D:

What would you consider if no urine passed out of the catheter?

RESPONSE D:

- It is possible that the catheter is blocked, either with jelly or particulate matter. I would try to flush this through with 5 to 10ml of saline.

- The tip of the catheter may be misplaced and not in the central lumen of the bladder.

- The bladder may simply have no urine in it; this is more likely in conditions such as acute renal failure.

Key points

- Urinary catheterisation is a core clinical skill; it is essential to be able to perform this using a sterile, non-touch technique. You will be asked to perform this on several occasions as a junior doctor.

- When catheterising to relieve acute or acute on chronic urinary retention, try to choose the smallest gauge catheter (size 12 or 14FG); this will reduce the likelihood of causing intra-urethral mucosal trauma and bleeding.

- Before inflating the balloon in a Foley catheter, ensure that the tip is well inside the bladder lumen (this is indicated by a good flow of urine in a full/moderately full bladder) thereby avoiding causing trauma by inflating the balloon in the urethra.

Clinical procedure 12:　　　　　　Level * *

Use of a bronchodilator

Mr Howard is a 55-year-old male who has attended your outpatient respiratory clinic today. He has been referred by his GP with a several-month history of wheeze with episodes of breathlessness. Peak flow analysis indicates that he is likely to have asthma. Advise him about his diagnosis and how he should use a salbutamol inhaler device.

QUESTION A:

How would you proceed?

RESPONSE A:

- INTRODUCTION: To begin with I would introduce myself. Check I am speaking to the right patient by eliciting his name and date of birth, and asking what his occupation is, as this can be related to his condition. At this stage I would try to establish a rapport and make him feel at ease.

- EXPLANATION: I might say 'Your symptoms, along with the peak flow result are highly suggestive that you may be asthmatic. Can you tell me what your understanding of asthma is?'

- Once the patient is allowed to indicate what his interpretation of the diagnosis is, then I should be able to elaborate according to his response.

  I might say: 'Asthma is a condition which causes patients to have difficulty in breathing. Asthmatics tend to have sensitive airways which become narrowed in response to irritant materials, this results in difficulty in air to move in or out of the lungs. For this reason we use bronchodilator devices which work by relaxing the airway passages in the lungs, allowing ease of the flow of air into the lungs.

  I would like to show you how to use one of these devices; the one most frequently used is that which contains the drug salbutamol.'

- CONSENT: Ask the patient if that is OK, and check with him if he has any questions or concerns.

- POSITION: The patient should be either be sitting up in a chair or standing.

- Show him how to shake the inhaler before use.

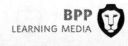

- Ask him to take a few deep breaths in and out. After the third expiration, I would indicate he should press the inhaler as he breathes in, hold the breath for a few seconds (around 10 seconds would be appropriate) before releasing the device gently.

- Ensure he understands the steps involved, ask him to demonstrate to me.

- Inform him that he should wait around one minute before taking another puff of the inhaler. This gives time for the drug to mix with the propellant.

- If the patient appears unconfident, I can arrange for further training at a later time, perhaps with the respiratory nurse.

QUESTION B:

What are the side effects of salbutamol administration?

RESPONSE B:

Salbutamol inhalers are generally quite safe, however, it would be prudent to keep an eye out for side effects such as headache, palpitations, fine tremor, a rapid heart rate (tachycardia) and dry mouth.

QUESTION C:

What drugs are you aware of that can be used in the treatment of asthma?

RESPONSE C:

- Salbutamol, the blue inhaler can be used as and when required. If a patient is finding he or she needs this frequently, for example, more than two puffs, four times a day, it may be appropriate to consider the use of other medications too.

- The brown inhalers, such as beclomethasone, are used to prevent attacks occurring; they will not treat an asthma attack that has already begun. This should be taken two puffs twice a day.

- When an acute attack has occurred, patients often find benefit from a short course of steroids. They are given for short periods, the dose being gradually tailed off. This is because they are not without their own side effects such as osteoporosis, weight gain and diabetes.

Key points

- Be able to clearly explain a diagnosis of asthma to a patient.
- Practice teaching patients how to use their asthma inhaler devices.
- There are side effects with every drug, note some of the hazards.

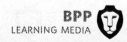

Clinical procedure 13: Level *

Venepuncture

Mr Williams has been admitted to the medical admissions unit with a presumed chest infection on a background of known renal failure. You are the FY1 doctor on call, and required to take some routine blood tests to assess his response to the treatment initiated.

QUESTION A:
How would you proceed?

RESPONSE A:

*   INTRODUCTION: To begin with I would introduce myself. Check I am speaking to the right patient by eliciting his name, date of birth and hospital number. At this stage I would try to establish a rapport and make him feel at ease.

*   EXPLANATION: I would explain the reasons for taking the blood test: 'Hello Mr Williams, my name is Peter Atkins. I'm the doctor covering the admissions unit today. I need to take some blood from you so we can check your blood count along with some other routine blood parameters; together this will help to give us an indication of how your kidneys and lungs are responding to the treatment we've given since your admission.'

*   CONSENT: I would now explain the procedure to the patient and obtain his verbal consent. 'I will apply a tourniquet to your arm, and then insert a needle into one of your veins, then I can withdraw some blood directly into a syringe. Is that OK? Do you have any questions?'

*   POSITION: The patient should be sitting or lying comfortably, it may help to have a pillow under his arm.

QUESTION B:

What equipment do you need to perform the venepuncture?

RESPONSE B:

I would have the following equipment to perform the procedure:

*   Syringe and blue/green needle. Alternatively I would use a vacutainer and blue/green needle, or even a butterfly needle.

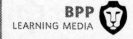

- Cotton wool or gauze
- Alcohol steret
- Tourniquet
- Sharps container
- The appropriate blood bottles, in this case a purple and yellow top bottle (some regional variations may exist)
- A pair of gloves

QUESTION C:

Please describe the procedure to me.

RESPONSE C:

- I would wash my hands with an appropriate disinfectant, then dry them.
- Put on a pair of gloves.
- Apply the tourniquet above the elbow and tighten it.
- Identify an appropriate vein to use, either by palpation and/or visually.
- I would indicate techniques that may help to accentuate the veins, such as asking the patient to repetitively open and close their fist, or gentle percussion over the venous site.
- Clean the area with an alcohol steret; to do this, I use a circular motion, moving from the centre to the periphery. Allow to air dry.
- Select the needle size, attach the needle to a syringe (or vacutainer).
- Warn the patient of an impending 'sharp scratch'. Retract the skin around the vein to achieve some tension, and insert the needle at an angle between 15° and 30° passing through the skin, subcutaneous fat and into the vein.
- Draw back on the syringe while advancing it, looking for a flashback at the base of the syringe indicating that the needle is in the correct position. There will be no flashback with a vacutainer.
- With the needle and syringe (or vacutainer) in place still in the arm, gently pull on the plunger of the syringe (or if a vacutainer is used, attach a blood bottle to it), until sufficient blood is obtained to fill the bottles required.

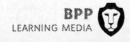

- Release the tourniquet.

- Place some cotton wool/gauze over the venepuncture site and remove the needle.

- Apply digital pressure with a finger over the cotton or gauze for about one minute. Once the bleeding has stopped, apply a plaster to the venepuncture site (checking beforehand that the patient is not allergic to the plaster material being used).

- Transfer the blood in the syringe into the blood bottles required. This step will not be required if a vacutainer has been used.

- Dispose the sharps into the sharps container, also dispose of my gloves and any soiled material appropriately.

- I would thank the patient and ask if he has any questions or concerns.

QUESTION D:

What would you do with the blood bottles once you have collected the blood?

RESPONSE D:

I would label the blood bottles clearly with the patient's details (name, date of birth, hospital number, date sample taken). I also need to complete the accompanying request forms, in this case for haematology and biochemistry. On the forms I would complete the relevant sections, usually this includes the name of the patient's consultant along with the relevant clinical details for performing the test.

Key points

- Venepuncture is often assessed in an OSCE using a model upper limb. It is a skill you will be called upon to perform on a very regular basis during your first couple of years as a junior doctor.

- In virtually every hospital, note that the clotting (blue-topped) bottle needs to be filled to the top (approximately 4 to 4.5ml).

- Also in every hospital the transfusion request bottle – often pink in colour (for group and save or cross match) needs to be hand-labelled and signed. The other bottles, for haematology and biochemistry, can often be labelled using a patient sticker containing the patient's details – it is important to check with your hospital policy, otherwise the blood specimen may not be processed.

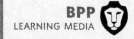

Clinical procedure 14:   Level *

Venous cannulation and IV infusion

Mr Evans is a 48-year-old male who has been admitted with a recent history of excessive vomiting and diarrhoea. He appears clinically dehydrated. You have been asked by the nurse taking care of him to insert an intravenous cannula (venflon) and commence him on an intravenous fluid infusion regime.

QUESTION A:

How would you proceed?

RESPONSE A:

- INTRODUCTION: To begin with I would introduce myself. I would check I am speaking to the right patient by eliciting his name, date of birth and hospital number. At this stage I would try to establish a rapport and make him feel at ease.

- EXPLANATION: I would explain the reasons for inserting a venflon. 'Hello Mr Evans, my name is Louise Smith. I'm the doctor covering the ward today. I have been asked to set up a drip to give you some fluids. To do this I would need to insert a venflon, which is a thin plastic tube, into a vein in your hand or arm. This will help us to keep you adequately hydrated.'

- CONSENT: I would ask the patient if that is OK, and check with him if he has any questions or concerns.

- POSITION: The patient should be sitting or lying comfortably. Select an arm and place a pillow underneath the arm to support it.

QUESTION B:

What equipment do you need to perform the venflon insertion?

RESPONSE B:

I would have the following equipment to perform the procedure:

- Venflon, a selection of sizes (18G green, 20G pink, 22G blue)
- Venflon cover
- Cotton wool or gauze
- Alcohol steret
- Tourniquet

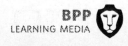

- Sharps container
- 10ml syringe
- 10ml 0.9% sodium chloride flush
- Three-way tap
- Bandage
- A pair of gloves

QUESTION C:

Can you describe the procedure to me?

RESPONSE C:

- I would wash my hands with an appropriate disinfectant, then dry them.

- Put on a pair of gloves.

- Apply the tourniquet above the elbow and tighten it.

- Identify an appropriate vein to use, either by palpation and/or visually.

- I would use techniques that may help to accentuate the veins, such as asking the patient to repetitively open and close their fist, or gentle percussion over the venous site.

- Clean the area with an alcohol steret; to do this, use a circular motion, moving from the centre to the periphery. Allow to air dry.

- Select the appropriate-sized venflon, based on the size of the vein. Remove the cap off the venflon.

- Retract the skin around the vein to achieve some tension, now warn the patient they will feel a 'sharp scratch' and insert the cannula (with the bevel facing upwards) at a shallow angle and look for a flashback in the flash chamber of the stylet.

- Once the flashback is seen, advance the cannula and needle by 2mm. Now keep the needle stationary and advance the plastic cannula only.

- Release and remove the tourniquet.

- Press over the vein at the tip of the cannula.

- Remove the needle and put it in the sharps container; attach the three-way tap to the end of the cannula.

- Flush the venflon with 5 to 10ml of 0.9% sodium chloride flush. Watch out for any localised swelling or leakage. Check with the patient that they are not in any pain on insertion of the saline.

- Secure the cannula with the adhesive plaster.

- Bandage the venflon to the arm.

- Dispose of my gloves and any soiled materials.

- Thank the patient and ask if he has any further questions or concerns.

Intravenous infusion

QUESTION D:

Now the venflon is inserted, and you have already obtained permission to commence a drip, how would you proceed to commence the infusion?

RESPONSE D:

- Check the fluid prescription chart; here the patient has been prescribed a 1-litre bag of normal (0.9%) saline to be run over eight hours.

- Look at the bag to check its expiry date, solution type and concentration.

- Make sure it is being given to the correct patient, by checking their identity – usually easily done by looking at the patient's identity bracelet.

- Ensure I am aware of the patient's allergies and that the fluid material does not contain anything that could cause them harm.

- Hang the fluid bag on a stand. Connect the giving set to the fluid bag (by removing the blue winged part and passing through the portal).

- Run the fluid through the tubing to remove any air bubbles. Then close the tap and clamp the connecting tubing to prevent any more fluid running through.

- Use an alcohol steret to clean one port of the three-way tap, allow to air dry for around 30 seconds.

- Attach the connecting tubing to the port. Open the three-way tap and unclamp the connecting tubing to allow the saline to run through the venflon.

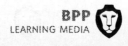

- Observe for any swelling over the point of venflon insertion, and ask the patient if he is in any pain or discomfort.

- Set the desired flow rate by adjusting the flow through the drip chamber.

- Record on the fluid chart the type of fluid commenced, its concentration, rate, date and time with my signature.

QUESTION E:

How do you adjust the flow rate running through the drip?

RESPONSE E:

- Well, in large drip chambers, you can consider that 10 drops is equivalent to 1ml.

- 10 drops/minute = 60ml/hour.

- 16 drops/minute = 96ml/hour.

- To adjust for a rate of 125ml/hour (ie 1 litre over 8 hours), I would adjust to 20 drops/minute.

University Hospital NHS Trust			SURNAME						
INTRAVENOUS INFUSION PRESCRIPTION			ADDRESS						
N.B. WHEN DRUGS ARE ADDED TO THE FLUID AFFIX A PINK ADDITIVE LABEL TO THE CONTAINER			DATE OF BIRTH		AGE	SEX		CIVIL STATE	
DATE	INTRAVENOUS FLUID	VOL	NAME & DOSE OF DRUG TO BE ADDED	RATE IN HOURS	TIME TO BE SET UP	SIGNATURE OF PRESCRIBER	TIME DRUG ADDED TO CON-TAINER	SIGN OF PERSON ADDING DRUG	TIME ACTUALLY SET UP

Figure 3.4: Example of an IV fluid prescription form

Key points

- Explain to the patient why he or she needs a venflon along with IV fluids and seek consent.

- Use the appropriate size cannula for the vein.

- Dispose of sharps carefully along with gloves and any soiled material.

- When attaching a drip to the venflon, always check the right fluid and concentration is being administered to the correct patient.

- Adjust the rate of fluid administration as per the clinical need.

- Document in the fluid prescription chart what has been given, the concentration, rate, along with date and time.

Clinical procedure 15:   Level * *

Suturing a wound

Mrs Taylor is a 53-year-old female has presented to A&E with a 6cm laceration to her left forearm following a fall. As the FY2 doctor attending her injury, your opinion is that the wound will require suturing. A mannequin is provided with a lacerated forearm; you will be asked to demonstrate your technique of wound closure on this.

QUESTION A:

How would you approach the patient in preparation to suture the wound?

RESPONSE A:

• I would start by introducing myself to the patient, eliciting her name, date of birth, hospital number and explaining what I would like to do, and obtaining her consent to proceed. 'Hello Mrs Taylor, my name is Tom Isles, I am the doctor on call in A&E today. I have had a look at the wound on your left forearm. I think it needs a few stitches to allow it to heal and prevent further bleeding and infection. I will use a local anaesthetic; you may feel some pulling and tugging as I carry the procedure out but it should not be painful. Is it OK for me to proceed?'

QUESTION B:

Would you like to perform any further clinical examination of the forearm or any investigations before you proceed with suturing the wound?

RESPONSE B:

• Well, I would thoroughly inspect the wound to look for any dirt or contamination which would require antiseptic cleaning and debridement before I can start suturing.

• I would also examine the patient's distal motor and sensory function in that limb, comparing it with the other, 'normal' side.

• Due to the nature of the injury, it would be appropriate to perform an X-ray of the distal forearm, AP and lateral views. This would not only identify any fracture, but may also show any foreign body contamination of the wound.

QUESTION C:

What items of equipment do you need to suture the wound?

RESPONSE C:

- A suture pack containing suture material and needle
- Betadine antiseptic
- Sterile cotton wool/gauze
- Two pairs of forceps, one toothed, one non-toothed
- A suture needle holder
- A pair of sterile gloves
- A selection of needles, blue (25G) and green (21G)
- A 10ml syringe
- Local anaesthetic in the form of 1% lignocaine
- A sharps container

QUESTION D:

Can you describe how you would suture the wound?

RESPONSE D:

- Commence by washing my hands.

- Open the suture pack on to a procedure trolley. On here I would also open the packets for, and place, the sterile gloves, sutures, the syringe and needles.

- Clean the wound with betadine solution. Clean from the centre of the wound, in a circular fashion to the periphery; I do not retract back to previously cleaned areas using the same swab.

- Infiltrate the wound with local anaesthetic using the syringe and 25G needle. Aspirate the needle before injecting to prevent inadvertent intra-arterial administration of the local anaesthetic. Do not exceed the maximum safe amount. Wait approximately five minutes for the anaesthetic to act. Test it has worked by prodding around the wound with a pair of forceps.

- Holding the needle holder with the thumb and index finger in the bows (as on holding a pair of scissors) it would be inserted no further than the distal phalynx, using my dominant hand. Now I grasp the needle two-thirds along its shaft from its tip.

- Hold the toothed forceps between the thumb and index finger of my non-dominant hand (left hand for a right-handed candidate) just as if holding a pencil. They should be used to manipulate the skin edges. *Note that toothed forceps are used for skin and tough tissues, non-toothed being used for blood vessels and bowel.*

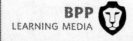

- Insert the needle at right angles to the skin, 0.5cm from the skin edge. I advance the needle through one skin edge, pick it up using the toothed forceps, and pass the needle full thickness through the skin, so that the suture also passes through, leaving only 3-4 cm of suture outside the wound. Re-mount the needle with the needle holder, pick up the opposite skin edge and pass the needle through, aiming once more to be 0.5cm from the skin edge on this side. Pull the suture through, leaving a small (3-4cm) length at the non-needle end.

- Apply a knot using an instrument tie, grab the needle end using the forceps, and wind two loops of the suture around the closed mouth of the needle holder. Now open the mouth of the needle holder and pull the short end of the stitch through the loops created. Pull the knot down on to the skin simultaneously opposing the two sides of the wound. Produce a tight knot which allows apposition of the skin edges ensuring no tension.

- With each suture insertion, the distance from the skin edge (0.5cm) should also be approximately equal to the thickness of the wound (0.5cm). I note that successive sutures should be applied equidistant, at a distance of twice the wound depth (in this case therefore 1cm apart).

- Continue with the above method of suture application until achieving wound closure, which should be without tension.

- Apply a dry dressing over the wound.

- Discard the sharps in the sharps container, and dispose of the remaining clinical waste.

QUESTION E:

What is the maximum safe dosage of lignocaine; could you also use adrenaline with the lignocaine?

RESPONSE E:

The maximum safe dosage of lignocaine is 3mg/kg without adrenaline and 7mg/kg with adrenaline. Yes, adrenaline can be used on a forearm laceration but it should not be used on digits, ie fingers and toes; this is because it has a peripheral vasoconstrictive effect which could result in ischaemia.

Body site	Suture type & size	Time of removal (days)
Scalp	non-absorbable, 3/0	7
Face	non-absorbable, 6/0	3-5
Trunk	non-absorbable, 3/0	10
Hands	non-absorbable, 5/0	10
Limbs	non-absorbable, 4/0	10

Table 3.2: Type & size of suture according to body site & length of time before removal

For skin & other superficial wounds, use monofilament non-absorbable sutures, eg Prolene or Nylon.

For deep wounds, use absorbable sutures eg Vicryl or Monocryl.

Key points

- Perform a thorough wound inspection before suturing any wound. Any contamination with foreign bodies or debris needs to be appropriately dealt with before closing the wound.

- Never add adrenaline to lignocaine when infiltrating local anaesthetic over a digit, such as a finger or toe. This can result in the development of ischaemia.

- On applying a suture, be wary of over-tightening a knot. The aim is to ensure adequate apposition of both edges of a wound in a tension-free manner.

- When suturing skin, choose a monofilament non-absorbable suture such as prolene or nylon.

Clinical procedure 16:
Level * *

Blood glucose measurement

As the medical FY1 doctor covering the diabetes and endocrinology firm, you have been asked to speak to Mr Kyle. He is a 41-year-old male who been newly diagnosed to have diabetes mellitus; it is your job to explain to him how he can self-monitor his blood sugar using a BM machine.

QUESTION A:

How would you proceed?

RESPONSE A:

- INTRODUCTION: To begin with I would introduce myself. Check I am speaking to the right patient by eliciting his name, date of birth and hospital number. At this stage I would try to establish a rapport and make him feel at ease.

- EXPLANATION: I would explain the reasons for checking his blood sugar. 'With diabetes it will be necessary to keep a strict control of your blood sugar. To monitor this when you are at home it would be best for you to learn how to check the readings for yourself using a blood glucose monitoring machine.'

- CONSENT: Obtain the patient's consent for you to take the blood sugar reading; in so doing, also teach him how he can do this when he is discharged.

- POSITION: The patient should be sitting or lying comfortably.

QUESTION B:

What equipment do you need to perform the blood sugar measurement?

RESPONSE B:

I would have the following equipment to perform the procedure:

- BM meter
- BM reagent test strip
- Lancet
- Cotton wool or gauze
- Alcohol steret
- Sharps container
- A pair of gloves

QUESTION C:

Can you describe the procedure to me?

RESPONSE C:

- I would ask the patient to wash his hands with an appropriate disinfectant and lukewarm water, then dry them.

- Ensure the patient is comfortable.

- Now I would wash my hands and put on a pair of gloves.

- Prepare the BM meter, by switching it on and inserting the BM reagent strip. Ensure compatibility by comparing the codes on the meter and reagent strip.

- Clean the patient's fingertip with an alcohol steret, choosing a finger on the non-dominant hand. Allow the alcohol to dry.

- Apply the spring-loaded lancet device to the side of the fingertip or the pulp. Warn him that he will feel a 'sharp scratch', then press firmly.

- Discard the lancet into the sharps container.

- Squeeze the finger from proximal to distal to express sufficient blood to perform the test. The droplet(s) of blood expressed should be transferred from the patient's finger directly to the BM reagent strip.

- Place a piece of cotton wool or gauze directly on to the fingertip and ask the patient to apply pressure to arrest the bleeding.

- If sufficient blood has been taken, the BM meter should count down to give an accurate reading of the capillary blood glucose.

- Appropriately dispose of the remaining clinical and soiled waste.

- Inform the patient of the blood glucose result.

- Ensure the reading is documented in the patient's notes along with the patient's own glucose levels diary if he has one.

QUESTION D:

What would you tell your patient is the correct range of blood glucose level they should aim to achieve? Also, what is the importance of keeping the BMs in this range?

RESPONSE D:

Different texts will quote slightly different levels of blood glucose per se, however, a good reference range for a diabetic to aim for would be a BM of around 4-7mmol/l before eating, and under 9mmol/l two hours after food. The importance of keeping within these limits is to help reduce the risk of complication of diabetes, namely preventing problems with sight, feet, kidneys and sensation.

QUESTION E:

How frequently would you advise your patient to check his blood sugars?

RESPONSE E:

As the patient has only recently been diagnosed, I would advise that he check his own BMs about three to four times a day. A reasonable regime would be before breakfast, two to three hours after lunch and last thing at night before sleeping. On discharge I would ask his GP to review his diabetic control; when he has shown he is achieving good control, he should be able to reduce the frequency of checks.

Key points

- Try to obtain sufficient blood for a BM reading using only a single prick of the lancet device.

- It would be useful for a patient to have their own BM diary, so they can monitor their blood glucose levels over time; suggest this to the examiner when mentioning you are documenting the results in the notes.

- Check the patient's understanding of the importance of keeping glucose levels within a tight range. Patients are more likely to compliance with checking BMs regularly if they are aware of the consequences of poor control.

Clinical procedure 17:   Level * *

Pleural aspiration

Mr Bacon is a 68-year-old male, known chronic smoker with a several years' history of heart failure. He has been admitted to the respiratory ward with a week's history of complaining of worsening cough and difficulty in breathing. As the FY2 doctor on the ward, you examine him to find he has dullness to percussion over the right-side mid and lower zones, with reduced air entry on auscultation. A chest X-ray confirms the presence of a pleural effusion.

QUESTION A:

State the indications for performing a pleural aspiration, also known as a pleural tap.

RESPONSE A:

There are two main reasons for performing a pleural tap:

- Diagnostic purposes:

    - If the total protein content of the fluid is >30g/l, or the pleural fluid total protein >50% of blood total protein, this indicates an inflammatory exudate, as found in, for example, infection or malignancy.

    - If the total protein content of the fluid is <30g/l, this indicates a transudate, an ultrafiltrate of plasma resulting from increased venous pressure as occurs in, for example, heart failure, or reduced colloid osmotic pressure, hypoalbuminemia, which can be found in liver failure (reduced albumin synthesis) or nephrotic syndrome (increased albumin loss).

    - If the amylase level is raised, this may be associated with pancreatitis.

- Therapeutic purposes:

    - For symptomatic relief of the pleural effusion.

    - For direct drug administration, such as antibiotics for infection or cytotoxic agents in cancer.

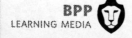

QUESTION B:

What equipment do you need to assemble to perform the procedure?

RESPONSE B:

I would obtain:

- A sterile dressing pack
- Cotton wool/gauze
- A pair of gloves
- Marking pen
- Three-way tap and sterile tubing
- Kidney dish
- Betadine antiseptic solution
- 5ml syringe
- 20ml syringe
- specimen bottles including those for specific tests (glucose, cytology)
- 21G (green), 22G (blue) and 25G (orange) needles
- Sharps container
- A vial of lignocaine 1%

QUESTION C:

Can you describe the procedure of pleural aspiration to me?

RESPONSE C:

- I would begin by introducing myself to the patient, eliciting his name, date of birth, hospital number and explaining what I am doing and why, and also obtain his consent.

- I would ask the patient to remove his shirt and get him in the correct position. He should be sat upright, leaning forwards with arms crossed. A table can be placed in front of him to lean on for support. I would check and ask to ensure the patient is comfortable. This position allows elevation of the scapulae, improving access to the posterior thorax.

- Now I would once more percuss the patient's thorax over the area of dullness caused by the effusion, and delineate the aspiration site below this level; this should ideally be at the level of the 8th to the 9th intercostal space in the posterior axillary line.

- Wash my hands, wear sterile gloves.

- Clean the aspiration site with the betadine antiseptic solution soaked in cotton wool, and create a sterile field around this site using drapes from the sterile pack.

- Infiltrate the skin around this site with 1% lignocaine using a 25G needle. Change to a 22G needle to infiltrate deeper to the pleura. On each occasion, aspirate before injecting the local anaesthetic to ensure a blood vessel has not been injected. Note that the neurovascular bundle runs along the lower border of the upper rib, hence as the needle is advanced I should aim for the upper border.

- Once a small volume of pleural fluid is aspirated, remove the needle, noting the depth it had been inserted to.

- Attach a 21G needle to a 20ml syringe, insert it perpendicular to the skin, following the same track as the local anaesthetic, aiming for the interspace just above the rib. On puncturing the parietal pleura, aspirate approximately 20ml of fluid.

- Withdraw the needle as I ask the patient to exhale; cover the entry site with a dry gauze dressing.

- Place the aspirate fluid into the appropriate specimen bottles, label and send to the lab for biochemistry including glucose, cytology, microbiology for gram stain culture and sensitivity.

- Dispose of needles in a sharps container as well as clinical waste appropriately.

QUESTION D:

What complications should you be wary of when performing a pleural aspiration?

RESPONSE D:

Conditions I need to be wary of when performing this procedure are development of:

- Infection
- Pneumothorax

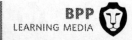

- Haemothorax

- Hypotension. This can occur as a consequence of hypovolaemia if too much fluid is removed, so generally I would try not to remove more than 1000ml at any one sitting.

- Mediastinal shift, for the same reason as above.

Key points

- The technique of pleural aspiration is done for both diagnostic and therapeutic purposes.

- An aseptic technique is paramount.

- When inserting a needle for local anaesthetic infiltration, as well as for the aspiration of fluid, note that the neurovascular bundle lies along the lower border of the upper rib in the interspace between the ribs, hence as you advance the needle aim for the upper border.

- On analysing the pleural aspirate, if the total protein content is >30g/l, this would indicate an inflammatory exudate as found in, for example, infection or malignancy. If the protein content is <30g/l this would indicate a transudate as found in, for example, heart or liver failure.

Clinical procedure 18:   Level * *

Administering drugs via a nebuliser

Mrs Gibson is a 42-year-old asthmatic who has been referred by her GP with a recent history of increasing shortness of breath, an audible wheeze and oxygen saturations of 88-90% on room air. She has had an arterial blood gas in A&E. Your registrar tells you she needs to be admitted and will benefit from salbutamol nebulisers.

QUESTION A:

What are the indications for nebuliser treatment?

RESPONSE A:

• In an acute setting, nebulisers can be used in the emergency treatment of acute asthma or chronic obstructive pulmonary disease (COPD).

• They can also be used as a form of long-term treatment in COPD.

• Through a nebuliser, antibiotics can be administered in, for example, lung disorders such as bronchiectasis or cystic fibrosis.

QUESTION B:

How would you make her feel at ease on arrival to the medical ward?

RESPONSE B:

• I would start by introducing myself, eliciting the patient's name, date of birth and hospital number.

• Check to make sure the patient has no allergies.

• The next step would be to explain what we are going to do and why. 'Due to the breathing problems you have been admitted with, I would like to try you on some medication (salbutamol) using a nebuliser. A nebuliser works by converting a drug which is dissolved in liquid into a fine aerosol mist; in this way it can pass directly to the lungs, where it can act to relax the airway passages and ease your breathing. You will have to wear a face mask. Be aware that, because the machine is connected to a pump to deliver the medication, it does make a bit of an annoying noise!'

• The next step would be to obtain the patient's informed verbal consent.

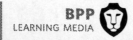

QUESTION C:

What equipment do you require for the procedure and how would you assemble it?

RESPONSE C:

There are a few components to the nebuliser:

- A face mask
- Nebuliser chamber, which converts the liquid drug (in this case salbutamol) into a gaseous mist
- A supply of oxygen or compressed air, which powers the nebuliser

Once I have all these parts available I can begin to assemble the nebuliser itself.

- Attach the air tubing from the compressor source to the nebuliser base.
- Connect the mask to the nebuliser.
- Check that I have the right drug, salbutamol (usually 5ml); read off the label and check the expiry date. Confirm the details with a nurse or another colleague.

QUESTION D:

Can you describe the procedure to me?

RESPONSE D:

- First ensure the patient is sitting upright and is comfortable.
- Place the mask to the patient's face, and tighten the elastic cord so it does not fall off.
- Switch on the compressor device to the recommended gas flow rate, usually at around 5 to 7l/min. Use air (if the patient is retaining carbon dioxide – as, for example, in patients with COPD) or oxygen, as the driving gas in acute asthma.
- Ask the patient to breathe normally into the mask until there is no longer any gaseous mist. Inform them that the procedure should last approximately 10 minutes.
- Sign, date and time the patient's drug chart to document the drug has been administered. I may need a nurse or colleague to countersign.

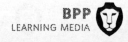

- Once the nebuliser stops producing mist, switch off the compressor device. Dismantle and clean the equipment.

- Give advice to the patient how to clean the mask and chamber to help reduce the risk of infection. Use warm soapy water to clean the various parts (except tubing). Rinse with warm water, shake off the excess water and clean with a dry cloth.

QUESTION E:

How would you assess if the nebuliser has been effective?

RESPONSE E:

I would ask the patient if she had felt there had been any improvement in her shortness of breath; I would also assess her clinically, by listening to her chest to observe if the wheeze had improved. Any improvement could be measured using a peak flow reading, and comparing this result to those on admission before the nebuliser treatment had been given.

Key points

- Note that a nebuliser can be used in an acute (asthma) or chronic (COPD) setting. Nebulisers can also be used to administer antibiotics.

- Explain clearly to the patient how you would go about performing the procedure and obtain his or her consent.

- To assess improvement in a patient's symptoms clinically you can ask if there has been a subjective improvement; listen to their chest; or, for a more accurate measurement, use a peak flow meter and compare this reading with one before the nebuliser administration.

Clinical procedure 19:   Level *

Taking a swab

Mrs Kay is a 47-year-old female who has noticed that the wound from her left knee replacement performed five days ago has opened up and is discharging some yellow offensive pus. Please take a bacterial wound swab.

QUESTION A:

How would you proceed?

RESPONSE A:

- **INTRODUCTION:** To begin with I would introduce myself. Check I am speaking to the right patient by eliciting her name, date of birth and hospital number.

- **EXPLANATION:** I would explain the reasons for taking the swab. 'Mrs Kay, I understand the wound from the operation you had a few days ago is oozing out pus. I would like to take a wound swab from the site; it should not be a painful procedure and will help us treat you with the right medication.'

- **CONSENT:** Obtain the patient's consent for you to take the wound swab.

- **POSITION:** The patient should be sitting or lying comfortably, preferably on a bed.

QUESTION B:

What equipment do you need to perform the wound swab?

RESPONSE B:

I would have the following equipment to perform the procedure:

- A pair of gloves
- Sterile swabs in an appropriate culture tube
- Gauze or another type of dry dressing

QUESTION C:

Can you describe how you would perform the procedure?

RESPONSE C:

- I would start by washing my hands and putting on a pair of non-sterile gloves.

- I'd open the outer sterile package, detach the cotton swab from its plastic tube, without allowing the swab to touch the sides of the container.

- Rotate the swab in the area to be cultured, ensuring that no area of the swab has been swabbed twice. If the wound site is large, it is appropriate to use more than one swab to swab a number of small areas.

- Replace the swab back in its plastic case, again avoiding touching the swab against the inner sides of the container.

- I wound redress the wound with the gauze provided, if required.

- Discard my gloves and any other clinical waste appropriately.

- Offer to sit the patient back up if they are lying down, and wash my hands.

QUESTION D:

What would you do with the swab taken to get it processed?

RESPONSE D:

- Label the swab container with the patient's name, date of birth, hospital number, the site from which the swab is taken (left knee) and the date taken.

- Fill in a microbiology request form, state the investigation required (gram stain, microscopy, culture and sensitivity), indication for taking the swab (infected post-operative wound), site from which swab is taken, and the names of any antibiotics the patient is currently on. Also I would put the date, name, signature and contact details of the requesting clinician. Ensure the swab is sent to the lab – I may need to contact a porter.

- Document the procedure in the patient's notes.

- Thank the patient and ask if she has any questions.

Key points

- Explain to the patient the necessity of performing a swab, namely it will help target which antibiotics they should be taking.

- When swabbing a wound, ensure that no area of the swab has been swabbed twice.

- If the wound is large, use more than one swab to swab a number of small areas.

- Label the swab container correctly with all the required information before sending it to the lab.

Clinical procedure 20:   Level * *

Recording an ECG

Mr Aitken is a 76-year-old male who has presented on the ward with new onset central chest pain. The nurse taking care of him has called you to perform an ECG.

QUESTION A:

How would you proceed?

RESPONSE A:

- INTRODUCTION: To begin with I would introduce myself. Check I am speaking to the right patient by eliciting his name, date of birth and hospital number.

- EXPLANATION: I would explain the reasons for the procedure. 'Mr Aitken, my name's Peter Sinha, I am the medical doctor on call this evening. I have been asked to perform an ECG tracing of your heart. I think it would be a good idea to do this, to help us identify if your chest pain is related to your heart. The ECG will allow us to have a recording of the electrical activity of your heart, including its rhythm. It is not a painful procedure, all I will need to do is to connect some sticky patches to your arms, legs and chest; these are then directly connected to the ECG machine. In a matter of seconds, we will be able to get an ECG trace. Is that OK?

- CONSENT: Obtain his consent.

- POSITION: Help the patient into a supine position, with adequate exposure of his arms, legs and chest.

PROCEDURE:

- Wash my hands or apply alcohol gel.

- Ensure I am familiar with the ECG machine to be used and that there is paper inside.

- Obtain the following equipment before proceeding:

  - Adhesive electrode pads
  - Alcohol sterets
  - Disposable razor blade

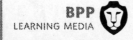

- Shave any chest hair that could interfere with the trace.

- Clean the lead attachment sites with the alcohol sterets.

- Limb leads: Attach the electrode pads, one to each forearm on the dorsal aspect, and one to each lower limb, proximal to the ankles. Attach the limb leads to these pads. It is often helpful to note that these are usually longer than the chest leads and are colour co-ordinated. In a clockwise fashion, right arm (red), left arm (yellow), left leg (green) and right leg (black).

- Chest leads, position these as follows:

  V1 4th intercostal space, right sternal edge
  V2 4th intercostal space, left sternal edge
  V3 midway between V2 and V4
  V4 5th intercostal space, left mid-clavicular line
  V5 5th intercostal space, left anterior axillary line
  V6 5th intercostal space, left mid-axillary line

- Turn the ECG machine on; check that it is set at a paper speed of 25mm/sec and calibrated to 10mm/mV. Press 'filter' followed by 'start' to print the ECG trace.

- Check the quality of the ECG trace and repeat if necessary. I may have to ask the patient to keep still, in order to reduce artefacts.

- Once I have the ECG printout, I would label it with the patient's name, date of birth and hospital number, along with the date and time the ECG was taken.

QUESTION B:

What would you do after obtaining the trace?

RESPONSE B:

- Remove the leads and electrode pads from the patient.

- Discard any clinical waste appropriately.

- Wash my hands with soap and water or use alcohol gel.

- Review and interpret the ECG; discuss your findings with the patient and construct a management plan.

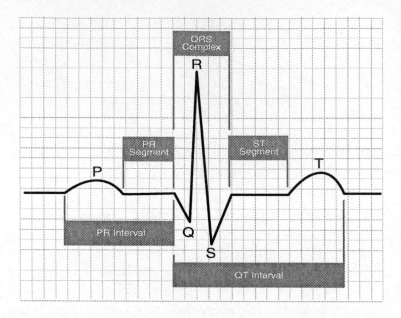

Figure 3.5: A 'typical' ECG trace

P wave:

- Represents depolarisation of the right and left atria.

- Should precede each QRS complex.

- Normal duration is less than 0.12 seconds, with amplitude of less than 2.5mm.

- Bifid P-wave (P-mitrale) occurs in left atrial hypertrophy.

- Peaked P-wave (P-pulmonale) occurs in right atrial hypertrophy.

- Absent P-wave may occur in atrial fibrillation, sino-atrial block, atrio-ventricular nodal rhythm.

QRS complex:

- Represents the time taken for right and left ventricle simultaneous depolarisation.

- Normal duration is less than 0.12 seconds.

- If duration is greater than 0.12 seconds, this suggests bundle branch block.

R wave:

- Is the first positive deflection.
- Tall R waves can indicate left ventricular hypertrophy.

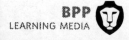

S wave:

- Is the negative deflection following the R wave.
- Deep S waves can indicate right ventricular hypertrophy.

T wave:

- Represents ventricular repolarisation.
- This is tented in hyperkalaemia and flattened in hypokalaemia.
- Although it is normally inverted in lead AVR, it is pathological if it is inverted in other leads. Inversion may be seen in conditions such as pulmonary embolism, left ventricular hypertrophy, subendocardial myocardial infarction along with left and right bundle branch block.

QUESTION C:

How would you go about interpreting the ECG trace?

RESPONSE C:

I would try to have a systematic way to read an ECG:

- Have a brief review of the ECG to see if there are any obvious glaring abnormalities.

- Identify the **rate**: Consider each large square to be a 0.2 second period. Each small square therefore becomes a 0.04 second period. The rate can be calculated by dividing the number of large squares between two adjacent R waves into 300. A normal rate is 60-100 bpm; bradycardia is <60 bpm; tachycardia is >100 bpm.

- Identify the **rhythm**: P-waves preceding each QRS complex indicate sinus rhythm. An absence of P-waves could suggest atrial fibrillation.

- Identify the **axis**: If the QRS complexes are, on the whole positive in leads I and II, the axis is normal. If the complex is positive in lead I, but negative in lead II this indicates left axis deviation. Right axis deviation is suggested by a negative QRS complex in lead I, regardless of lead II.

- Observe the QRS complex, assess its duration, and look for pathological Q waves.

Key points

- Take every opportunity to interpret the ECG of all patients admitted to your ward.

- There are some abnormal examples of ECGs that you may commonly be shown in your exam. In particular, be able to identify ECG patterns which show: atrial fibrillation; acute myocardial infarction; left ventricular hypertrophy; ventricular fibrillation; heart block.

- Have your own systematic way which allows you to read an ECG trace, such as the one described in this scenario.

BPP
LEARNING MEDIA

Clinical procedure 21:   Level *

Taking blood cultures

Mr Walsh is a 68-year-old male who has been admitted with an apparent chest infection. His nurse calls you to let you know his temperature has risen to 39.5°C. As the doctor on call, you have also been asked to take some blood cultures from him as part of a septic screen.

QUESTION A:

How would you proceed?

RESPONSE A:

- INTRODUCTION: To begin with I would introduce myself. Check I am speaking to the right patient by eliciting his name date of birth and hospital number.

- EXPLANATION: I would explain the reasons for taking the blood cultures: 'Mr Walsh, I am the medical doctor on call today and have been asked to take a sample of blood from your arm. The procedure itself is the same as taking blood for routine blood tests. It will help us to identify the type of infection you have.'

- CONSENT: Obtain the patient's consent to take the blood tests for culture.

- POSITION: The patient should be sitting or lying comfortably with their arm horizontal and elbow extended; support the arm with a pillow.

QUESTION B:

What equipment do you need to obtain the blood culture?

RESPONSE B:

I would have the following equipment to perform the procedure:

- A pair of gloves
- Blood culture bottles, aerobic and anaerobic
- Alcohol steret
- Gauze or another type of dry dressing
- Three green/blue needles
- 20ml syringe
- Tourniquet

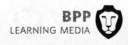

QUESTION C:

Can you describe how you would perform the procedure?

RESPONSE C:

- I would start by washing my hands and putting on a pair of non-sterile gloves.

- With the patient's arm fully extended, I apply the tourniquet above the antecubital fossa.

- I identify an appropriate vein and clean the skin over this with the alcohol steret, and wait for around 30 seconds for the alcohol to evaporate.

- Attach a green (21G) needle to the 20ml syringe.

- Insert the needle at an angle of between 15 and 30 degrees through the skin into the vein. Aim to venesect 10-20ml of blood.

- Release the tourniquet, apply pressure over the venepuncture site with gauze (or cotton wool) until the bleeding has stopped.

- Dispose of the needle in a sharps box, and the clinical waste appropriately.

- Apply a new sterile 21G needle on to the syringe.

- Remove the caps off the culture bottles and clean the rubber tops with another alcohol steret, this helps to ensure sterile access into the culture medium.

- Inject 5 to 10ml of blood into the anaerobic culture bottle, and then the same amount into the aerobic culture bottle. Replace and apply a new needle before injecting into each bottle.

- Dispose of all needles in the sharps box and the clinical waste in the appropriate waste bags.

QUESTION D:

What would you do with your blood culture bottles at this point?

RESPONSE D:

- Label the blood culture bottles with the patient's name, hospital number and date of birth, along with the date and time the sample was taken.

- Fill in a microbiology request form, state the investigation required (microscopy, culture and sensitivity); indication for taking the test (pyrexial with an apparent chest infection); site from which sample was taken (eg left arm); date, name and contact details of the requesting clinician; and the names (along with dosages) of any antibiotics the patient is already taking.

- Ensure the swab is sent to the lab – I may need to contact a porter.

- Document the procedure in the patient's notes.

- Thank the patient and ask if he has any questions.

If asked you can state that a preliminary report of the results can usually be obtained after about 24 hours. The full culture results including, antibiotic sensitivities, will take at least 48 hours and may take up to 3 to 5 days.

Key points

- Explain to the patient the importance of taking the blood cultures.

- Blood cultures should ideally be taken before antibiotics are commenced.

- For each set of blood cultures an aerobic and anaerobic bottle is required.

- If a patient has a central line in situ, the blood should also be taken from the line.

Clinical procedure 22: Level * * *

Ankle brachial pressure index measurement

Mr Mendoza is an 82-year-old male who is complaining of pain in his legs at rest. He is known to be hypertensive, an insulin-dependent diabetic and has suffered from angina in the past. As the surgical FY2 doctor on the ward, you have been asked by your registrar to measure his ankle brachial pressure index (ABPI).

QUESTION A:

How would you proceed?

RESPONSE A:

- INTRODUCTION: To begin with I would introduce myself. Check I am speaking to the right patient by eliciting his name date of birth and hospital number. At this stage I would try to establish a rapport and make him feel at ease.

- EXPLANATION: I would explain the reasons for taking the ABPI measurement and how I would proceed. 'Hello Mr Mendoza, my name is David Davies, I am the surgical doctor on the ward today. Due to the symptoms you have been having I would like to measure the blood pressure in your arms and legs. I will be using a blood pressure cuff and a something called a Doppler device to do this. It is not a painful procedure and is simple to perform.'

- CONSENT: Ask the patient if that is OK, and check with them if they have any questions or concerns.

QUESTION B:

What equipment do you need to perform the ABPI measurement?

RESPONSE B:

I would have the following equipment to perform the procedure:

- A sphygmomanometer
- A Doppler device
- Calculator
- Lubricating jelly
- Gauze swabs/cotton wool

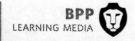

QUESTION C:

Can you describe the procedure to me?

RESPONSE C:

*   The patient should be comfortable, lying flat with their feet and arms exposed for the procedure.

*   It would, perhaps, lead to a more accurate reading if the patient is at rest for 15 to 20 minutes. This allows for any pressure changes recorded to be more likely to be secondary to arterial disease rather than patient movement.

*   **Brachial** pulse: I would place the cuff around the patient's arm. Identify the brachial pulse on the anteromedial aspect of the antecubital fossa and apply lubricating jelly over the skin covering this region.

*   Hold the Doppler device such that the probe is at a 45° angle to the direction of blood flow in the artery. (I may have to move the probe around until a good signal is achieved.)

*   Now inflate the cuff until the signal disappears. At this stage, slowly deflate the cuff (at no greater than a rate of 2mmHg/second). The aim is to accurately record the pressure at which the blood flow signal returns.

*   Note the pressure reading, which is the brachial systolic pressure.

*   Repeat the procedure on the other arm. The higher of the two values should be used to calculate the ABPI.

*   Use the gauze swabs or cotton wool to wipe off the lubricating jelly.

*   **Ankle** pulse: Identify the dorsalis pedis pulse and apply lubricant jelly. Using the Doppler device take the ankle systolic pressure as described for the brachial pulse. Document the result.

*   Repeat the technique for measurement of the posterior tibial pulse.

    You can tell the examiner that you could also measure the peroneal pulse, but in practice you will probably have insufficient time in the exam to do this. Document the results for each measurement.

*   The highest reading between the pulses should be used to calculate the ABPI for that ankle. Repeat the same steps for the other ankle.

*   Remember to wipe off the lubricating jelly from the skin of the patient at each site as well as the Doppler probe.

*   Wash my hands.

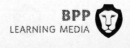

QUESTION D:

How would you calculate the ABPI once you have the individual readings, and what is your interpretation of the results?

RESPONSE D:

I would calculate the ABPI by dividing the ankle pressure by the brachial pressure. Obtain a separate ABPI reading for each leg. I remember to use the highest systolic pressure reading between the dorsalis pedis artery, posterior tibial artery (and peroneal artery if also calculated) for each leg. I would also use the highest systolic reading of the left and right arm brachial artery. I would use the following equation:

$$ABPI = \frac{\text{Highest ankle Doppler pressure (for leg in question)}}{\text{Highest brachial Doppler pressure (for both arms)}}$$

Hence two separate ABPI readings are obtained (one for each side). The ABPI is a measurement which aids in the diagnosis of peripheral vascular disease; if found to be the case, it is also used as a means of assessing the severity of this condition.

- Normal index is greater than or equal to 1.

- In a patient with peripheral vascular disease, as the perfusion of the leg begins to decrease, the ratio (index) also falls.

- Individuals with intermittent claudication have an index of approximately 0.5-0.8.

- Individuals with critical ischaemia have an index of approximately 0.1-0.4. An absolute pressure of less than 50mmHg at the ankle is also indicative of critical ischaemia.

- In diabetics the ABPI may be falsely elevated. In this situation the ankle systolic pressure reading is often high because of calcification of the wall of the blood vessel which results in a greater resistance to compression.

Key points

- The ABPI is used as a means to diagnose and assess the severity of peripheral vascular disease.

- An ABPI value between 0.1-0.4 indicates critical ischaemia, 0.5-0.8 indicates intermittent claudication; a value greater than or equal to 1 is normal.

- Patients with diabetes may have a falsely elevated ABPI due to calcification of the blood vessel wall.

Clinical procedure 23:   Level * *

Sizing and applying a hard collar

Mr Billing is a 23-year-old cyclist involved in a road traffic accident. You are at the scene of the accident, having seen him been knocked down by an oncoming car. The paramedics are with you and have asked if you can immobilise his cervical spine.

QUESTION A:

State the indications for immobilising a cervical spine.

RESPONSE A:

- If the patient is unconscious and there has been a history of trauma.

- In the conscious patient with:
    - Multi-system trauma
    - Trauma and unexplained hypotension
    - Blunt injury above the clavicle
    - Neck pain and or tenderness
    - Neurological deficit
    - A reduced range of neck movements
    - Significant mechanism of spinal injury, such as a fall from more than 3 metres

QUESTION B:

How would you proceed and apply a hard collar?

RESPONSE B:

- INTRODUCTION: I would introduce myself to the patient if he is conscious.

- EXPLANATION: I would explain what I would like to do. 'My name is Dr Amy Clarke; I am the doctor working with the paramedic crew today. I would like to place a collar round your neck to help protect your spine from injury.'

- As long as the patient is conscious and able to verbally communicate with me, it is likely that the airway is patent and not likely to be in any immediate danger.

 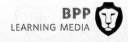

- CONSENT: It may not be practical or appropriate to obtain consent in an emergency situation like this. It should be considered that I am acting in the patient's best interests.

- I would take universal precautions to protect myself and the staff around me from any danger.

- Ask a member of the paramedic crew to maintain in-line immobilisation, keeping the patient's neck held in a neutral position.

- Ask for a one-piece hard collar, (I measure the size of the collar required by measuring from the angle of the mandible (jaw) to the top of shoulder/trapezius using my hand).

- On the hard collar itself, I measure from the bottom of the rigid plastic to the 'measuring post'. This should correspond to the above measurement.

- The flat-sided one-piece hard collar is applied by sliding it under the patient's neck and fastening it from the front.

- Three-point fixation is necessary to achieve a neutral cervical spine alignment and immobilisation. To do this, I would apply sandbags on either side of the patient's head, tape the sandbags to the head and spinal board (or trolley) on either side.

QUESTION C:

What X-ray views of the cervical spine would you perform? If these images do not identify any injury, would you be happy to remove the immobilisation?

RESPONSE C:

I would need to perform AP, lateral and odontoid peg X-ray views of the cervical spine. I would not be happy to remove the immobilisation on X-ray radiological clearance of injury alone. The patient must be cleared clinically as well as radiologically before the immobilisation can be taken off. If there is still a high suspicion of neck injury I would also request a CT scan of the cervical spine.

Key points

- A one-piece hard collar forms part of the initial management of patients with suspected cervical spine injury. It must be applied in all unconscious patients where there has been a history of trauma, and in conscious patients if there is any suspicion of injury following trauma.

- Immobilisation should only be removed when the patient is cleared clinically, as well as radiologically, from cervical injury.

- All cervical spine X-rays in the trauma setting should contain AP, lateral and odontoid peg views.

Clinical procedure 24:   Level *

Pulse oximetry

Mrs Min is a 48-year-old female admitted to the respiratory ward following an acute exacerbation of asthma. As the FY1 doctor on the respiratory firm you have been asked by the nurse taking care of her to measure her oxygen saturation using pulse oximetry.

Pulse oximetry is a non-invasive method of allowing the monitoring of the oxygenation of a patient's haemoglobin levels. An oximetry device comprises of a sensor placed on a thin part of the patient's body, usually a fingertip or earlobe, or, in the case of an infant, across a foot. Two light-emitting diodes (LEDs) emit light with red wavelengths and light with infrared wavelengths which are sequentially passed from one side to a photo detector on the other side. A microprocessor unit displays a waveform, oxygen saturations and heart rate. The light absorption at each wavelength is determined by the degree of oxygen saturation of haemoglobin.

QUESTION A:

How would you proceed?

RESPONSE A:

- INTRODUCTION: To begin with I would introduce myself. Check I am speaking to the right patient by eliciting her name, date of birth and hospital number. At this stage I would try to establish a rapport and make her feel at ease.

- EXPLANATION: I would explain the reasons for taking the pulse oximetry and also state how it is performed. 'The procedure will give us an indication of the levels of oxygen in your blood. It does not hurt and is very easy to perform; all I have to do is place a probe on your fingertip.'

- CONSENT: Ask the patient if that is OK, and check with them if they have any questions or concerns.

- Before proceeding I would wash my hands/apply the alcohol gel.

QUESTION B:

Can you describe the procedure to me?

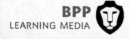

RESPONSE B:

- I would check that the pulse oximeter is switched on to the mains or the battery power is acceptable.

- On switching the machine on, I would have to allow it to calibrate.

- Now I would ask the patient to ensure she has clean hands, also free from nail varnish. I can then apply the correct size probe and place it on a fingertip. The fingers are the most common sites to be used but if, for any reason, they are not suitable the nose and ear lobe can also be used.

- I would then simply wait for the pulse oximeter to give a digital electronic reading of the patient's heart rate and oxygen saturation.

- To verify the reading is accurate, I would check that a waveform is displayed on the machine.

QUESTION C:

What would you do once you have a reading of the results?

RESPONSE C:

- I would document the heart rate and oxygen saturation in the patient's notes.

- Inform the patient what the results mean and what, if any, further course of action is required.

- Finally, I would ask the patient if they have any concerns and answer any questions they may have.

QUESTION D:

Are you aware of any factors that may result in false or inaccurate measurements?

RESPONSE D:

- Nail varnish

- Bright lights

- Shivering, or someone who is having seizures or tremors

- Carbon monoxide and cyanide poisoning

- Conditions causing peripheral vasoconstriction eg hypovolaemia, hypotension, hypothermia

QUESTION E:

How accurate is pulse oximetry at assessing a patient's respiratory status?

RESPONSE E:

Pulse oximetry measures only the oxygenation levels of haemoglobin; it does not give an indication of a patient's ventilation. It does not give us a value for the arterial oxygen concentration, PaO_2 or the CO_2 concentration.

Arterial blood gases (ABGs) should be done to assess a patient's ventilation; they would give an indication of base deficit, CO_2 levels, bicarbonate concentration and blood pH levels. The results of pulse oximetry and ABGs should be reviewed in the context of the patient's clinical condition.

Key points

- Pulse oximetry is a non-invasive method of allowing the monitoring of the oxygenation of a patient's haemoglobin levels. It does not give an assessment of a patient's ventilation.

- Some factors which can influence the accuracy of pulse oximetry readings include nail varnish, bright lights, shivering, seizures and also conditions causing peripheral vasoconstriction.

- Interpret the results of pulse oximetry and arterial blood gases in the context of the patient's clinical condition.

Clinical procedure 25:   Level * *

Ascitic tap

Mrs Wallbank, a 55-year-old female, known to be an alcohol dependent, presents to the surgical assessment unit with gross ascites. As the FY2 surgical doctor on call, you have been asked by your consultant to perform an ascitic tap.

QUESTION A:

Name some of the indications for performing an ascitic tap, also known as paracentesis.

RESPONSE A:

- It can be performed for diagnostic purposes to determine the aetiology of the ascites, to differentiate a transudate from an exudate, and also to detect the presence of cancerous cells or bacterial peritonitis.

- It can be a therapeutic procedure. It can be used to relieve respiratory distress or abdominal pain or pressure secondary to ascites.

QUESTION B:

In what situations is an ascitic tap contraindicated?

RESPONSE B:

- Coagulopathy
- Pregnancy
- Skin infection at the proposed puncture site

QUESTION C:

What equipment do you require to perform the procedure?

RESPONSE C:

- Dressing pack
- Several gauze swabs
- 21G (green) needle
- 20ml syringe
- 2% lignocaine

- Betadine
- Specimen culture bottles
- Mepore sterile dressing

QUESTION D:

Can you explain the procedure to me?

RESPONSE D:

- I would start by INTRODUCING myself to the patient, EXPLAINING what I would like to do and seeking her CONSENT. 'Hello Mrs Wallbank, my name is Dr White. I am the surgical doctor on call today. I would like to extract some of the fluid in your abdomen, if that is OK. It will allow me to send a sample off to the laboratory to help identify why your abdomen has become distended. It should not be a painful procedure, as I will use some local anaesthetic and it should not take more than a few minutes to perform. Is that OK, and do you have any questions?

- Before proceeding I would check the patient's blood results, in particular the clotting result. If there was any problem, this would need to be reviewed and corrected before carrying on.

- I would ask the patient to empty her bladder and then ask her to lie flat on the couch or bed on her back.

- Expose the patient's abdomen fully and percuss the ascitic fluid.

  Demonstrate shifting dullness and a fluid thrill. Mark, with a pen, the point of drainage. If she has had previous abdominal surgery, I must avoid old surgical scars as the bowel may show adhesions here.

- Scrub and gown up.

- Clean the skin with betadine-soaked gauze swabs.

- Infiltrate the skin over the drainage site with 2% lignocaine.

- Give the local anaesthetic 2 to 3 minutes to act.

- Attach the 21G needle to the 20ml syringe, and gently advance the needle through the skin at the marked site while aspirating the ascitic fluid.

- Take the needle out and apply a mepore sterile dressing over the drainage site.

- Inform the patient the procedure is over; tell her that I will be sending the fluid off for analysis, and ask her if she has any questions and if she would like any pain relief.

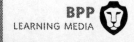

- Place the fluid in the specimen culture bottles and send for microbiology (culture and sensitivity), cytology (looking for malignant cells), biochemistry – looking at the protein count, amylase, glucose and lactate dehydrogenase (LDH) levels.

- Document the procedure in the patient's notes.

- When ascitic fluid is being removed for therapeutic purposes, I shouldn't take off more than 500ml in the first 10 minutes, or 1 litre in one sitting, due to the increased risk of developing hypotension.

Key points

- An ascitic tap can be performed for diagnostic or therapeutic purposes.

- The procedure is contraindicated in the presence of a coagulopathy, pregnancy and localised infection over the puncture site.

- Excessive amounts of ascitic fluid taken off at one sitting (more than one litre or greater than 500ml in 10 minutes) can be associated with developing hypotension.

Clinical procedure 26:   Level *

Administering an intramuscular injection

Mr Newton is a 42-year-old male admitted with an episode of renal colic. He has been prescribed diclofenac 50mg IM three times a day. You have been asked by the sister on the ward to administer the injection intramuscularly as prescribed. Explain how you would perform the procedure.

QUESTION A:

How would you proceed?

RESPONSE A:

- INTRODUCTION: To begin with I would introduce myself. Check I am speaking to the right patient by eliciting his name, date of birth and hospital number. At this stage I would try to establish a rapport and make him feel at ease.

- EXPLANATION: I would explain the reasons for giving the medication. 'I have been asked to give you a painkiller drug called diclofenac, you may have heard of it; it is also called Voltarol. This should help the pain of renal colic you are experiencing. It is very effective when given by an intramuscular route. Do you have any questions?'

- CONSENT: I would obtain verbal consent from the patient and warn him of some of the more common possible side effects of the drug (diclofenac) such as stomach cramps, nausea and diarrhoea.

- POSITION: The patient should be sitting or lying comfortably.

QUESTION B:

Explain how you would prepare the equipment for performing the procedure, including preparing the drug itself.

RESPONSE B:

- I would start by checking the patient's drug chart to verify the name of the drug, the route of administration (intramuscular in this case), date and time to be given and the signature of the requesting clinician – ie the validity of the prescription.

- Check to ensure the patient has no contraindications to the drug prescribed; in this case, ensure there is no history of gastric ulcers or renal problems.

- Clarify if the patient has any drug allergies, and specifically to the drug to be administered.

- Check the British National Formulary (BNF) to see if the drug and dose are appropriate.

- Wash my hands using a disinfectant, dry thoroughly and put on a pair of gloves.

- Other equipment I would have include a 5ml syringe, a couple of 21G (green) needles and a steret (alcowipe).

- Check the name, strength and expiry date of the drug in the ampoule or vial with a nurse or colleague.

- Once the checks are performed, I can then prepare to give the injection. I would attach the needle to the syringe and draw up the correct amount of drug from the vial.

- An additional point to remember is that when a drug is in the form of a dry powder, it needs to be diluted. Therefore check the name, strength and expiry of the sterile water solution. Use the BNF or the manufacturer's guidelines to determine the appropriate amount of solvent to dilute the drug. The solvent can now be injected into the vial, and shaken vigorously until all the solid has been dissolved.

QUESTION C:

What body sites could you use to perform an intramuscular injection, and what considerations do you need to bear in mind before carrying it out?

RESPONSE C:

Possible sites for performing an intramuscular injection include:

- Body of the deltoid muscle: Inject lateral to, and a few centimetres below, the acromion process, in this way avoiding the radial nerve. This site has a very good blood supply, hence ensuring a rapid rate of uptake. It is also the most accessible intramuscular site.

- Gluteus muscle: Inject into the upper outer quadrant to avoid the sciatic nerve and the superior gluteal artery. A useful landmark is posterior to, and above, an imaginary line drawn from the anterior superior iliac spine to the greater trochanter, bounded superiorly by the iliac crest.

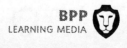

• Vastus lateralis muscle (a component of the rectus femoris group): Inject into the antero-lateral aspect of the thigh. This is safe, and good for oil-based (depot) preparations as well as narcotics and sedatives. It can be more painful due to the overlying fascia lata.

QUESTION D:

Please describe the procedure, using the mannequin arm and the equipment provided.

RESPONSE D:

• With the patient in a comfortable position, either sitting or lying, I would clean the injection site with a steret.

• With the drug in the syringe and a new 21G needle attached (discarding the needle used to draw up the medication), with one hand I would stretch the skin taut at the injection site.

• Hold the needle and syringe in the other hand, inform the patient of a 'sharp scratch', then inject with the needle at 90° to the patient's skin.

• Insert the needle in a smooth, quick motion to approximately 3mm below the hilt. Draw back on the plunger of the syringe to check that a blood vessel has not been accidentally entered; if this has occurred and blood is aspirated, the injection site should be changed.

• Inject the drug slowly, according at the rate stated in the BNF.

• Once the drug has been fully given, wait 10 seconds before removing the needle and applying pressure over the injection site with a gauze swab.

• Discard sharps and clinical waste appropriately.

• Document that I have administered the drug in the drug chart along with the time and date of administration, and sign.

Key points

- Before administering any drug, it is paramount that some basic checks are performed; this includes the patient's identity, any allergies, the drug, its dosage, strength, dilution, expiry date and method of administration. Mention that you would check the drug with a nurse or colleague before administering it.

- Explain to the patient why they need the drug and seek their consent to administer it.

- Administer the IM injection at the correct rate, as stated in the BNF.

- Document in the drug chart that the drug has been administered, along with the date and time, and sign.

Clinical procedure 27: Level *

Administering a subcutaneous injection

Mr Curtis is a 56-year-old male who has recently been diagnosed with a deep vein thrombosis (DVT) after a period of immobility following orthopaedic surgery. He has been prescribed 15,000 units of heparin by subcutaneous injection every 12 hours. The nurse taking care of him has asked you to administer the injection.

QUESTION A:

How would you proceed?

RESPONSE A:

- INTRODUCTION: To begin with I would introduce myself. Check I am speaking to the right patient by eliciting his name, date of birth and hospital number. At this stage I would try to establish a rapport and make him feel at ease.

- EXPLANATION: I would explain the reasons for giving the medication. 'I have been asked to give you an injection of a clot-busting drug called heparin. This will help combat the DVT in your leg, and in particular it will help prevent the clot from dislodging and passing to your lung.'

- CONSENT: I would obtain verbal consent from him and warn him of some of the more common possible side effects of the drug (heparin) such as pain, redness or irritation at the injection site. I would also ask him to watch out for prolonged bleeding from cuts on the gums.

- POSITION: The patient should be sitting or lying comfortably.

QUESTION B:

Explain how you would prepare the equipment for performing the procedure including preparing the drug itself.

RESPONSE B:

- I would start by checking the patient's drug chart to verify the name of the drug, the route of administration (subcutaneous in this case), date and time to be given and the signature of the requesting clinician – ie the validity of the prescription.

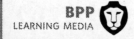

- I would check to ensure the patient has no contraindications to the drug prescribed, including no history of haemophilia and other haemorrhagic disorders.

- Clarify if the patient has any drug allergies, and specifically to the drug to be administered.

- Check the British National Formulary (BNF) to see if the drug and dose are appropriate.

- Wash my hands using a disinfectant, dry thoroughly and put on a pair of gloves.

- Gather appropriate sized needles, 23 to 25G, and a steret (alcowipe).

- Check the name, strength and expiry date of any dilutant with a nurse or colleague.

- Once the checks are performed, I can prepare the correct volume of the heparin, diluting according to the manufacturer's instructions, and draw it up into a syringe. However, I note that in most hospitals, heparin usually comes in a pre-prepared syringe.

- Attach the needle to the syringe containing heparin, expel any excess air.

QUESTION C:

What body sites could you use to perform a subcutaneous injection and what considerations do you need to bear in mind before carrying it out?

RESPONSE C:

I would use an injection site where there is a large amount of fatty tissue in the subcutaneous layer, between the skin and muscle, such as the thighs, abdomen or upper arms.

- I would rotate the injection sites, so that the same site is only used once every 6 to 7 weeks. Repeated injections in the same area can cause scarring and hardening of fatty tissue, which can interfere with the absorption of the medication. Rotating injection sites in immunocompromised patients, such as those with diabetes, reduces the risk of fat necrosis.

- I would consider using a body chart for injection sites, marking each site each time it is used.

- Areas to avoid include sites of infection, joints or other bony prominences and scars.

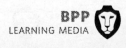

QUESTION D:

Please describe the procedure, using the mannequin arm and the equipment provided.

RESPONSE D:

- With the patient in a comfortable position, either sitting or lying, I would clean the injection site with a steret, and allow the area to dry for approximately 30 seconds.

- Remove the needle cap, holding the syringe barrel like a pencil.

- With the other hand, pinch a fold of skin between my thumb and index finger.

- Hold the syringe at a 45° angle about 1 inch from the skin surface.

- Insert the needle rapidly into the patient, give him a warning beforehand ('You will feel a sharp scratch'). The needle should go all the way into the skin.

- Pull back on the plunger of the syringe a little; if blood is identified in the syringe, do not inject the drug solution. If this happens, remove and discard the syringe and try again at a different site.

- If there is no blood in the syringe, slowly push the plunger to inject the drug solution.

- Apply cotton wool or gauze swab over the injection site (but not pressing down yet); I'd remove the needle and press down on the swab over the injection site for 10 seconds. Apply a mepore or other dry dressing over the site.

- Discard sharps and clinical waste appropriately. Wash my hands.

- Document that I have administered the drug in the drug chart along with the time and date of administration, and sign.

- Check that the patient is comfortable after the procedure. Inform him that it has been performed successfully and ask him if he has any questions or concerns.

Key points

- Before administering any drug, it is paramount that some basic checks are performed: this includes the patient's identity, their allergies, the drug, its dosage, strength, dilution, expiry date and method of administration. Always mention that you would also check the drug with a nurse or colleague before administering it.

- Explain to the patient why he or she needs the drug and seek their consent to administer it.

- Remember to rotate the site of subcutaneous injection; a body chart for injection sites may be useful for this purpose.

- Document in the drug chart that the drug has been administered, along with the date and time, and sign.

Clinical procedure 28:   Level *

Use of surgical drains

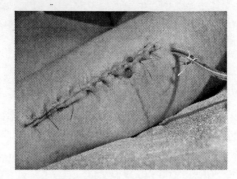

Figure 3.6: Instrument identification A

QUESTION A:

Identify what this is, and state the indications for its use.

RESPONSE A:

This is a surgical drain; it can be used in a variety of settings.

- To allow the drainage of a collection. This could be blood, other fluid, infective collections such as pus from an abscess or also air.

- Abolition of a dead space.

- To remove a potential collection, eg seroma following hernia surgery.

QUESTION B:

Do you know of any methods to classify surgical drains?

RESPONSE B:

- Surgical drains can be classified as either active or passive systems.

- Both of these subtypes can be further divided into open and closed systems.

- Less commonly, they are grouped according to the material from which they are made. In this regard, they can be made of PVC, latex, silastic or polyurethane.

QUESTION C:

How do the different types of drain work?

RESPONSE C:

Drains can be classified as either active or passive systems. In both categories, the drain may either be open or closed.

Active System Drains include:

Closed system drains (eg Redivac drain). These:

- Function by creating a vacuum, which drains fluid into a reservoir chamber
- Have a reservoir capacity of approximately 300ml
- Have non-return valves, which prevent reflux from occurring
- Are disposable
- Have a relatively low infection risk
- Can achieve a low-pressure suction of around 100mmHg

Open system drains (eg Sump drain). These:

- Are usually more efficient than closed suction drains
- Comprise an inner tube under suction, which is protected from blockage by an outer irrigated or vented tube
- Offer irrigation and aspiration

Passive System Drains include:

Closed system drains (eg Robinson drain):

- Drainage is dependent on fluid moving down a pressure gradient into a collecting bag.

Open system drains (eg Stoma bag):

- Drainage of fluid relies on gravity or a capillary action. For this reason the position and site the drain is placed is important.

QUESTION D:

What complications can occur with the use of surgical drains?

RESPONSE D:

Complications can be divided into:

- Those that occur at the time of drain insertion, such as bleeding at the insertion site. Damage or perforation of adjacent structures is also possible.

- Problems that can occur in the early post-operative period include displacement of the drain, or blockage/occlusion of the drain. Infection can also occur if a drain remains in situ for too long. In most circumstances, drains are usually removed within five days or when the output is less than 50-75ml/hour.

- Late problems that can arise include damage to the blood supply of adjacent tissue, causing ischaemia and/or necrosis.

Key points

- Surgical drains can be inserted to drain a collection, remove a potential collection or to abolish a dead space.

- Drains can be classified into Active and Passive systems, and these can be further divided into Open and Closed systems.

- Complications that can occur with surgical drain insertion include bleeding, perforation of adjacent structures, blockage and infection.

Clinical procedure 29:   Level * *

Diagnostic peritoneal lavage (DPL)

You are the FY2 trainee working in A&E. A 48-year-old male involved in a road traffic accident has been brought to the resuscitation room by the ambulance crew. He is unconscious and has been identified to be hypotensive. Your registrar asks you to perform a diagnostic peritoneal lavage (DPL).

QUESTION A:

What do you understand by the term DPL and what are the indications for performing this procedure?

RESPONSE A:

DPL is a procedure that can be performed when intraperitoneal bleeding is suspected, usually secondary to trauma. In a haemodynamically unstable patient, with a high risk mechanism of injury, peritoneal lavage is the quickest, most reliable method of determining if there has been a concomitant intra-abdominal injury requiring laparotomy.

Indications

- The indication for performing DPL in trauma is when intra-abdominal bleeding is suspected, thereby providing the clinician a means of rapidly diagnosing whether or not an intra-abdominal injury requires a laparotomy.

Contraindications

- The only absolute contraindication would be if there is already a clear need and indication for performing a laparotomy.

- Relative contraindications, which could make the procedure risky and perhaps more challenging to perform, include those patients with medical concerns such as liver cirrhosis, the morbidly obese and those with a coagulopathy. Previous abdominal surgery and operator inexperience are also relative contraindications.

QUESTION B:

Now can you explain how to perform the procedure?

RESPONSE B:

As the patient is unconscious, the procedure of DPL would be regarded as being in the patient's best interests to perform, hence I would obtain and fill in a two-doctor consent form.

Initially I would gather the equipment required to do the procedure:

- Betadine antiseptic
- Some local anaesthetic, a vial of 10ml 1% lignocaine
- 26G needle and a couple of 10ml syringes
- A sterile procedure pack
- A suture and needle-holder pack
- Peritoneal dialysis catheter
- A one-litre bag of normal saline

I would ensure the patient is positioned correctly, namely supine on his back.

A urinary catheter and a nasogastric tube should already be in situ to ensure the bladder and stomach are decompressed respectively.

I would then move on to the procedure itself:

- To start with, I would scrub up, put on gloves and gown.

- Prepare the entire abdomen, using the betadine solution to create a sterile field.

- Apply sterile drapes to expose the abdomen.

- Inject local anaesthetic (1% lignocaine) into the skin and subcutaneous tissues, one-third of the distance between the umbilicus and the pubic symphysis, using the 26G needle and syringe.

- In the anaesthetised area, make a vertical skin incision for about 2cm, the dissection is carried down to the fascia.

- At this point, the linea alba is grasped between forceps and gently pulled upwards and the incision is further deepened to get into the peritoneal cavity.

- The dialysis catheter is passed through the opening in the peritoneal cavity and advanced towards the hollow of the pelvis.

- I would attach a syringe to the free end of the dialysis catheter and aspirate.

- If no blood is aspirated, connect the dialysis catheter to the bag of warmed normal saline via a connecting tube.

- The fluid inside the abdomen is now swished around by gentle agitation of the abdomen.

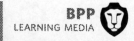

- Once the fluid has entered the peritoneal cavity, it should be allowed to stay for up to 10 minutes; it should then be siphoned off by bringing the fluid bag or bottle down to the floor.

- On collecting the fluid, a sample should be sent to the lab for analysis of the white and red blood cell counts.

- The dialysis catheter is removed and the wound would be dressed.

QUESTION C:

What would indicate a positive DPL result?

RESPONSE C:

- More than 100,000mm3 red blood cells.

- More than 500mm3 white blood cells.

- If gross intestinal contents such as bile, faeces or frank blood are identified.

- I note that a negative result does not exclude a retroperitoneal injury eg to the duodenum or pancreas.

QUESTION D:

What are the complications associated with DPL?

RESPONSE D:

- Injury to the urinary bladder, if not emptied well.

- Wound infection.

- Peritonitis can occur secondary to intestinal perforation whilst performing the procedure and from the catheter itself.

- A false positive result may occur due to haemorrhage from the incision site.

Key points

- DPL can be performed when intra-abdominal trauma has occurred, there is a suspicion of intraperitoneal bleeding and the examination of the patient is unreliable or equivocal.

- The only absolute contraindication to performing DPL is where there is already a clear need and indication for performing a laparotomy. Relative contraindications include patients with medical problems such as liver cirrhosis, coaguloapathy, morbid obesity, previous abdominal surgery and operator inexperience.

- A positive DPL result is indicated by more than 100,000mm3 red blood cells, and/or more than 500mm3 white blood cells and/or the presence of gross intestinal contents such as bile, faeces or frank blood.

Clinical procedure 30:   Level *

Performing a Papanicolaou (Pap) smear

Mrs O'Neil is a 31-year-old female referred by her GP for a routine cervical smear test. You are the FY2 doctor in Obstetrics & Gynaecology and have been asked to perform the test.

QUESTION A:

How would you approach the patient in preparation to perform the test?

RESPONSE A:

- I would start by INTRODUCING myself to the patient, EXPLAINING what I would like to do and obtaining their CONSENT: 'Hello Mrs O'Neil, my name is Dr Kumar. I understand you have come to have a cervical smear test today. Is it OK for me to proceed to perform the examination?'

- I would also inform her that the procedure is generally safe, and that bleeding and perforation are the main complications that can arise. However, I would reassure her that neither of them is common.

- I would ensure I have a female chaperone with me.

QUESTION B:

How would you position the patient and prepare for the procedure?

RESPONSE B:

- I would ask the patient to lie flat on her back with her knees flexed, feet together and the thighs slightly apart.

- Check that the patient is comfortable, with her underwear off; I would have a blanket to help keep her modesty until the procedure is performed.

- Then I would wash my hands and put on a pair of gloves.

- Ensure the lighting in the room is satisfactory.

- I would have all the equipment required at hand. This includes a vaginal speculum, cervical spatula (also known as an Ayre's spatula), histology slides and alcohol fixatives.

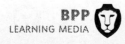

QUESTION C:

How would you perform the examination?

RESPONSE C:

- I would tell the patient I will keep her informed during each step of the procedure. It should not be painful, but if she is in discomfort then I can pause what I am doing.

- I would inspect the perineum for warts and ulcers.

- Gently separate the labia and carry on with my inspection; this includes the clitoris, vestibule of the vagina, along with the vaginal orifice (looking for prolapse or discharge).

- Next, I would warm the blades of the speculum with warm water.

- Then use my left hand to part the labia minora and insert the speculum at a 45° angle to the horizontal.

- As I open the speculum I can inspect the cervix and vagina for cysts, masses or other swellings.

- I would rotate the Ayre's through 360° around the external os to obtain cells from the squamo-columnar junction.

- Then I would smear the cells obtained on to a histology slide and fix it with the alcohol fixative.

- Now I can place the tip of the cervical brush into the external cervical os and rotate it through 360°, ensuring that it is always in contact with the cervix.

- I would then also smear these cells onto a histology slide, using the alcohol fixative.

- I carefully remove the speculum from the vagina.

- Ask if the patient requires any assistance with their clothing.

- Dispose of any clinical waste.

- Label the slides with the patient's name, date of birth and hospital number.

- Wash my hands.

- I would also document the procedure in the patient's notes.

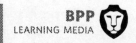

- This is part of the national screening programme to look for *the presence of markers indicative of cervical pre-malignant disease, also known as cervical intra-epithelial neoplasia (CIN).*

- The sample of cells sent for analysis will be examined to look for *their degree of abnormality or dyskaryosis.*

- Dyskaryosis can be classified as mild (in which case the smear *should be repeated), or moderate or severe (in which case colposcopy is recommended).*

- Women are generally invited for screening from the age of 25; *up to the age of 50, three-yearly screening is indicated, between the ages of 50 to 65, women are screened at 5-yearly intervals.*

- If a woman is regarded as high risk, annual screening should be *performed.*

Table 3.3: Papanicolaou smear examination

Key points

- The Pap smear is part of the national screening programme to look for the presence of markers indicative of cervical pre-malignant disease.

- Have some understanding of the interpretation of a patient's results.

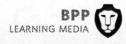

Clinical procedure 31:

Level * *

Performing a dressing change

Mr Mohan is a 66-year-old male who has undergone a hip replacement three days ago. His surgical wound dressing appears to have soaked through; as the attending FY1 doctor in the orthopaedic firm you have been asked to change the dressing.

QUESTION A:

How would you proceed?

RESPONSE A:

- INTRODUCTION: To begin with I would introduce myself. Check I am speaking to the right patient by eliciting his name, date of birth and hospital number. At this stage I would try to establish a rapport and make him feel at ease.

- EXPLANATION: I would explain the reasons for changing the dressing: 'Mr Mohan I understand from the nursing staff that your wound dressing appears to be soaked through. I would like to review the wound and put another, clean and sterile dressing in its place.'

- CONSENT: I would obtain the patient's verbal consent for me to proceed and ask if he has any questions or concerns.

- ANALGESIA: Ask the patient if he is in any pain; if so, it may be appropriate to give him some analgesia before the dressing change is performed.

- INFECTION: Identify if the patient has any infection risks such as clostridium difficile or MRSA, accordingly take relevant precautions.

QUESTION B:

How would you position and prepare the patient?

RESPONSE B:

- POSITION: The patient should be lying comfortably in the supine position.

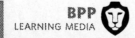

- I would have the curtains drawn around his bed space to ensure privacy and expose the hip wound.

- I would then create a sterile field; on a procedure trolley I would open a sterile dressing pack. On this there should be a small gallipot from which I can pour some sterile saline, or a chlorhexidine solution.

- In the dressing pack there should also be some cotton gauze, a pair of sterile gloves along with a waste disposal bag. This bag I would open and attach to the side of my procedure trolley.

QUESTION C:

Can you describe the procedure to me?

RESPONSE C:

- I would remove the patient's old dressing, and discard this into the waste disposal bag.

- Then I would review the wound, looking to assess:

    – presence of wound sutures or surgical clips
    – presence of erythema
    – inflammation and swelling
    – discharge
    – if the wound has a pungent smell
    – wound healing, if there is any dehiscence
    – scar formation

- If the wound is open or there are features suggestive of ulcer formation, then I would also look to assess:

    – the size of the defect in relation to the wound size
    – the shape and edge (smoothness and regularity) of any ulcer
    – base (is there any evidence of necrosis, granulation tissue formation?)
    – margins between the wound site and surrounding tissues, eg does it appear clean and healthy, or aggressive and inflamed?

- Before applying a new clean dressing over the wound site, I would wash my hands, place the new dressing on the sterile field (or ask my assistant to do so), then put on the pair of sterile gloves.

- If there is any evidence of wound discharge, then it would be appropriate to obtain a wound swab at this stage.

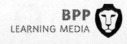

- Then I would clean the wound with saline (or chlorhexidine) soaked cotton gauze. It is important to clean the wound from the centre and move towards the outside. I would clean in a circular fashion from the middle of the wound, in this way avoid re-applying the same swab on to a previously cleaned site.

- Now I can apply the new dressing over the wound site, if necessary keeping it in position with some overlying mepore tape.

QUESTION D:

How would you complete the procedure?

RESPONSE D:

- Well, I would tell the patient the procedure is over, asking him if he has any questions.

- I would dispose of any waste appropriately, disinfect the procedure trolley with an alcohol steret.

- Wash my hands.

- Then I would document the procedure on the patient's notes.

- If any wound swab was taken, I would label this appropriately and fill in the microbiology request form, asking for a gram stain, culture and sensitivity.

Key points

- The examiner will be looking out to see whether you can adequately describe the wound and perform a dressing change with a sterile field and good technique.

- Remember to consider wound infection in this setting. A wound swab should be taken if there is any suggestion of discharge from the wound site.

Clinical procedure 32:

Level *

Removing skin clips and sutures

Mr Lennon is a 64-year-old male who has come to the general surgical ward 10 days after having an exploratory laparotomy for the removal of an abdominal mass. As the FY1 doctor on the ward you have been asked to remove the abdominal surgical skin clips.

QUESTION A:

How would you proceed?

RESPONSE A:

- INTRODUCTION: To begin with I would introduce myself. Check I am speaking to the right patient by eliciting his name and date of birth. At this stage I would try to establish a rapport and make him feel at ease.

- EXPLANATION: I would explain the reasons for removing the clips 'Mr Lennon, I understand that you have had recent surgery on your abdomen. The wound site should have healed well enough now for me to remove the skin clips (staples).'

- CONSENT: I would obtain the patient's verbal consent for me to proceed and ask if he has any questions.

- ANALGESIA: I would ask the patient if he is in any pain; if so, it may be appropriate to give him some analgesia before the clips are removed.

QUESTION B:

How would you position and prepare the patient?

RESPONSE B:

- POSITION: The patient should be lying comfortably in the supine position.

- I would have the curtains drawn around his bed space to ensure privacy and expose the abdominal wound.

- I would then create a sterile field: on a procedure trolley I would open a sterile dressing pack. On this there should be a small gallipot from which I can pour some sterile saline, or chlorhexidine solution.

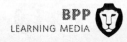

- In the dressing pack there should also be some cotton gauze, a gallipot, a pair of sterile gloves and sterile drapes, along with a waste disposal bag. This bag I would attach to the side of my procedure trolley. I would also open a staple remover and put this on the sterile field.

- On removing and discarding the wound dressing, I would inspect the wound, making sure there are no features to suggest infection such as erythema (redness), discharge (including presence of pus), warmth and tenderness (on gentle palpation).

- Also, I can see whether surgical clips or insoluble sutures have been used on the skin.

QUESTION C:

Can you describe the procedure to me?

RESPONSE C:

- I would wash my hands, place the new dressing on the sterile field (or ask my assistant to do so), then put on the pair of sterile gloves.

- Look to see if there is any evidence of wound discharge; if so, it would be appropriate to obtain a wound swab at this stage.

- Then I would clean (prep) the wound with saline (or chlorhexidine) soaked cotton gauze. It is important to clean the wound from the centre and move towards the outside. I would clean in a circular fashion from the middle of the wound, and in this way avoid re-applying the same swab onto a previously cleaned site.

- On prepping the wound, I would use the sterile drapes in the dressing pack to create a sterile field around the abdominal wound

- Now I would remove each skin clip (staple) in turn by placing the staple remover's jaws carefully between the patient's skin and the clip to reduce any patient discomfort. Then, by squeezing the two handles of the staple remover, this should loosen the staple allowing easy removal. A pair of toothed forceps can be used to pick the staple up and be discarded into the gallipot. Work my way from one end of the wound to the other.

- If the patient has insoluble sutures instead of skin clips, first I would see if interrupted stitches have been used or whether a continuous stitch is in situ.

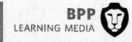

- If interrupted sutures are in place, then with a pair of toothed forceps I would pick up each knot and cut only one end of the stitch adjacent to the skin. I should then be able to remove the stitch with my forceps.

- Where a continuous suture is in place, I would cut the suture at one end, then by gently pulling the stitch at the other end, the stitch should release and come out freely.

- Once all the stitches have been removed, apply butterfly adhesive strips or steristrips to approximate and support the wound edges. Over this I would reapply a clean, new mepore dressing.

QUESTION D:

How would you complete the procedure?

RESPONSE D:

- Well, I would tell the patient the procedure is over, asking him if he has any questions.

- I would dispose of any waste including sharps appropriately, and disinfect the procedure trolley with an alcohol steret.

- Wash my hands.

- Then I would document the procedure in the patient's notes.

- If any wound swab was taken, I would label this appropriately and fill in the microbiology request form, asking for a gram stain, culture and sensitivity.

Key points

- When practising removing skin clips or sutures, try to avoid applying too much tension on releasing and removing the material. This should help limit any pain to your patient.

- Continue to look for signs of infection when you first review a wound; and also as the skin clips or sutures are removed.

Clinical procedure 33:   Level *

Insertion of a tracheostomy tube

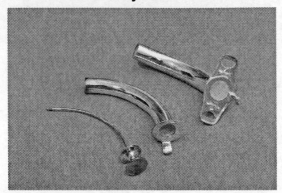

Figure 3.7: Instrument identification B

QUESTION A:

Can you identify what this is, and what are the indications for its use?

RESPONSE A:

This is a tracheostomy tube, it is used in a variety of settings:

*   Emergencies: To secure the airway in cases of maxillofacial trauma, laryngeal oedema (eg secondary to anaphylaxis or burns), or when there is obstruction of the airway secondary to a foreign body.

*   Elective: In head and neck surgery

*   To facilitate ventilation: This can be to reduce the physical work of breathing and dead space, eg due to chronic obstructive pulmonary disease (COPD) and to enable an effective respiratory lavage. Tracheostomies are also used to facilitate ventilation in patients with debilitating neurological disorders (eg motor neurone disease) that can lead to paralysis of the respiratory muscles.

QUESTION B:

Can you describe how you would perform the procedure of tracheostomy insertion?

RESPONSE B:

- I would start by INTRODUCING myself to the patient, EXPLAINING what I would like to do, including the risks and benefits involved, and seeking his written CONSENT. If the patient is unconscious or for some other reason unable to give consent, it would be appropriate to speak to, and obtain consent from, his next of kin, if they are available.

- I would perform the procedure in sterile conditions in an operating theatre, with the patient under a general anaesthetic and with endotracheal intubation in situ.

- The patient should be positioned lying supine on his back with his neck hyperextended. To help achieve this position I would place a sandbag between the shoulder blades.

- I would prepare for the procedure by scrubbing up and putting on a gown and gloves.

- I would prepare the skin of the neck with betadine solution and then apply sterile drapes to produce a sterile field around this incision site.

- Apply local anaesthetic over the incision site using 15ml of 2% lignocaine and adrenaline (1:100,000) solution.

- Now make a transverse skin incision at the midpoint between the cricoid cartilage and sternal notch.

- Below the skin, the incision is deepened to divide the platysma muscle. Once the strap muscles are seen, place a self-retaining retractor to gently move these, and expose the trachea and thyroid isthmus.

- Divide the thyroid isthmus.

- Now make a transverse incision over the trachea from the second to the fourth tracheal cartilage, to allow the insertion of the tracheostomy tube.

- Speak to the anaesthetist, asking if they can withdraw the endotracheal tube; now I can insert the tracheostomy tube. Inflate the cuff and suture the tissues around the tube and apply ties around the tube to keep it secured in position.

- The tube can be changed in 24 hours.

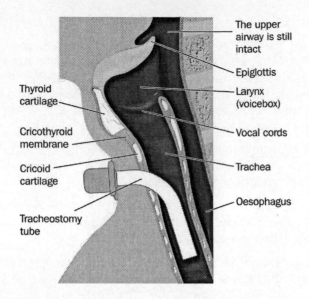

The upper airway is still intact

Epiglottis

Larynx (voicebox)

Vocal cords

Trachea

Oesophagus

Thyroid cartilage

Cricothyroid membrane

Cricoid cartilage

Tracheostomy tube

Figure 3.8: Tracheostomy tube placement

QUESTION C:

What complications can occur with this procedure?

RESPONSE C:

Complications can be divided into intra-operative complications, early post-procedural and late post-procedural complications.

- Intra-operative complications:

    - Neuro-vascular injury: excessive bleeding can occur
    - Oesophageal injury including perforation
    - Subcutaneous emphysema

- Early post-procedural complications:

    - Displacement of the tube
    - Blockage
    - Aspiration
    - Infection (organisms most commonly involved include E.coli, Pseudomonas species and Staphylococcus aureus)

- Late post-procedural complications:

    - Tracheal stenosis
    - Tracheo-innominate artery fistula

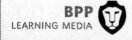

Key points

- Tracheostomy tubes are inserted in emergencies to help secure an airway, along with elective head and neck surgery, and also to facilitate ventilation, to help reduce the physical work of breathing.

- The skin incision required to perform the procedure should be transverse and extend at the midpoint between the cricoid cartilage and sternal notch.

- Complications associated with the procedure can be divided into intra-operative complications and early and late post-procedural complications.

Clinical procedure 34:   Level * * *

Methods of oxygen delivery

Mrs Hussein is a 58-year-old female who has had a hip replacement. She is on your ward and appears to have developed reduced oxygen saturations; a chest X-ray identifies atelectasis. As the foundation trainee working on the ward, the patient's nurse has called you to assess her oxygen requirements.

QUESTION A:

Can you describe how you would go about doing this?

RESPONSE A:

- I would start by INTRODUCING myself to the patient, and checking her identity by eliciting her name, date of birth and hospital number.

- I would then EXPLAIN the requirement to give her supplemental oxygen and obtain her verbal CONSENT to proceed. 'Hello Mrs Hussein, my name is Dr Thomas. I am the surgical doctor working on the ward today. I have been informed that your oxygen saturations are a little on the low side; this is not uncommon after an operation. It's something that we can help you with by giving some supplemental oxygen for a brief period, is that OK?

- I would then POSITION the patient so that she is sitting upright in bed and make sure she is comfortable.

- The first part of the procedure involves assessing her oxygen requirements. To do this, I would need an up-to-date oxygen saturation result, arterial blood gas (ABG) result, as well as a chest X-ray.

- Then I can decide on a suitable amount of oxygen to be given and prescribe this on the drug chart.

- I would need to select an appropriate oxygen delivery device. This could be, for example, a face mask, reservoir bag or nasal cannulae. This should also be clearly documented on the drug chart.

- I can then connect the oxygen delivery device to the oxygen tubing, the other end of the tubing to be connected to an oxygen cylinder.

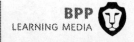

- According to the patient's saturation, I would alter the oxygen flow rate, apply the delivery device (eg face mask/nasal cannulae) to the patient and check with her that she is comfortable.

QUESTION B:

Please describe, or even draw a table detailing, the methods of oxygen delivery device you are aware of, along with the percentage of oxygen each can provide – as well as difficulties that can be encountered with each.

RESPONSE B:

Method of oxygen delivery (device used)	Percentage oxygen delivered (FiO$_2$)	Flow rate	Difficulties with delivery device
Reservoir bag – attached to face mask	95%	15 litres per minute	–
Venturi mask (providing a fixed-volume delivery)	24%, 28%, 35%, 40%, 60%	Flow variable according to mask	Maximum oxygen delivery 60% FiO2
Hudson face mask	40%	15 litres per minute	Face mask performance is variable
Nasal cannulae	30-40%	4-6 litres per minute	Oxygen delivery is variable according to a number of factors, including the patient's respiratory rate, tidal volume, whether respiration through nose or orally

Table 3.4 Methods of supplementary oxygen delivery

QUESTION C:

If the patient has Type II respiratory failure, eg secondary to chronic obstructive pulmonary disease, how would this influence how you deliver oxygen?

RESPONSE C:

In Type II respiratory failure, in an emergency setting I would give the patient maximal oxygen therapy. If, however, it is a chronic problem with no acute deterioration in oxygen levels, the oxygen delivered should be titrated up as tolerated, as hypercapnia (high pCO_2) develops. Hypercapnia should be assessed by measuring ABGs.

QUESTION D:

What would you tell the patient and nursing staff on finishing the procedure?

RESPONSE D:

I would inform the patient and nursing staff:

- Regular monitoring of the oxygen saturations should be performed, with an oxygen saturation monitor to be placed on a fingertip.

- ABG measurements will need to be performed each time the oxygen flow rate and/or method of delivery is changed. Normally we would wait around 20 to 25 minutes after modifying the oxygen therapy to check the ABG, to obtain a more accurate result (to allow a steady arterial oxygen level to be achieved).

- The supplemental oxygen will only be given for a temporary period; once the saturations are acceptable at a given oxygen concentration, the supplemental oxygen will slowly be weaned off to eventually stop.

- Specifically request the nursing staff to monitor the oxygen saturations at regular hourly intervals (this frequency of monitoring can be increased, depending on the clinical need).

- I would also document the procedure, detailing the management plan in the patient's notes.

Key points

- The method and percentage of oxygen delivery should be determined by how acute the indication is and what oxygen delivery device a patient can tolerate.

- In patients with Type II respiratory failure, in an acute emergency setting, maximal oxygen therapy should be given. If, however, the patient has a chronic respiratory disorder with no acute deterioration in oxygen levels, the oxygen delivered should be titrated up as tolerated, as hypercapnia develops.

Clinical procedure 35:   Level * *

Use of airway adjuncts

In patients with a reduced conscious level (reduced GCS), the ability to protect the airway will be also be affected. The tongue can fall backwards causing obstruction of the pharynx. Manual airway manoeuvres including a chin lift and jaw thrust can be used to combat this. Subsequently the airway can be temporarily maintained using simple airway adjuncts.

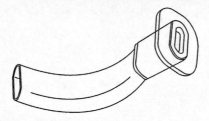

Figure 3.9: Instrument identification C

QUESTION A:

Please identify this and describe how you would use it.

RESPONSE A:

This is an oropharyngeal tube, also known as a Guedel airway.

- I would prepare for the procedure by washing my hands and putting on an apron and gloves.

- To identify the correct size of Guedel airway, I would assess this by placing it against the patient's face with one end at the tragus of the ear, the other at the angle of the mouth. A good fit would extend between these structures, not beyond or short.

- Open the patient's mouth, using a chin lift; insert the Guedel airway into the mouth in a reverse position.

- As the airway is gently moved towards the back of the mouth, I would rotate the airway into its correct position. However, if the patient is an infant, the airway should be advanced into the mouth in the correct position (not reverse as with an adult).

- The correct position for the airway is for it to lie between the teeth.

- Once in situ, the patient can be ventilated with a bag and mask device.

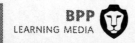

QUESTION B:

In what circumstance would you not use a Guedel airway?

RESPONSE B:

This should not be used in a conscious patient in whom the gag reflex is intact. This is because there is a risk of vomiting and aspiration.

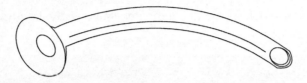

Figure 3.10: Instrument identification D

QUESTION C:

Can you identify what this is, and can you describe in what circumstances it is used – and when it should be avoided?

RESPONSE C:

This is a nasopharyngeal tube.

*   It is used in patients who have an intact gag reflex.

*   It is contraindicated when there is suspicion of a fracture of the base of the skull. This may be suspected if the patient has blood or CSF coming out of his nose or ears. It should also not be used if the patient has obstruction of the nasal pathways, eg secondary to blood or polyps.

QUESTION D:

Can you describe how you would insert the nasopharyngeal airway?

RESPONSE D:

*   I would prepare for the procedure by washing my hands and putting on an apron and gloves.

*   To identify the correct size of nasopharyngeal airway, I would find an airway which has a lumen diameter the same as the diameter of the patient's finger.

*   Now I would lubricate the tip of the airway with some KY jelly.

- Insert the tip into the nostril and gently advance downwards towards the nasopharynx. Continue to advance the airway until the flange sits on the patient's nostril. I note that the flange has a safety pin which prevents the airway from being advanced too far into the nostril.

- Whilst inserting the airway, if there is any resistance felt, then I would stop, take the tube out and attempt to insert it in the other nostril.

- Once in situ, the patient can be ventilated with a bag and mask device.

Key points

- Airway adjuncts including an oropharyngeal (Guedel) airway and nasopharyngeal airway can be used when there is a likelihood that a patient is unable to protect his or her own airway. A Guedel tube should only be used in unconscious patients; it should not be used if the gag reflex is intact, due to a risk of vomiting and aspiration.

- A nasopharyngeal tube is used in patients who have an intact gag reflex. It is contraindicated when there is suspicion of a fracture of the base of the skull or if there is obstruction to the nasal pathways, ie secondary to blood or polyps.

Further reading

Useful papers for clinical procedural skills:

(2008), *Policy for the insertion of a naso-gastric tube in adults*, Birmingham East and North NHS primary care trust.

Caruana, MF, Bradbury, AW and Adam, DJ. The validity, reliability, reproducibility and extended utility of ankle to brachial pressure index in current vascular surgical practice. *European Journal of Endovascular Surgery* 2005; 29(5):443–451.

Davies, CWH, Gleeson, FV and Davies, RJO. BTS guidelines for the management of pleural infection. *Thorax* 2003; 58:ii18-ii28.

Ginès, P and Arroyo, V. Paracentesis in the Management of Cirrhotic Ascites. *Journal of Hepatology* 1993; 17 Suppl 2:S14–8.

Hampton, JR (2008) *The ECG Made Easy*. 7th edition. Oxford: Churchill Livingstone.

Harris, C et al. Urinary catheterisation and catheter care. *Best Practice Statement* 2004; June.

Holt, T and Kumar, S (2010) *ABC of Diabetes*. 6th edition. Oxford: Wiley Blackwell.

Hutton, P and Clutton-Brock, T. The benefits and pitfalls of pulse oximetry. *BMJ* 1993; 307:457.

Kikuchi-Numagami, K et al. Irritancy of scrubbing up for surgery with or without a brush. *Acta Dermato-Venereologica* 1999; May; 79(3):230–2.

Liew, SC and Hill, DA. Complication of hard cervical collars in multi-trauma patients. *Australia and New Zealand Journal of Surgery* 1994; 64(2): 139–140.

O'Driscoll, BR et al. Nebulisers for chronic obstructive pulmonary disease, Thorax 1997.

Seupal, R. How do I perform a lumbar puncture and analyze the results to diagnose bacterial meningitis. *Annals of Emergency Medicine* 2007; 50(1):85–87.

Shore, A and Sandoe, J. Blood cultures. *Student BMJ* 2008; 16: 294–336.

Taylor, CJ et al. Changes in practice and organisation surrounding blood transfusion in NHS trusts in England 1995–2005. *BMJ Quality & Safety* Aug 2008; 17(4):236–237.

Whitehouse, JS and Weigelt, JA. Diagnostic peritoneal lavage: a review of indications, technique, and interpretation. *Scandinavian Journal of Trauma, Resuscitation and Emergency Medicine* 8 Mar 2009; 17:13.

Zuber, TJ. Knee joint aspiration and injection. *American Family Physician* 15 Oct 2002; 66(8): 1497–1501.

Chapter 4

Data interpretation

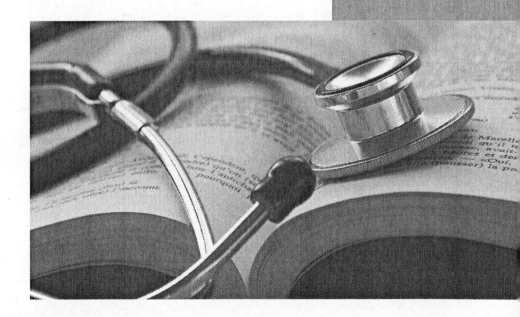

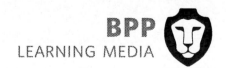

Data interpretation 1:   Level: * *

Interpretation of an abdominal X-ray

This plain abdominal X-ray has been taken of a 48-year-old male with a four-day history of what he describes as colicky abdominal pain along with several episodes of vomiting.

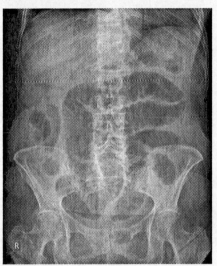

Figure 4.1: Plain abdominal X-ray

QUESTIONS:

A) What position was this X-ray taken in?

B) How would you describe the salient features of this X-ray?

C) With the history stated and radiological features identified, what would be your diagnosis?

D) Describe your management for this patient.

RESPONSES:

A) This is a plane film radiograph of the abdomen, taken in the supine position.

B) There is dilatation of the stomach, ileum and jejunal loops. It is clear that this is the small and not large intestine as the folds of the mucous membrane run transversely for about two-thirds of the circumference of the gut; these are called valvulae conniventes and indicate small bowel involvement.

C)   Small bowel intestinal obstruction.

D)   The management should comprise:

- Commence patient on intravenous (IV) fluids. Patients are likely to be dehydrated and will require aggressive fluid resuscitation.

- Insert a urinary catheter to monitor urine output. Boluses of fluid should be administered until a satisfactory urine output is produced (0.5-1ml per kg per hour). Note that if the patient is elderly with a history of cardiac disease, then fluid resuscitation should be performed with central venous pressure monitoring, to help avoid the risk of fluid overload.

- Insert a nasogastric tube to aspirate the increased intraluminal fluid secretion.

- Take blood tests to assess the serum urea and electrolyte concentration, this should help to direct the IV fluid replacement therapy.

- Commence the patient on regular intramuscular and/or intravenous analgesia along with anti-emetics.

Key points

- The cardinal features of small bowel obstruction are: abdominal pain (often described as colicky in nature), constipation, vomiting and abdominal distension.

- The most common physical findings of small bowel obstruction are associated with dehydration (namely dry skin turgor), dry tongue, a low grade fever and slight tachycardia.

- In adults, postoperative adhesions are the most common cause of small bowel obstruction (up to two-thirds of all cases). The next most common cause is an incarcerated hernia (up to a fifth of all cases) and neoplasms. Less common causes are gallstone ileus, diverticulitis and inflammatory bowel disease.

- Radiologically, the differentiation between large and small bowel can be identified by the presence of haustra (in large bowel), and valvulae conniventes. The haustral markings of obstructed large bowel are rounded and usually much further apart than the valvulae conniventes of the jejunum (along with remaining small bowel), and do not cross its full diameter. The large bowel is located more peripherally in the intestine, the small bowel being central.

Data interpretation 2:   Level: * *

Interpretation of a chest X-ray

As the FY2 trainee working in a surgical firm, you have been asked to review a chest X-ray of a 63-year-old male awaiting elective surgery.

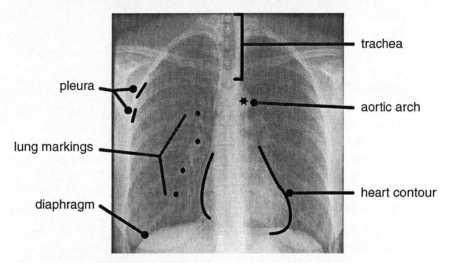

Figure 4.2: Erect chest X-ray

QUESTION A:

How would you approach interpreting a chest X-ray in general?

RESPONSE A:

*   I would start by looking at the film to verify the patient's name, date of birth, hospital number, along with the date the X-ray has been taken. I would then check out the technical components of the radiograph (X-ray).

*   Position of the side marker (left or right): check this against features such as the apex of the heart and stomach air bubble. A misplaced marker is more common than dextrocardia (a congenital defect where the heart is situated on the right side of the chest).

*   Posture: For normal films the posture is erect, supine usually being for patients who are confined to bed. This should be stated on the label on the radiograph. A way of detecting this is also to

look at the position of the gastric air bubble: in an erect film this is clearly in the fundus with a clear fluid level; if supine, it is in the antrum. The significance of this is that in a supine film blood will flow more to the apices of the lungs than when the patient is erect. Failure to detect this can lead to a misdiagnosis of pulmonary congestion.

- Rotation: this should be minimal. This can be assessed by comparing the medial ends of the clavicles to the margins of the vertebral body at the same level between them. The medial ends should be equidistant from the spinous process of that vertebra.

- Penetration: A good way of detecting this is to look at the position of the lower aspect of the cardiac shadow; at this level the vertebral bodies should just be visible.

- Inspiration: A chest X-ray (CXR) should be taken in full inspiration (an exception being when looking for a small pneumothorax, which is best seen on full expiration). Some people, however, may have difficulty in holding a full inspiration. A CXR in full inspiration should have the diaphragm at the level of the 6th rib anteriorly; the liver pushes it up a little higher on the right than on the left side.

- Orientation: Posteroanterior (PA), Anteroposterior (AP) or, less commonly, lateral. Most are PA projections, AP being usually for patients confined to bed. If in doubt, look at the relationship of the scapulae to the lung margins. A PA view will show the scapulae clear of the lungs, whereas in AP they will overlap. The heart also looks bigger on an AP view.

I would carry out a systematic search for pathology:

- Trachea: The trachea should be central. Where this is shifted, it may represent some pathology causing the trachea to lie deviated.

- Mediastinum: Look at the mediastinal contours, first the left then the right side, the aortic arch is the first structure on the left, followed by the left pulmonary artery. The branches of the pulmonary artery branch out through the lung.

- Heart: Observe the cardiothoracic ratio (CTR): The width of the heart should be no more than half the width of the chest. Approximately a third of the heart should lie to the right of the centre and two-thirds to the left. Also note that the heart looks larger on an AP film; for this reason you cannot comment on the presence or absence of cardiomegaly (an enlarged heart) on an AP radiograph.

- Borders: Look at the heart borders. The left border consists of the left atrium which lies above the left ventricle. The right border comprises only the right atrium; above this is the border of the superior vena cava. As the right ventricle is anterior, it does not have a border on a PA CXR film. It may be visible on a lateral view.

- Lung hilum: The pulmonary arteries, veins, lymph nodes along with the main bronchi originate from the left and right hila. The left hilum should be slightly higher than the right (by approximately 1cm). Enlarged lymph nodes (eg bilateral hilar lymphadenopathy seen in sarcoidosis or lymphoma) or lung tumours may give the hilum a bulky appearance.

- Lung fields: Compare left with right sides; they should be of equal translucency. Identify the position of the horizontal fissure in the right lung.

  Observe to see that the surface of the hemidiaphragms curve downwards, and that the costophrenic and cardiophrenic angles are not blunted. Presence of blunting implies an effusion. An extensive effusion or lung collapse would result in an upward curve of the hemidiaphragm.

  Look for free air under the hemidiaphragms; this can occur in bowel perforation, but is also seen after a laparotomy or laparoscopy.

- Diaphragm: The right hemidiaphragm is normally higher than the left (by 3cm), due to the presence of the liver below the right diaphragm. Look for a flat or raised diaphragm. A flattened diaphragm may indicate emphysema. A raised diaphragm may indicate an area of airspace consolidation as occurs in pneumonia.

- Soft tissues and bones:

  In females look to see if both breast shadows are present.

  Is there any evidence of a fractured rib? If so, take a closer look to see if there is a pneumothorax.

  Look at the scapulae and vertebrae: is there any evidence of damage to these structures?

QUESTION B:

When would you perform a lateral film?

RESPONSE B:

As an X-ray is a two-dimensional shadow, a lateral film helps to identify a lesion in three dimensions. The usual indication is to confirm a lesion seen on a PA film. However, it is useful to note that in a lot of hospitals where a PA film is suspicious of any lesion, it is common to proceed to performing a CT scan of the chest.

Key points

- When asked to interpret any image, including a CXR, it is good practice to begin by verifying that you are looking at the right image, ie check the patient's name, date of birth, hospital number, along with the date the X-ray has been taken.

- Have your own system for interpreting a CXR. A useful way to proceed is to talk about the technical components of the film, namely position, posture, rotation, penetration, inspiration and orientation, as indicated above.

- When looking for pathology, remember to comment on the trachea, mediastinum, the cardiothoracic ratio, the heart borders, the lung hilum, the lung fields, diaphragm along with soft tissues and bone.

Data interpretation 3:   Level: *

Conducting a primary survey following a road traffic collision (RTC)

Two patients have been admitted to A&E resuscitation in your hospital after having been involved in a road traffic accident. You are the FY2 doctor working in the A&E department.

By ticking the appropriate statements as true or false, indicate how you would conduct a primary survey of their injuries.

OPTIONS	True	False
a) Identify if they are able to mobilise		
b) Assess their breathing and ventilation		
c) Immediately categorise the patients to minor, intermediate or major injuries		
d) Identify each patient's mechanism of injuries		
e) Assess each patient's neurological status		
f) Undress each patient completely		
g) Take a concise history of each patient's recollections of the events leading to their A&E admission		
h) Provide each patient with warm blankets and warmed intravenous fluids to help protect them from hypothermia		

RESPONSE:

True Answers: b, e, f, h

False Answers: a, c, d, g

- Note that in the presence of severely injured trauma patients immediate measures should comprise a rapid primary evaluation and immediate resuscitation of vital functions. Once these are stabilised a more detailed secondary assessment is required before definitive care is instituted.

- The initial part of the assessment of patients presenting with trauma is called the primary survey. At this time, life-threatening injuries are identified and, simultaneously, resuscitation commences. A simple mnemonic, ABCDE, is used as a method of memorising the order in which problems should be addressed.

  - **A:** Airway and cervical spine control

  - **B:** Breathing and ventilation

  - **C:** Circulation with haemorrhage control

  - **D:** Disability with neurologic evaluation

  - **E:** Exposure and environmental control – this requires completely undressing the patient, but also protecting against hypothermia

Key point

Note the ABCDE approach for carrying out a rapid primary survey.

Data interpretation 4:   Level: * * *

Gastrointestinal abnormalities

The following six patients have all attended the gastroenterology OPD clinic. Match the patient histories with the most likely full blood count result and diagnosis.

Patient history	Full blood count	Diagnosis
1) A 75-year-old female with a known background of hypothyroidism and a history of collapse	A) Hb 11.0, MCV 69, WBC 11.7, Plt 660	a) Pernicious anaemia
2) A 60-year-old male with an eight-month history of weight loss and constipation	B) Hb 9.4, MCV 103, WBC 4.9, Plt 350	b) Alcoholic liver disease
3) A 30-year-old male with an 18-month history of treated episodic bloody diarrhoea and passage of mucus P.R	C) Hb 7.7, MCV 105, WBC 4.1, Plt 66	c) Inflammatory bowel disease
4) A 34-year-old male with a background of chronic liver disease and a raised cell transketolase	D) Hb 3.8, MCV 123, WBC 2.3, Plt 31	d) Colonic carcinoma
5) A 25-year-old female with a 12-month history of weight loss, lethargy and steatorrhoea	E) Hb 9.8, MCV 68, WBC 10.5, Plt 300	e) Peptic ulcer disease
6) A 29-year-old male with a recent history of epigastric pain and malaena	F) Hb 9.0, MCV 86, WBC 6.6, Plt 220	f) Coeliac disease

Your responses:

1) ____   ____
2) ____   ____
3) ____   ____
4) ____   ____
5) ____   ____
6) ____   ____

RESPONSES:

1) D   a
2) E   d
3) F   c
4) C   b
5) B   f
6) A   e

1)   D a

Pernicious anaemia is associated with several autoimmune disorders, particularly hypothyroidism. The macrocytosis can be secondary to the hypothyroidism or the vitamin B_{12} deficiency of pernicious anaemia. Severe vitamin B_{12} deficiency, as in this example, causes bone marrow suppression resulting in a pancytopenia. This can occur over a long period of time and can result in a suppressed haemoglobin, which may be surprisingly well tolerated. Management should include thyroid replacement therapy, vitamin B_{12} injections and upper GI endoscopy as these patients are at increased risk of gastric carcinoma.

2)   E d

All causes of lower and upper GI bleeding can present with a microcytic anaemia. However, acute bleeding is often associated with a thrombocytosis. A change in bowel habit in a patient over the age of 40 requires further investigation, in this case with a colonoscopy.

3)   F c

Inflammatory bowel disease commonly results in a normochromic, normocytic anaemia. If there is associated GI blood loss, it may cause a microcytic anaemia and, less commonly, a terminal ileal Crohn's disease may lead to vitamin B_{12} deficiency.

4)   C b

Patients with alcohol-related liver disease may present with a pancytopenia, as in this example, due to the direct toxic effects of alcohol on bone marrow. Macrocytosis may be secondary to the liver disease or direct effect of the alcohol.

5)   B f

Coeliac disease causes malabsorption within the jejunum, resulting in a folate deficiency, hypoalbuminemia, hypomagnesaemia and a hypocalcaemia. Any individual in this age group with a macrocytic anaemia should be screened for the presence of coeliac disease. This involves a duodenal biopsy, which shows a pattern of subtotal villous atrophy. Anti-endomysial antibodies are the specific immune markers associated with this condition.

6)   A e

This patient has a microcytic anaemia which indicates a chronic bleeding problem; however, this example is associated with a raised platelet count (thrombocytosis) and malaena, both of which are indicators of acute blood loss. The patient should have an urgent GI endoscopy.

Key points

- Note that pernicious anaemia is associated with several autoimmune disorders including hypothyroidism.

- Coeliac disease causes malabsorption within the jejunum resulting in a folate deficiency, hypoalbuminemia, hypomagnesaemia and a hypocalcaemia. Look out for a macrocytic anaemia.

Data interpretation 5:

Level: * *

Hyponatremia

The following five patients have all attended the endocrinology OPD clinic. Match the patient histories with the most likely hyponatremia associated diagnosis.

Patient history	Diagnosis
1) A 30-year-old male, with a background of long-term usage of steroids, presents with postural hypotension and multiple pigmented scars	a) Diuretic usage
2) A 23-year-old male presents with a week-long history of fever, malaise and a dry, non-productive cough	b) Atypical pneumonia with associated SIADH
3) A 67-year-old female presents with a three-week history of constipation, generally feeling lethargic and more recently having a croaky voice	c) Addison's disease
4) A 73-year-old male presents with cardiac failure	d) Psychogenic polydipsia
5) A 39-year-old female is feeling very thirsty (polydipsia) recently; she has been drinking around 6 litres of water daily over the past two weeks. Her blood glucose result is 5.5	e) Primary hypothyroidism

Your responses:

1) ____
2) ____
3) ____
4) ____
5) ____

BPP
LEARNING MEDIA

RESPONSES:

1) c
2) b
3) e
4) a
5) d

1) c

A long-term usage of steroid results in a suppression of endogenous steroid production; this is the commonest cause of Addison's disease. Patients usually present with non-specific symptoms; in the severest cases coma may occur. In a patient presenting with coma and hyponatremia, Addison's must be in the differential diagnosis. Where no cause is identifiable, steroids should be given – such as 100 to 200mg of IV hydrocortisone every 4 to 6 hours. The dose and frequency can be adjusted according to clinical response.

2) b

Atypical pneumonias, including secondary to mycoplasma infection, are a known cause of Syndrome of Inappropriate ADH (SIADH) secretion. Other causes can be divided into cranial (such as head injury), meningitis, encephalitis and tumours. Malignant tumours can arise, for example, from the thymus (thymoma), pancreas and prostate. Lung abnormalities that can cause SIADH include pneumonia, lung cancer, abscesses and tuberculosis. Several drugs have also been implicated; these include carbamazepine, chlorpropamide and some types of chemotherapy drugs.

3) e

When hyponatremia occurs due to hypothyroidism, there is usually an associated macrocytosis. Hyponatremia itself occurs due to increased ADH secretion and a reduction in water elimination. The macrocytosis is secondary to thyroid disease or to an associated pernicious anaemia (lack of absorption of vitamin B_{12}).

4) a

In the older age group, the most common cause of hyponatremia is the use of diuretics. Furosemide and other loop diuretics are also associated with other side effects, such as hypokalaemia, hypomagnesaemia and pre-renal impairment (which can, in turn, cause an increase in urea and creatinine concentrations).

5)   d

Common causes of the combination of polydipsia and polyuria are diabetes mellitus and diabetes insipidus. Psychogenic polydipsia is an uncommon cause of hyponatremia. In this setting there is an associated low serum osmolality and low urine osmolality. To confirm the diagnosis, a water deprivation test is performed.

Key points

- A long-term usage of steroid results in a suppression of endogenous steroid production; this is the commonest cause of Addison's disease.

- When hyponatremia occurs due to hypothyroidism, there is usually an associated macrocytosis.

- In the older age group, the most common cause of hyponatremia is the use of diuretics.

Data interpretation 6:   Level: * *

Disorders of potassium concentration

The following conditions are associated with disorders in potassium concentration. Please group them according to whether they cause a **hypokalaemia** (low potassium level) or **hyperkalaemia** (high potassium level):

1) Addison's disease
2) ACE inhibitors
3) Acute renal failure
4) Ectopic ACTH secretion
5) Cardiac failure with secondary hyperaldosteronism
6) Furosemide infusion
7) Conn's syndrome
8) Cushing's disease
9) Fanconi's syndrome
10) Spironolactone
11) Type I Renal Tubular Acidosis (RTA)
12) Type IV Renal Tubular Acidosis (RTA)

Hypokalaemia (<3.5mmol/l)	Hyperkalaemia (>5.5mmol/l)

RESPONSES:

Hypokalaemia (<3.5mmol/l)	Hyperkalaemia (>5.5mmol/l)
• Cardiac failure with secondary hyperaldosteronism • Conn's syndrome • Cushing's disease • Ectopic ACTH secretion • Fanconi's syndrome • Furosemide infusion • Type I Renal Tubular Acidosis (RTA)	• Addison's disease • ACE inhibitors • Acute renal failure • Spironolactone • Type IV Renal Tubular Acidosis (RTA)

Note:

Both Cushing's disease (pituitary dependent) and Cushing's syndrome (eg ectopic ACTH production) cause a hypokalaemia. Ectopic ACTH secretion most commonly occurs with malignant carcinoma, particularly a small-cell lung carcinoma. With ectopic ACTH secretion, a severe hypokalaemia can result in association with a metabolic alkalosis.

Addison's disease can cause a hyperkalaemia along with a hyponatremia and a metabolic acidosis.

Some groups of diuretics such as loop (eg Furosemide) and thiazide (eg Bendrofluazide) cause a hypokalaemia. Potassium-sparing diuretics, including spironolactone, result in potassium retention. ACE inhibitors, including ramipril, cause a relative hyperkalaemia through their effect on the renin-angiotensin system.

Type I RTA, along with Fanconi's syndrome (associated with a Type II RTA), cause a hypokalaemia. In contrast, a Type IV RTA is associated with a hyperkalaemia.

Primary hyperaldosteronism (Conn's syndrome), along with secondary hyperaldosteronism, cause a hypokalaemia with an associated metabolic alkalosis. Secondary hyperaldosteronism can arise secondary to, for example, cardiac, liver or renal failure. Patients often develop dependent oedematous states in this setting.

Key points

- Loop and thiazide diuretics are a very common cause of hypokalaemia (as well as hyponatremia) in clinical practice, remember to look at a patient's drug chart to identify if they have been prescribed.

- Addison's disease (also known as primary adrenal insufficiency) is associated with a combination of hyperkalaemia and hyponatremia.

- Primary hyperaldosteronism (Conn's syndrome), along with secondary hyperaldosteronism, cause hypokalaemia.

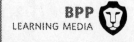

Data interpretation 7:

Level: * * *

Disorders of thyroid function

Using the information below, match the correct diagnosis for each patient:

Normal range:

Thyroid stimulating hormone (TSH)	0.2-4.0miu/L
Total serum triiodothyronine (T₃)	0.9-2.5nmol/L
Free serum thyroxine (T₄)	10-20pmol/L

Patient	TSH (miu/L)	T₃ (nmol/L)	T₄ (pmol/L)	Diagnosis
1	65.0	0.7	0.8	
2	0.06	9.0	54.5	
3	1.0	0.7	8.0	
4	0.07	41.2	13.3	
5	3.1	2.3	18	

Diagnosis:

A) Thyrotoxicosis
B) Primary hypothyroidism
C) Sick euthyroid syndrome
D) Euthyroid
E) T₃ thyrotoxicosis

RESPONSES:

1   B – Primary hypothyroidism

Here the results show a high TSH level, with low levels of T₃ and T₄. This occurs post-thyroidectomy, radioactive iodine therapy and irradiation for thyrotoxicosis. It is also associated with Hashimoto's disease (autoimmune disorder) and iodine deficiency states.

2   A – Thyrotoxicosis

Here we have a suppressed TSH level, with high T₃ and extremely high T₄ levels. This combination is the most common presentation in thyrotoxicosis. Causes include malignant and benign thyroid disease and autoimmune thyrotoxicosis, as well as a multinodular goitre.

3   **C – Sick euthyroid syndrome**

At times of an acute illness, including systemic disease states, it is possible to have an abnormal production of thyroid hormones and transport proteins. This can lead to an abnormal, non-obvious set of biochemical results. Here, with low T_3 and T_4 levels, the data initially suggests a hypothyroidism. However, the TSH is also low (at the lower end of reference range) which suggests a problem with the hypothalamic/pituitary function or the sick euthyroid syndrome. At times of less acute disease states or moderate illness, the thyroxine levels (T_4) may be raised, with a normal or raised TSH level.

4   **E – T_3 thyrotoxicosis**

In this situation the patient presents clinically with the symptoms and signs of thyrotoxicosis. However, the T_4 lies in the normal range, with the T_3 elevated. This is an uncommon cause of thyrotoxicosis.

5   **D – Euthyroid**

The thyroid function tests, TSH, T_3 and T_4 are within the normal range.

Key points

- Primary hypothyroidism can be identified by a high TSH level, with low levels of T_3 and T_4.
- The most common presentation of thyrotoxicosis is associated with a suppressed TSH level, with high T_3 and extremely high T_4 levels.

Data interpretation 8:

Level: * *

Full blood count analysis

A 68-year-old female is next to be seen in your consultant outpatient clinic. As the FY2 doctor in the clinic, you have been asked to explain to her the results of the blood tests she has had. The patient has been referred by her GP after some abnormalities were found in her full blood count (FBC) result performed as part of a routine check-up.

Full blood count analysis (FBC)	
Haemoglobin (Hb)	72g/l
White cell count (WCC)	6 x 109/l
Platelets (Plt)	210 x 109/l
Packed cell volume (PCV)	0.30
Mean cell volume (MCV)	64fl
Mean cell haemoglobin (MCH)	21pg
Mean cell haemoglobin concentration (MCHC)	25g/dl

QUESTION A:

What abnormalities are present in the FBC result?

RESPONSE A:

The patient has an iron deficiency anaemia, as identified by the low haemoglobin (Hb), packed cell volume (PCV), mean cell volume (MCV) – as well as the low mean cell haemoglobin concentration (MCHC).

QUESTION B:

What should you ask the patient to help establish the cause, and what physical examinations would you perform?

RESPONSE B:

I would have to ask her if she has any abdominal pain or any other gastrointestinal symptoms such as a recent change in her bowel habit, appetite and weight. I would also specifically ask her if she has noticed any bleeding on opening her bowels.

I would perform a complete gastrointestinal examination including a rectal examination.

In a woman of this age, the likely cause is gastrointestinal blood loss, which could be a presenting feature of a bowel carcinoma. In a younger female, I would consider excessive menstrual blood loss.

QUESTION C:

What tests can you perform to help confirm your diagnosis?

RESPONSE C:

I would request biochemical tests, namely serum ferritin levels (although note that, as ferritin is an acute phase reactant, in inflammatory disorders this marker is raised) or serum iron and iron binding capacity. It would not be of any benefit to assess for faecal occult blood.

I would arrange for appropriate imaging of the gastrointestinal tract in the form of GI endoscopy and/or barium studies.

Method of interpreting FBC

1) Review patient details:

   Male or female, what is their age? This will assist in the differential diagnosis: for example, in a younger female, blood loss may be secondary to increased menstrual bleeding; in an older patient you need to consider more sinister causes, such as carcinoma of the colon.

2) Check that the basic blood parameters are within the normal range, ie Hb, WCC and platelet count.

3) If any of these parameters are abnormal, identify to what extent it is lower or higher than the reference range; attempt to determine if there are any associations between these. For example, a low Hb, WCC and platelets may indicate an aplastic anaemia.

4) Look the erythrocyte sedimentation rate (ESR). If this is raised, it may indicate an infective or inflammatory disorder.

5) Try to identify patterns in the red cell count indices:

   • Microcytosis (low mean cell volume) or macrocytosis (high mean cell volume)

   • Low mean cell haemoglobin concentration (in iron deficiency anaemia)

   • Raised packed cell volume (as occurs in erythrocytosis)

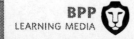

6) Try to identify patterns in the white cell count indices:

- Is the neutrophil count raised (neutrophilia) or reduced (neutropenia)?

- Is the lymphocyte count raised (lymphocytosis) or reduced (lymphopenia)?

Key points

- Note the FBC patterns for some of the more common disorders used in OSCE stations: iron deficiency anaemia, megaloblastic anaemia, aplastic anaemia and leukaemia.

- To aid in your differential diagnosis, you will need to consider the patient's details and match these with their blood results: for example, in a young female with low Hb and a microcytosis, menstrual blood loss should be high as a cause in your differential.

Data interpretation 9:

Level: * *

Urea and electrolytes

The following 74-year-old female patient's biochemistry results are available. You are the foundation trainee looking after her.

Biochemistry	
Sodium (Na)	142mmol/l
Potassium (K)	3.1mmol/l
Urea	18.7mmol/l
Creatinine	198μmol/l
Bicarbonate	26mmol/l
Chloride	99mmol/l

QUESTION A:

What do you think is the most likely cause?

RESPONSE A:

The combination of raised urea and creatinine, along with a low potassium level, is likely to be secondary to overtreatment with a diuretic. Another cause for the low potassium level could be secondary to steroid treatment (eg hydrocortisone or prednisolone).

QUESTION B:

This patient is known to have stable heart failure, as well as rate-controlled atrial fibrillation; the blood tests have been performed because she is complaining of feeling nausea and has vomited on a few occasions. Another complaint she has is of feeling unsteady and a little dizzy on waking up in the mornings. What do you think is the most likely reason for these symptoms?

RESPONSE B:

As stated the patient is likely to be having an overtreatment with a diuretic (if not more than one), this can also be responsible for producing a postural hypotension, causing unsteadiness and dizziness on getting up. The patient is likely also to be on digoxin to control the atrial fibrillation. The deteriorating renal function can result in a reduced excretion of digoxin; this can cause a subsequent toxicity.

QUESTION C:

What physical examination would you perform, and what would you look for? The patient is taking the loop diuretic furosemide 40mg once daily, along with digoxin at a dosage of 125µg (micrograms) once daily. How would you aim to manage this?

RESPONSE C:

As my differential here is overtreatment with diuretics, and digoxin toxicity, I would like to perform a full cardiovascular examination. This would include assessment of the patient's blood pressure (including postural), pulse rate (radial and apex) and capillary refill.

Accordingly, I would like to institute an appropriate fluid replacement regimen; stop the digoxin temporarily; reduce the dose of the diuretic and commence potassium replacement therapy. I would also consider starting the patient on a potassium-sparing diuretic, such as spironolactone, along with an ACE-inhibitor such as ramipril.

Method of interpreting urea and electrolytes

1) Review patient details:

   Male or female, what age (note that renal function deteriorates with age, with loss at a rate of approximately 1ml GFR per year)

2) Check the basic indices, such as sodium, potassium, urea, creatinine, bicarbonate and chloride.

3) If both urea and creatinine are elevated, this would suggest renal impairment. This would require further investigation in the form of creatinine clearance (renal function). Try to determine if there is pre-renal, renal or post-renal failure.

4) If urea alone is raised (but not creatinine to the same level) this would suggest a GI bleed (protein overload), or reduced renal blood flow secondary to volume depletion or excessive diuretic therapy (for heart failure).

5) If urea alone is low (not common), this can be seen in liver failure.

6) High potassium (hyperkalaemia) is most commonly seen in renal failure.

7) Low potassium (hypokalaemia) is most commonly seen with diuretics.

8) High sodium (hypernatremia) is most commonly seen in dehydrated states, ie insufficient fluid intake.

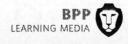

9) Low sodium (hyponatremia) is most commonly seen as a
    side effect of some drugs (eg diuretics such as furosemide,
    ACE inhibitors such as enalapril or anti-convulsants such as
    carbamazepine) or fluid therapy with intravenous dextrose
    solution.

10) Bicarbonate, if raised, would indicate an alkalosis; if low, an
    acidosis.

Key points

- A common cause of abnormalities in urea and electrolytes levels
  is secondary to therapy with certain drugs. Be familiar with the
  more common drugs that cause a high and low sodium and
  potassium level.

- Where volume depletion is suspected, a full cardiovascular
  examination should be performed.

BPP
LEARNING MEDIA

Data interpretation 10:   Level: * *

Interpretation of orthopaedic X-rays

As the FY2 trainee working in an orthopaedic firm, you have been asked to review a hip X-ray of a 59-year-old female.

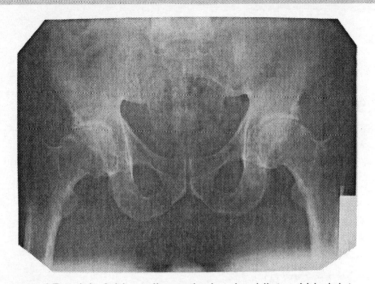

Figure 4.3: AP pelvis & hip radiograph showing bilateral hip joint osteoarthritis

QUESTION A:

How would you approach interpreting an orthopaedic X-ray, in general?

RESPONSE A:

- I would start by looking at the film to verify the patient's name, date of birth, hospital number, along with the date the X-ray was taken.
- I would then consider the technical components of the radiograph (X-ray) and any obvious abnormalities:
    - Orientation of the radiograph (do we have AP and lateral views?)
    - Quality of the radiograph
    - Bone quality, commenting on density (does it look osteoporotic?)
    - Bone abnormalities: fractures, subluxation or dislocations

- I would then make a systematic examination of the X-ray, to look for pathology, whilst looking at both the AP and lateral views:

  - Are there any fracture lines (these would appear as a lucent line)?
  - Cortical abnormalities, trace the outline of the cortex. Is there any bulging or deformity in the integrity of the bone?
  - Joint spaces
  - Cartilage
  - Soft tissue swelling

Be able to succinctly present your findings and give a diagnosis.

QUESTION B:

If you suspect a patient has osteoarthritis, what salient features would you look for on an X-ray to confirm this?

RESPONSE B:

- **S**ubchondral sclerosis at the joint margins
- **C**ysts (bone cysts) close to the joint margins
- **O**steophyte formation
- **L**oss of joint space

Remember the mnemonic: SCOL

Key points

- When asked to interpret any image, including an orthopaedic X-ray, it is good practice to begin by verifying that you are looking at the right image: check the patient's name, date of birth, hospital number, along with the date the X-ray was taken.

- Have your own system for interpreting an orthopaedic X-ray. A useful way to proceed is to talk about the technical components of the film (namely the orientation – ensure there are AP and lateral views available – and quality of the radiograph), then proceed to examining the bone quality and look for bone abnormalities including fractures.

- In osteoarthritis, remember the mnemonic SCOL.

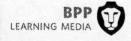

Chapter 5

Prescribing and writing skills

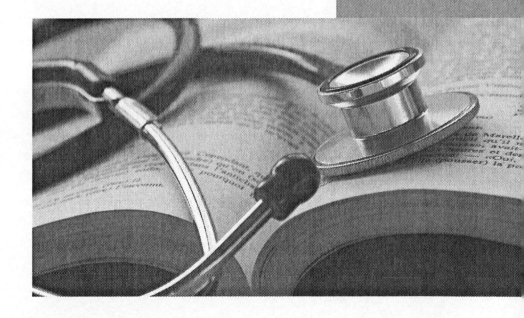

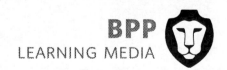

Prescribing and writing skills 1:   Level: * *

Patient with an asthma attack

Mr Cox is a 37-year-old male who has been brought into A&E by ambulance, with an acute exacerbation of shortness of breath. He is known to be an asthmatic and has had five previous hospital admissions, including being admitted to ITU on one occasion. As the A&E doctor on call you see him in resus. You note that he has difficulty speaking; his oxygen saturation is 91% on room air, pulse rate 110 beats per minute and regular, blood pressure is stable at 130/70. On auscultating his chest, you note that he has a generalised expiratory wheeze. He has no known drug allergies.

You have been asked to write the patient's drug chart using the information given below stating the patient's normal repeat prescription. Also prescribe what you feel is appropriate to deal with the acute asthma attack.

Mr Matthew Cox	Amlodipine 5mg od
Hospital number: C45786	Paracetamol 1gm qds
DoB: 04/07/76	Beclomethasone 2 puffs (200µg) bd
	Salmeterol 1 puff (50µg) od

QUESTION:

What components of the drug chart do you need to fill, and how would you do so?

RESPONSE:

- Apply a patient label on the front of the chart which should contain the following information. Alternatively I can manually write the information required:

  1. Name (Forename and surname)
  2. Hospital number
  3. Date of birth

- Allergies: I'd fill this in appropriately, with the name of the drug(s) the patient is allergic to. If there are no known allergies, I would also document this on the front of the chart as NKDA (No Known Drug Allergies).

Then I would prescribe the appropriate medications to deal with the acute medical emergency:

1.   Oxygen: In the regular section, 8 to 15 litres (36-60%) via a partial rebreather oxygen mask, to be given continuously over 24 hours.

2.   Salbutamol 5 to 10mg as a nebuliser, in the stat section.

3.   Hydrocortisone 100mg i.v., also in the stat section.

Then I would prescribe medication to deal with his continuous medical management:

1.   Continuous salbutamol nebulisers, 5mg, five to six times a day.

2.   Prednisolone orally, 50mg to be given daily for 7 days; this should then be slowly weaned off over the next few days.

Also prescribe his regular medications:

3.   Analgesia, regular paracetamol, oral, 1gm four times a day

4.   Salmeterol inhaler, 1 puff (50mcg) once daily

5.   Beclomethasone, 2 puffs (200mcg) twice daily

6.   Amlodipine 5mg, once daily

Then I would prescribe in the 'As Required' section (PRN):

1.   Salbutamol nebuliser 5mg, two to four hourly

2.   Codeine phosphate 30 to 60mg, six hourly

3.   Peak flow meter

KNOWN SENSITIVITY OR INTOLERANCE *Drug/Substance (generic)* *Type of reaction (e.g. Rash)*	WARD	PATIENT ID NUMBER
		NHS NUMBER	AFFIX
	WEIGHT	NAME	PATIENT
		DATE OF ADMISSION	LABEL
Signature, print name and bleep number Date	Date weighed	DATE OF BIRTH

MEDICINES CHART

St. Peter's NHS Trust **NHS**
Surrey, UK

CHART NUMBER _____ OF _____

ADDITIONAL CHARTS IN USE

FLUID ☐   TPN ☐   INSULIN ☐   OTHER ☐

ONCE ONLY DRUGS

DATE	DRUG (approved name)	DOSE	ROUTE	TIME TO BE GIVEN	Prescriber Signature, Print Name and Bleep Number	Administration Time given	Given by	Pharmacy

OXYGEN PRESCRIBING

OXYGEN PRESCRIBING				Date		Date		Date		Date		Date		Date		Date	
Drug Approved Name **OXYGEN**	Initially administered via: Nasal specs / mask (circle)		Time (circle)	Rate	Sign	Rate	Sign	Rate	Sign	Rate	Sign	Rate	Sign	Rate	Sign	Rate	Sign
			08:00														
Date	Target oxygen saturation (circle) (88 - 92%) (94 - 98%) (Other _____%) Indication:_____	Initial flow rate: ———— Duration (circle) PRN / Continuous	12:00														
			18:00														
Signature, Print Name and Bleep Number	Pharmacy		22:00														

for prn prescriptions the code "A" should be used to signify when a patient is receiving air

ORAL ANTICOAGULANT ↓ circle or amend			DATE →											
Approved Name			INR →											
			Dose →											
	Time	1800	Drs signature →											
Signature, Print Name and Bleep Number	Pharmacy		Given →											

Figure 5.1: Front page of a drug chart

Key point

Be aware of the medications along with dosages required to deal with an acute asthma attack. As the doctor dealing with the situation, the nursing staff will expect you to state what to give the patient. If you are in any doubt, check in the British National Formulary (BNF).

Prescribing and writing skills 2:   Level: * *

Patient with a gastrointestinal bleed

Mr Crooks is a 59-year-old male who has been brought into A&E by ambulance, with a background history of abdominal pain, feeling nauseous and haematemesis (vomiting blood). His blood pressure is 100/60, heart rate of 110bpm, with saturations of 96% on room air. On examination he is noted to have a tender epigastrium; p.r. examination has identified black tarry stools (malaena). He has been admitted to a medical ward after being diagnosed with GI bleed. As the foundation doctor on the ward you have been asked to write a drug chart for him. The patient's wife tells you he is allergic to penicillin, stating it has resulted in him having a rash last time he was given it. She also gives you a repeat prescription form that contains a list of his regular medications.

You have been asked to write the patient's drug chart, using the information given below with the patient's normal repeat prescription. Also prescribe what you feel is appropriate to deal with the GI bleed.

Mr Damien Crooks	Diclofenac 75mg bd
Hospital number: E37943	Aspirin 75mg od
DoB: 01/08/54	Amitriptyline 20mg od

QUESTION:

What components of the drug chart do you need to fill and how would you do so?

RESPONSE:

- Apply a patient label on the front of the chart which should contain the following information. Alternatively I can manually write the information required:

  1. Name (Forename and surname)
  2. Hospital number
  3. Date of birth

- Allergies: I would fill this in appropriately with the name of any drug the patient is allergic to and the reaction associated with the allergy (rash in this case).

  Then I would prescribe the appropriate medications to deal with the acute medical emergency:

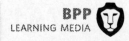

1. An IV proton pump inhibitor (PPI), eg pantoprazole i.v. 40mg, to be given stat (as a once-only prescription ASAP) and then regularly on a daily basis.

2. Prescribe i.v. anti-emetic, eg cyclizine 50mg tds

3. Analgesia: this should be prescribed in more than one form – if the patient is vomiting he cannot take it orally. Paracetamol 1gm qds, i.v./p.o. Codeine phosphate 30 to 60mg i.m./p.o. This gives the option to the nursing staff to administer intravenous or intramuscular analgesia if the patient cannot take it orally.

4. Also obtain a fluid chart and prescribe some colloids to help with fluid replacement as well as the blood pressure, eg i.v. gelofusine 500ml stat, this can then be followed with a bag of normal saline 1000ml over 6 to 8 hours, with or without potassium chloride (KCL) 20mmol (or 40mmol) in the bag, depending on the patient's blood results.

Then I would prescribe medication to deal with his continuous medical management:

*   Continue with his regular amitriptyline prescription, noting that he may not be able to take it temporarily if the nausea and vomiting persists.

*   Stop aspirin. This has an antiplatelet mechanism which can inhibit thrombus formation, and in this way encourage bleeding to occur.

*   Stop diclofenac. This is a non-steroidal anti-inflammatory drug (NSAID) which can also predispose to GI bleeding and peptic ulceration.

Then I would prescribe in the 'As Required' section (PRN): Another anti-emetic, eg Ondansetron 2 to 4mg, i.v. or i.m.

*   More analgesia, eg oramorph 2.5-5mg; this is an oral solution. Alternatively, i.v. morphine can be given instead, morphine sulphate 5 to 10mg every 4 to 6 hours as needed.

Key points

*   Note that the key components to prescribe in a patient with a GI bleed are an i.v. PPI, anti-emetics, analgesia and i.v. fluids.
*   Look carefully at what a patient takes normally, to see if there is anything that could exacerbate their current problem, eg aspirin or NSAIDs in a patient with a GI bleed.

Prescribing and writing skills 3:   Level: * *

Patient with acute heart failure

Mrs Logan is a 68-year-old female who has been brought to A&E by ambulance with acute shortness of breath. She is known to suffer from hypertension. Her husband informs you that over the past few months she has been complaining of feeling generally weak and lethargic; he has also noticed her ankles swelling up. On examination there is a raised JVP, she has widespread crackles on auscultation and bilateral ankle swelling. She is waiting to be admitted to a medical ward. As the foundation trainee in A&E, you have been asked to write her drug chart. You have been given her repeat prescription chart and have been informed that she has no known allergies.

What components of the drug chart do you need to fill and how would you do so?

Mrs Jenny Logan	Atenolol 50mg bd
Hospital number: T37170	Aspirin 75mg od
DoB: 05/08/1945	Ramipril 5mg od
	Paracetamol 1gm qds

RESPONSE:

- Apply a patient label on the front of the chart which should contain the following information. Alternatively I can manually write the information required:

  1. Name (Forename and surname)
  2. Hospital number
  3. Date of birth

- Allergies: Fill this in appropriately, with the name of the drug(s) the patient is allergic to. If there are no known allergies, this should also be documented on the front of the chart as NKDA (No Known Drug Allergies).

Then I would prescribe the appropriate medications to deal with the acute medical emergency:

- Oxygen: In the regular section, 8 to 15 litres (36-60%) via a partial rebreather oxygen mask to be given continuously over 24 hours.

BPP
LEARNING MEDIA

- Furosemide: This is a loop diuretic used in the treatment of congestive heart failure and oedema. This should be prescribed as a stat dosage of 40-80mg i.v. Then prescribe this also in the regular part of the chart at a dosage of 20mg bd p.o.

- Opiate analgesia: Diamorphine, this can be prescribed as a stat dosage of 2.5 to 7.5mg i.v.

- Anti-emetic: Either cyclizine 50mg i.v. stat, or eg ondansetron 2 to 4mg i.v.

- Glyceryl trinitrate (GTN) infusion: this can be given stat at a dosage of 50mg GTN in 50ml of normal saline. Instruct that this should be given to titrate between 2ml to 10ml/hour, with the nursing staff to keep an eye on the patient's blood pressure and aim for the systolic blood pressure to remain greater than 110mmHg.

Then I would prescribe medication to deal with her continuous medical management:

- Continue with regular atenolol (beta blocker) 50mg bd p.o.
- Continue with aspirin 75mg od p.o.
- Continue with ramipril 5mg od p.o.
- Continue with paracetamol 1gm qds p.o.

Then I would prescribe in the 'As Required' section (PRN):

- Another anti-emetic, eg metoclopramide 10mg, i.v. or i.m.

- More analgesia, eg oramorph 2.5-5mg, this is an oral solution. i.v. morphine can be given instead, morphine sulphate 5 to 10mg every 4 to 6 hours as needed.

Key points

- When dealing with a patient with heart failure, note that this also manifests as peripheral oedema secondary to fluid overload. This should be treated with a diuretic: Furosemide at a stat dosage of 40 to 80mg i.v. followed by a regular prescription of 20mg bd p.o can be used as an appropriate regime.

- Other pharmacological agents commonly used in the treatment of heart failure include the use of an ACE inhibitor (ramipril being the example in this case), beta blocker (eg atenolol) and glyceryl trinitrate in the form of an infusion.

- Patients should also be given strong and effective opiate analgesia.

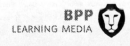

Prescribing and writing skills 4: Level: * *

Patient with a myocardial infarction

Mr Bradley is a 58-year-old male who has been brought to A&E by ambulance with acute shortness of breath and chest pain. His chest pain appears to have improved with the opiate analgesia, and oxygenation improved with high flow oxygen therapy. An ECG shows ST elevation in several leads and his troponin level has also come back raised. As the medical foundation trainee on call, you have been informed by your registrar that he is to be admitted under medical care. You have his repeat prescription chart and have been informed that he has no known allergies. Please complete his inpatient drug chart.

What components of the drug chart do you need to fill in, and how would you do so?

Mr Julian Bradley
Hospital number: C37058
DoB: 02/09/1955

Aspirin 75mg od.
Paracetamol 1gm qds/prn

RESPONSE:

- Apply a patient label on the front of the chart which should contain the following information. Alternatively I can manually write the information required:

    1. Name (Forename and surname)
    2. Hospital number
    3. Date of birth

- Allergies: Fill this in appropriately, with the name of the drug(s) the patient is allergic to. If there are no known allergies, this should also be documented on the front of the chart as NKDA (No Known Drug Allergies).

Then I would prescribe the appropriate medications to deal with the acute medical emergency:

- Oxygen: In the regular section, 8 to 15 litres (36-60%) via a partial rebreather oxygen mask to be given continuously over 24 hours.

- Glyceryl trinitrate (GTN) spray: Give the patient two puffs of GTN spray.

BPP
LEARNING MEDIA

- Thrombolysis: Streptokinase as a single dosage of 1.5 million units in a solution of normal saline (100ml of 0.9%) over one hour.

- Beta blocker: atenolol 5mg i.v. to be given slowly at a rate of 1mg/minute

- Opiate analgesia: diamorphine, this can be prescribed as a stat dosage of 2.5 to 7.5mg i.v.

- Anti-emetic: Either cyclizine 50mg i.v. stat, or eg ondansetron 2 to 4mg i.v.

Then I would prescribe medication to deal with his continuous medical management:

- Regular atenolol 25mg od p.o.
- Regular aspirin 75mg od p.o.
- Regular ramipril 2.5mg bd p.o.
- Regular statin therapy eg simvastatin 20mg od p.o.

Then I would prescribe in the 'As Required' section (PRN):

- Another anti-emetic, eg metoclopramide 10mg, i.v. or i.m.

- More analgesia, eg oramorph 2.5-5mg, this is an oral solution. i.v. morphine can be given instead, morphine sulphate 5 to 10mg every 4 to 6 hours as needed.

- GTN spray, two puffs as required.

Key points

- Slight variations may exist between hospital trusts as to the preferred drugs used following myocardial infarction. While doing attachments on medical wards become familiar with those used in your trust.

- If you are in doubt about interactions between new drugs you are prescribing for a patient with those they are already taking, check the BNF; you can also ask the ward pharmacist for more information.

Prescribing and writing skills 5: Level: * *

Prescribing antibiotics for a lower respiratory tract infection

You are a foundation trainee working in a General Practice. You have seen Mr Kyle, he is a 48-year-old male who has had a sore throat, productive cough and felt feverish for the past five days. On examining him your diagnosis is that he has a lower respiratory tract infection (LRTI). You have been asked to take a concise history, inform him what your impression is, and prescribe appropriate antibiotics.

QUESTION A:

How would you introduce yourself to him and what questions would you ask?

RESPONSE A:

- INTRODUCTION: To begin with I would introduce myself. Check I am speaking to the right patient by eliciting his name and date of birth. At this stage I would try to establish a rapport and make him feel at ease.

- PERSONAL DETAILS: In addition to his name and age, I would identify his occupation and ethnic origin.

- PRESENTING COMPLAINT:

  - Fever: 'How long has the fever being going on for? Have you checked your temperature; if so, how high does the temperature go? Is there any history of night sweats?'

  - Sore throat: 'How long has this been going on for? Does it cause any pain, do you have any problems with shortness of breath or other breathing difficulties?'

  - Cough: 'How long has this been going on for? How frequent is it now? If it is productive, what colour is the sputum?'

  - Associated features: 'Any history of poor appetite, weight loss, do you feel weak and or lethargic? Any history of rashes?'

- PAST MEDICAL HISTORY: Is there any history of respiratory problems such as asthma, COPD or tuberculosis? Have you been admitted to hospital for these or any other medical problems?

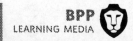

- DRUG HISTORY AND ALLERGIES: Common drug groups which can precipitate a cough include anti-hypertensives such as ACE inhibitors and beta blockers, also some types of analgesia such as NSAIDs.

  I would ask the patient if he has been given any anti-coughing drugs such as chlorpromazine (this belongs to a group of drugs called phenothiazines, which are also used as anti-emetics), or even tried codeine (also used as an analgesic).

QUESTION B:

How would you explain, in simple terms, your diagnosis and method of treatment?

RESPONSE B:

- EXPLANATION AND TREATMENT

  I would say: 'Mr Kyle, having taken a brief history from you and having examined your chest, I believe you have a mild form of pneumonia, or what is also called a lower respiratory tract infection. Due to the nature of your symptoms, you may well have contracted a bacterial infection. The way we tend to deal with this is with a course of antibiotics. Fortunately I don't think you need to be admitted into hospital for an intravenous course, we can start you on oral antibiotics in the first instance. I would like for you to take a full seven days' course and to see you again after that time; if you don't appear to be improving, then we may consider referring you to consider whether you do need admission. Obviously if your symptoms worsen in the interim please arrange an appointment to come in to the practice and see me sooner.'

  I would also give him a sputum pot, and say: 'Next time you cough up any sputum, please collect it in this pot and return it to the practice nurse. This will allow us to target your antibiotic regime in case you don't respond to the antibiotics we give you today.'

- PRESCRIPTION FORM

  I would obtain the correct form, a green FP10 form. I'd fill in the patient's details correctly, including their name, age, date of birth and address.

  I'd fill in the correct antibiotic and dosage: there may be slight variations from one region to the next, but for a community-acquired pneumonia, an example would be to use: Amoxicillin 500mg three times a day (tds). I'd request that the patient should have seven days' supply of this medication.

I'd consider if the patient has any allergies, and if so, alter my prescription accordingly.

I'd write my own name, sign and date it.

Key points

- There will often be several antibiotic options for a particular condition. Once you have established a likely diagnosis, look at your hospital/trust guidelines to prescribe the best option. Note that this may change once microbiological results are available.

- Look out for allergies which can result in you having to modify your preferred course of treatment.

- Only the mildest forms of pneumonia can be treated with oral antibiotics at home. If a patient is clinically unwell, consider referring him or her for hospital admission to have a chest X-ray and IV antibiotics.

BPP
LEARNING MEDIA

Prescribing and writing skills 6:   Level: * *

Prescribing controlled drugs

You are a foundation trainee working in Trauma & Orthopaedics. Mr Watts is a 59-year-old male who is due to be discharged six days after having a total knee replacement. He is still in considerable pain following the procedure, despite taking a combination of paracetamol 1gm four times a day and tramadol 100mg four times a day. Your consultant has asked you to prescribe him a course of morphine tablets 5mg every four hours for 3 weeks to help with the pain.

How would you prescribe morphine sulphate for the patient to be discharged with?

RESPONSE:

- INTRODUCTION: To begin with I would introduce myself. Check I am speaking to the right patient by eliciting his name, date of birth and hospital number.

- PRESCRIPTION:

    - Obtain the correct form, ie the blue FP10 form.
    - I'd use indelible ink, such as a black ballpoint pen.
    - Fill in the patient details, which includes name, age, date of birth, address.
    - I'd prescribe morphine sulphate tablets: 5mg, six times a day for 21 days.

    I would:

    - Indicate the correct dosage of each tablet, ie 5mg.
    - State the form of the medication, ie morphine sulphate 5mg tablets.
    - Write the total quantity in words and figures of the drug supply for that period, ie 630mg (six hundred and thirty milligrams) as total amount. [5 multiplied by 6 (for each day) multiplied by 21 (for the 21-day period)].
    - Write my own name, sign and date the prescription.
    - Write legibly throughout.

Patient details: *d.o.b.* 04/06/1954
Mr John Watts   Age: 59
2 West Close
Bromley,
BR1 6QB

Medication
(ensure number of days and dosage is stated):

      Morphine sulphate five milligram (5mg) tablets

      Take six (6) times a day, for twenty-one (21) days

      Please supply six hundred and thirty milligrams (630mg)
      morphine sulphate in total

Prescriber's signature: _____
      Dr Smith

Date: 21/07/2013

St. AnyWhere's Hospital,
5 DuCane Street,
Bromley,
BR2 2QQ

Figure 5.2: Sample form for a controlled drug prescription

Key points

- The most common controlled drugs you are likely to have to prescribe are opiate analgesia such as morphine.

- Other examples of controlled drugs include diamorphine, fentanyl, methadone and oxycodone.

Prescribing and writing skills 7:   Level: *

Completing an X-ray request form

Throughout your medical career you will be asked to request X-rays for your patients. As a result, you share the responsibilities for medical radiation exposure (as the referring clinician) with the radiologist (practitioner) and the radiographer (operator). Hence, it is of the utmost importance that, when filling out an X-ray request form, sufficient clinical information is given to indicate to the practitioner that it will be justified to proceed. Where practical (if the patient is alert and orientated), a patient's consent, either verbal or written, must also be obtained.

The scientific unit of measurement for radiation dose, commonly referred to as 'effective dose' is the millisievert (mSv). As different organs and tissues in the body have varying sensitivities to radiation exposure, the actual radiation risk to different parts of the body from an X-ray procedure varies.

A chest X-ray will result in an effective radiation dose of 0.05 mSv; an abdominal X-ray, 0.7 mSv; a skull X-ray, 0.02 mSv. When computed tomography (CT) imaging is used, the effective radiation exposure can increase in excess of a factor of 80 times that of a simple chest X-ray. Children have a three to five times larger radiation-induced cancer mortality risk than adults. If practical, imaging techniques that do not expose patients to ionising radiation (eg MRI or ultrasound) should be the preferred choice, particularly in children.

QUESTION A:

What information should you include in an X-ray request form?

RESPONSE A:

Request forms will vary from location to location, but I would ensure that the following issues, at least, were addressed:

- Apply a patient label on the front of the request form which should contain the following information (or alternatively I can manually write the information required)
  - Name (Forename and surname)
  - Hospital number
  - Date of birth
  - Address
- I'd identify the patient's consultant, together with information on the patient's location and ability to get to the X-ray (ie whether he or she was an in or outpatient, and ambulatory or confined to wheelchair or bed, etc)

- I'd note any known allergies and, for female patients, if there was any possibility of pregnancy.

- I'd note the reason for requesting the X-ray, with relevant clinical history and the issue to be addressed.

- Technically, I may need to identify if contrast is required and, if so, the date and detail of the most recent EGFR.

- Finally, the urgency of the request should be identified, together with my own details and signature.

Name (Forename and surname):
Hospital number:
Date of birth:
Address:
Patient's consultant:

| **Location** | Inpatient: | <> | Ward: | <> |
| | Outpatient: | <> | | |

Transport	Bed	<>
	Trolley	<>
	Chair	<>
	Walk	<>

....

Known allergies:

Is contrast required: Y ☐ N ☐
  If contrast required most recent EGFR & date taken
  EGFR: Date taken:

X-ray (state body part):

If female patient: any possibility of pregnancy: Y ☐ N ☐

Reason for request:

Please state the relevant clinical history and the question to be answered:

Urgency of request: Urgent ☐ Routine ☐
Please note if urgent, inform the radiologist on call

Referring clinician:
Name of Doctor: Bleep/contact number:
Grade:
Date of request: Clinician's signature:

Figure 5.3: Request for X-ray

QUESTION B:

What is the significance of checking a patient is pregnant when requesting X-ray imaging?

RESPONSE B:

In pregnancy, ionising radiation should be avoided due to the risk of developing childhood cancers and effect on cognition. If this is unavoidable, then a maximum dose of 1mSv should not be exceeded during the entire pregnancy.

In females of child-bearing age, if clinically feasible where there is a possibility of pregnancy, all X-ray requests of the lower abdomen and pelvis should be restricted to the first 10 days following the onset of the last menstrual period (LMP), due to the lower risk of pregnancy during this period.

Key points

- Be able to give sufficient and concise clinical information to justify requesting any imaging investigation, particularly when a patient is to be exposed to ionising radiation.

- In female patients of child-bearing age, remember to ask if there is a possibility of pregnancy.

Prescribing and writing skills 8:

Completing blood forms

Level: *

> As a junior doctor on the wards, you will be asked to order a variety of blood tests for your patients. Hence, blood forms will need to be completed accurately to ensure the right test is performed.
>
> What information should you include in a blood test request form?

RESPONSE:

- I'd apply a patient label on the front of the request form which should contain the following information, or alternatively, write the information required using a black indelible pen:

  - Name (Forename and surname)
  - Hospital number
  - Date of Birth
  - Address

- I'd identify the patient's consultant, and indicate the location and status of the patient (ie inpatient or outpatient).

- I'd state the indication for performing the test, and then identify the test(s) required.

- I'd need to indicate if this were a routine or urgent investigation and remember to contact the relevant laboratory – particularly important when required out of hours.

- Finally, I'd indicate the date and time the sample was taken, sign the form leaving my contact or bleep number so urgent requests could easily be communicated to me.

- I'd then place each blood bottle and form in the correct collection bag, likely to vary from location to location.

Tests required

Haematology requests: This includes a blood transfusion request which is a separate form; here you can request a group and antibody screen (G&S) and crossmatch – if this is needed, state the number of units required. In virtually every NHS trust, blood for blood transfusion is collected in a separate bottle (often coloured pink) that needs to be labelled with a pen – ie you cannot apply a patient label to the bottle.

As part of haematology, using another form you can request a full blood count (FBC), clotting screen which includes an international normalised ratio (INR), activated partial thromboplastin time (APTT), fibrinogen levels and D-Dimer.

BPP
LEARNING MEDIA

Biochemistry requests: Urea and electrolytes (U&E), liver function tests (LFTs), thyroid function tests (TFTs), glucose, c-reactive protein (CRP), lactate, Troponin T, tumour markers.

Microbiology request: Blood cultures – microscopy, culture and sensitivity (M, C&S)

Name: (Forename and surname)   **Hospital number:**

Date of birth:
Address:

Name of patient's consultant
Location: Inpatient, ward:
                             Outpatient:

....

Clinical details:

Tests required:

Urgency: Urgent ☐   Routine ☐

If urgent please contact the relevant laboratory, especially if required out of hours.

....

Sample date/time:

Referring clinician:

Name of Doctor: Bleep/contact number:

Grade:

Date of request: Clinician's signature:

Figure 5.4: Blood tests request form

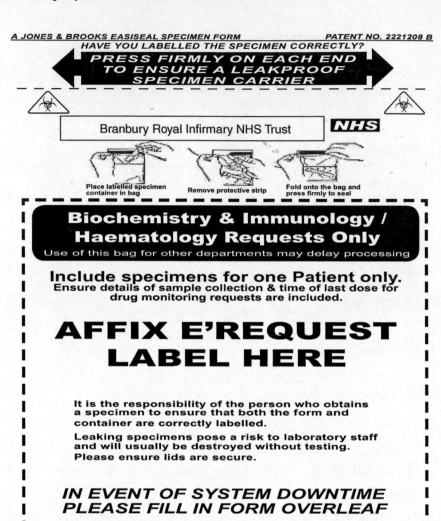

Figure 5.5: Blood bottle collection bag

Key points

- Be able to give sufficient and concise clinical information to justify requesting a blood test.

- Note that when requesting blood for blood transfusion, the sample needs to go in a separate pen-labelled bottle in a blood transfusion request form.

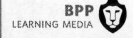

Prescribing and writing skills 9:   Level: *

Writing a discharge summary

As a junior doctor, whichever specialty you are working in, you will often be responsible for writing a discharge summary for patients leaving the ward. This is more often than not the only form of communication between the hospital and the patient's GP, hence it is of the utmost importance for this to be completed promptly and fully, with all the relevant information to ensure continuity of care and written legibly.

Most NHS trusts have their own standard template for a discharge summary; this is often called the TTO (To Take Out) or TTA (To Take Away) form. On this there is a section which also serves to act as a prescription form. Once completed, a copy of the discharge summary stays in the patient's notes, another copy is given to the patient and another copy is sent to the GP.

What information should you include in a patient's discharge summary?

RESPONSE:

- I should apply a patient label on the front of the request form or, alternatively, write the information required using a black indelible pen.

- I should identify the GP, the patient's consultant, the primary specialty/department during admission and the dates of admission and discharge.

- Reasons for admission and the presenting complaint(s) should be identified, and the diagnosis on discharge.

- I'd include a detailed list of:

  - Operations and/or procedures performed
  - Any problems or complications during hospital admission
  - Relevant investigations and results

- I should also include ongoing or aftercare issues, such as outstanding issues and investigations and details of any appointments (for example, stitches to remain in situ for seven days post-op, for removal at general practice; appointments for chest X-ray in 2 weeks, OP appointment at 10:30 a.m. on 7th August)

- I'd identify medication on discharge, indicating for each drug the name, dose, frequency, route of administration and duration.

- I'd confirm whether or not the drug needs to continue to be prescribed by the GP and, if so, for how long.

- Finally, I'd print my name and sign the form with my grade (designation), bleep/contact number and the date.

St.Nowhere's Hospital   NHS Trust

Patient Details	Admission and GP Details	
Surname	Discharging Consultant	
Forename	Discharging Speciality/ Department	
M / F/	Method of Admission	
Date of Birth	Date of Discharge	
NHS/ Hosp No.	Date of Discharge	
Address	GP Details: Name	
	GP Address:	
Tel No.		
Diagnosis at Discharge	**Operations and Procedures**	
Reason for Admission and Presenting Complaint(s)		
Clinical Narrative including any complications		
Relevant Investigations and Results		
Discharge Destination		
Information given to patient and/or authorised representative (including eg see GP in 2 weeks)		
Physical Ability & Cognitive Function : **At Discharge**	**On Admission**	
Physical		
Cognitive		
Other		
Advice, recommendations and future plans (including results awaited and outstanding investigations) GP Actions (Date)		
Strategies for potential problems		

Discharge summary   USE BLACK INK ONLY

BPP
LEARNING MEDIA

Actions and Outstanding Investigations			
	Action	Person Responsible	Date
Hospital (eg OP Appt) /Investigations			
Community & Specialist Services (eg nursing, therapy)			
Follow up:			

Medications Stopped/ Changed		Yes/ No		Allergies/ Risks & Warnings		
If yes please give details:						

Discharge Medications	Dose	Frequency	Route	Duration	Quantity Supplied (Pharmacy used)	GP to continue (state length)

Supplying Pharmacy

Pharmacy dispensed by	Checked by	Date

Details of Discharging Doctor

Print Name_____   Doctors Signature _____

Date _____ Grade FY/ ST< 3/ ST> 3/ SpR/ Con _____ Bleep No. _____

Figure 5.6: Sample discharge summary

Key points

- This is often the only form of communication between the hospital and the patient's GP, so it is of the utmost importance for this to be completed promptly and fully.

- When completing the list of medications a patient takes on discharge, be sure to include for each drug, its name, dose, frequency, route of administration, duration and whether or not the GP should continue the drug (if so, for how long).

Prescribing and writing skills 10: Level: *

Writing a transfer letter

Mr Shergill is a 34-year-old male who has been treated in your hospital under your consultant's care. He is now due to be transferred from your ward to the referring hospital. You have been asked by your consultant to write a transfer letter for the receiving medical team.

QUESTION A:

What essential details do you need to include in your letter?

RESPONSE A:

- Patient details: I would include the full name of the patient, date of birth, gender, home address, NHS number if known, hospital number used in my trust can also be included, but note that this is not always very helpful as it will vary from one trust to the next.

- Who the patient is going to: I would state the name of the accepting consultant, along with their specialty. Also I would give the name and specialty of the consultant the patient has been under the care of in my unit.

- When the decision for transfer was made. Also, the date when transfer was accepted and by whom (often this is done by a telephone conversation – it is useful to make a note of the individual who has accepted the patient on the consultant's behalf.) Also state the date of admission to the referring hospital.

- Why is the patient being transferred to the referring hospital. Is it, as in this case, for repatriation? Other reasons could include for specific medical or surgical management in a tertiary centre. Is it a one-way transfer or is the intention to bring the patient back to your hospital? Is it an elective or emergency transfer?

QUESTION B:

What other information would you include in the main stem of your letter?

RESPONSE B:

- I would give a brief summary of the patient's presentation, the presenting complaint, the investigations performed and management initiated in my unit, both surgical and medical.

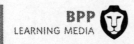

- Medication history, including allergies.

- State any complications or setbacks in management that have occurred whilst under my consultant's care.

- Identify and outline any outstanding issues, medical, surgical or social that need to be addressed when the patient is transferred back to the referring centre.

QUESTION C:

How would you conclude your letter; is there any other information that should go with the patient?

RESPONSE C:

- I would sign the letter, state my name and position. Also include contact details such as my bleep number.

- Ensure that a copy of all the patient's notes and drug charts are included, as well as results of investigations such as blood results, imaging results and, where possible, hard or soft copies should be sent – eg a CD, containing all the X-rays and CT scans.

Key points

- You may be given a brief summary of a patient and asked to write a transfer letter for them. Write legibly.

- Remember that the information you provide may be the only summary of the time they have spent in your hospital: be precise and succinct.

- Divide your letter into:
  - An introduction, containing information on the patient's personal details,
  - A main stem summarising their stay, including investigations and management strategies employed, both medical and surgical.
  - Contact details – your name and contact details.

- Include copies of the patient's notes, as well as drug charts and results of investigations (give copies of imaging if appropriate).

Prescribing and writing skills 11:   Level: *

Referring a patient

You are a FY2 doctor in a General Surgical firm; your consultant has asked you to refer an inpatient for review by another specialty to help optimise his medical care whilst he still remains in your hospital.

QUESTION A:

What methods are you aware of for referring a patient from one specialty to another?

RESPONSE A:

There are two practical ways to refer a patient to another specialist to seek an opinion: either by writing a referral letter to the relevant consultant (or a member of their team), or by contacting the person (or member of their team) directly, usually by a telephone conversation. If this method is used, it should still be done in conjunction with a referral letter.

QUESTION B:

What salient information should you aim to include in your referral letter?

RESPONSE B:

- Patient details: This should include the full name of the patient, date of birth, gender, home address and hospital number.

- The name of the consultant the patient is currently under the care of, their specialty along with the name of the consultant to whom the referral request has been made along with their specialty.

- The location of the patient, namely if he is an inpatient (and which ward) or outpatient.

- Reason for the referral request, stating the question or questions that you would like answers to.

- A brief summary of the patient's current presentation.

- Relevant features of the patient's past medical history.

- What medication the patient is taking, and any allergies.

- Salient features of the patient's examination.

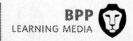

- What investigations have been performed to date, and what the results of these are.

- Are there any outstanding issues that need addressing, eg completion of an antibiotic course for a respiratory tract infection?

- How urgent is the referral? If it is, indeed, urgent for a particular consultant to see the patient, it would be prudent to ensure his registrar or another member of his team are also aware.

- Sign the referral letter, stating name and position. Also include contact details such as bleep number.

CONSULTATION REQUEST FORM

Dr./Ms. .... Date ....
would be grateful for

Dr./Ms. .... Date ....
to see/take over

> Mr./Mrs./Miss ....
>
> Forename(s) ....
>
> Hospital No. ....
>
> **IMPORTANT: COMPLETE NAME AND
> NUMBER, OR USE A BANDA LABEL**

Hospital.. Ward ....

Diagnosis

Signed ....

Figure 5.7: Request for consultation form

Key points

- Note there are essentially two methods of referring a patient: either by a referral letter to the consultant, or by direct contact such as a telephone conversation (with the consultant or a member of their team).

- You may be given a brief summary of a patient and asked to write a referral letter for them. Write legibly.

Chapter 6

Medical ethics

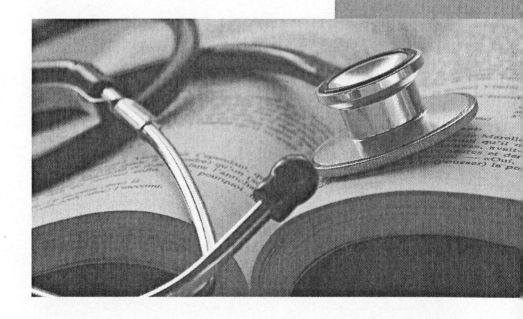

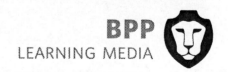

Medical ethics 1:

Level: *

Brainstem death testing

QUESTION A:

What do you understand by the term 'brainstem death'?

RESPONSE A:

Brainstem death can be defined as a clinical syndrome associated with the absence of reflexes along with the appropriate pathways through the brainstem, in a deeply comatose, ventilator dependent patient. The brainstem itself is the part of the brain which connects the spinal cord to the mid-brain, cerebellum and cerebral hemispheres.

QUESTION B:

What criteria are you aware of before a diagnosis of brainstem death can be made?

RESPONSE B:

- There should be no doubt that the patient's condition, deeply comatose and requiring an artificial form of ventilation, is due to irreversible brain damage of a known cause.

- There should be no doubt that the patient's condition is not due to depressant drugs.

- Primary hypothermia (temperature <35°C) should also be excluded.

- Potentially reversible metabolic and endocrine causes should be excluded.

- Potentially reversible causes of apnoea (dependence on the ventilator) such as the use of muscle relaxants or a spinal cord injury should be excluded.

QUESTION C:

That is fine with regards to verifying the relevant exclusion criteria have been met. Can you state the definitive clinical criteria that confirms brainstem death?

RESPONSE C:

- Pupils must be fixed in diameter and should not show a pupillary response to light.

- No corneal reflex.

- Absent vestibulo-ocular reflex: no eye movements following the injection of at least 50ml of ice-cold water into each ear in turn (the caloric reflex test). A normal response is deviation of the eye to the syringed ear.

- No facial response to a supraorbital stimulus.

- No cough or gag reflex.

- Perform the apnoea test: Pre-oxygenate the patient with 100% oxygen for 10 minutes. Check that the $PaCO_2$ value is in the normal, reference range (4.5 to 6.0kPa). Disconnect the ventilator and provide the patient with an adequate oxygen source (6 litres/minute), via the endotracheal tube. For approximately 8 minutes, the patient's chest and abdomen are observed for respiratory movements. If no movements are seen, a new blood gas is drawn. The apnoea test is positive if the $PaCO_2$ is greater than 6.0kPa (6.5kPa in patients with chronic carbon dioxide retention).

- Two doctors of specified status and experience, namely more than five years of clinical experience each (one doctor should be a consultant) are required to diagnose death on these criteria; the tests must be performed on two separate occasions. Neither of the doctors should be part of the hospital's transplant team.

Key points

- You may be asked to state the tests required to diagnose brainstem death.

- Have a good understanding of the caloric reflex test and the apnoea test.

- Note that in practice two doctors (one a consultant) with at least five years of clinical experience will need to diagnose death on these criteria, on two separate occasions.

Medical ethics 2:   Level: * *

Do Not Attempt Resuscitation (DNAR) orders

Mr Lee is an 88-year-old male who has been on your medical ward for the past four weeks with worsening heart failure and COPD. His condition has deteriorated considerably over the past 48 hours, despite maximal medical therapy. At the end of your ward round, your consultant informs you and the rest of the team that it may be appropriate to discuss a DNAR order with the patient and his family.

What salient features do you need to keep in mind when dealing with, and discussing, a DNAR order with a patient and/or family members?

RESPONSE:

- A DNAR order should only be discussed in a situation where the probability of an unsuccessful outcome is high, namely one that is likely to lead to death or leave a patient in a severe vegetative state.

- The decision to issue a DNAR order should come from a consultant.

- Where possible, I would involve the patient's family/next of kin as much as I could in the decision-making process.

- Make sure the family are fully aware that the presence of a DNAR order does not mean that I am withholding active forms of treatment, for example, non-invasive methods of ventilation or the administration of IV fluids or antibiotics if appropriate.

- The nursing staff should be kept up to date with the management plan on a regular basis.

- On a routine and regular basis an assessment of the patient's respiratory and cardiovascular status should be performed and documented in the patient's notes.

- A DNAR order form needs to be completed and signed by the consultant or senior registrar.

- The DNAR order status needs to be reviewed on a regular basis, definitely before the order expires and also if there is noted to be any clinical improvement in the patient's general health.

- Information should be documented clearly in the medical notes on when the order has been put in place, when it has been reviewed and reinstated or if it has been withdrawn. Also clearly state in the notes any discussion with the patient's family and the outcome of this.

DO NOT ATTEMPT CARDIOPULMONARY RESUSCITATION

Adults aged 16 years and over

Name ______________________

Address ______________________

Date of birth ______________________

NHS or hospital number ______________________

Newbury Park Royal NHS

Date of DNACPR order:

/ /

DO NOT PHOTOCOPY

In the event of cardiac or respiratory arrest no attempts at cardiopulmonary resuscitation (CPR) will be made. All other appropriate treatment and care will be provided.

1 **Does the patient have capacity to make and communicate decisions about CPR?** YES/NO
If "YES" go to box 2

If "NO", are you aware of a valid advance decision refusing CPR which is relevant to the current condition?" If "YES" go to box 6 YES/NO

If "NO", has the patient appointed a Welfare Attorney to make decisions on their behalf? If "YES" they must be consulted. YES/NO

All other decisions must be made in the patient's best interests and comply with current law.
Go to box 2

2 **Summary of the main clinical problems and reasons why CPR would be inappropriate, unsuccessful or not in the patient's best interests:**

3 **Summary of communication with patient (or Welfare Attorney). If this decision has not been discussed with the patient or Welfare Attorney state the reason why:**

4 **Summary of communication with patient's relatives or friends:**

5 **Names of members of multidisciplinary team contributing to this decision:**

6 **Consultant/ST3 or above completing this DNACPR order:**

Name ______________ Position ______________

Signature ______________ Date ______________ Time ______________

7 **Review and endorsement by Consultant:**

Signature ______________ Name Date

Review date (if appropriate)

Signature ______________ Name ______________ Date ______________

Signature ______________ Name ______________ Date ______________

Figure 6.1: DNAR form

Key points

- A DNAR order is a consultant decision but should be made in consultation with the patient (if he or she is able to communicate) and the family/next of kin if possible.

- The status of the DNAR order needs to be reviewed on a regular basis, particularly in the light of any clinical improvement.

Medical ethics 3: Level: * *

Confirmation of death

Mr Douglas is a 73-year-old male who has been in the care of the elderly ward for the past three days, battling a severe chest infection. It appears he has lost his fight. You are the medical foundation trainee on call, and have been called by his nurse at 3 a.m. to confirm that he has died.

QUESTION A:

What would you do on arriving at the patient's ward?

RESPONSE A:

- I would speak to the nurse, asking her the time that death occurred and if there were any witnesses.

- I would want to see the patient's hospital notes to identify the patient's diagnosis, past medical history, drug history and if there is any stated resuscitation status.

- From this I would try to ascertain if the death was expected, and who found the patient and at what time.

- Then I would ask the nurse to accompany me to the patient.

QUESTION B:

Using this mannequin, please describe what you would do.

RESPONSE B:

- Well, I would start by drawing the curtain around the patient's bed, to have some privacy and maintain the patient's dignity.

- I would confirm the patient's identity by looking at their wrist band which should have his name and hospital number.

- Observe the patient's general appearance, including a lack of physical movement and general colour. I would also call out close to his ear, 'Can you hear me, Mr Douglas?' As I do so, I can look, listen and feel for any respiratory effort for one minute.

- With a pen torch I would then assess the pupillary response in both eyes, which should show bilateral unreactive and dilated pupils. There should not be a direct or consensual light reflex.

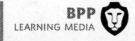

- Using a wisp of cotton wool, I would assess for a corneal reflex on both sides.

- Using an ophthalmoscope, I would examine the fundi for rail roading.

- I would then perform a sternal rub or apply pressure over the supra-orbital region (painful stimulus) and observe if there is a response.

- I would then palpate the major pulses, the carotids and femoral arteries on both sides, for one minute, noting their absence.

- With my stethoscope I would then auscultate over the precordium, listening for heart sounds for one minute, noting their absence.

- I would also listen at the lungs, both the front and back of the chest, for breath sounds for three minutes.

- Once these observations and my clinical examination have been performed confirming there are no signs of life, the patient can be pronounced dead.

- I would then document in the notes the time and place of death. I would include my clinical examination, including presence of unreactive, dilated pupils, no respiratory effort, no palpable pulses, no heart or breath sounds. I would date this, state the time, sign and leave my bleep number.

- I would request the nurse to arrange for the next of kin to be contacted, so that I can make them aware if they did not know already, and for the body to be moved to the mortuary as soon as is practical to do so.

QUESTION C:

Is there anything else that you need to do, or anyone else that needs to be informed that the patient has died?

RESPONSE C:

- Well, I would also check, as part of my external examination, that the patient does not have a pacemaker. I would also offer to write the death certificate.

- I would offer to speak to the patient's family or next of kin, informing them that death has occurred.

- If the cause of death is not clear, I would discuss the case with the coroner, who should be able to tell me whether or not a post mortem will be required.

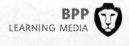

Key points

- Be systematic in your clinical examination when confirming death. In clinical practice, do not assume that, just because a nurse has informed you the patient looks like they have died, that this is the case until your examination is performed.

- Don't forget to say you would speak to the patient's family or next of kin on confirming death. In cases where there is doubt over the cause, state you would discuss the case with the coroner.

Medical ethics 4:

Level: *

Death certification

Mr Rickman is an 89-year-old male who died on your ward last night, following a stroke last week. As the foundation trainee working for his consultant, you have been asked to write his death certificate.

- *You can only complete a death certificate if you are a doctor who has been attending a patient during their most recent illness and have seen them at least two weeks prior to death or soon after their death.*

- *If, for example, you are the doctor who has been asked to verify a patient's death (commonly the case if you are the on-call doctor), but have not been involved in their care during their most recent illness, you are not permitted to fill in the death certificate.*

- *A death certificate is required for undertakers to remove a body from the hospital mortuary.*

- *A death certificate is a legal document which is required by law to register a death by the Registrar for Births, Deaths and Marriages.*

QUESTION:

What salient information do you need to include in the death certificate?

RESPONSE:

- Name of the deceased patient
- Age at death
- Date, time and place at which death occurred
- The date when the patient was last seen alive by me or the attending doctor
- Cause of death: I will need to correctly fill in, and in the correct order the relevant parts, ie:
    - 1a) Disease or condition directly leading to death
    - 1b) Other disease or condition leading to 1a)
    - 1c) Other disease or condition leading to 1b)

2)   Other disease or significant conditions that may have contributed to or accelerated death, but are not related to the disease or condition causing it

If I am in doubt as to the cause of death, I can discuss this with the senior members of my team including the registrar or consultant.

- I will need to tick the relevant box if I feel the death was related to the patient's employment; this may include any industrial disease-related process. In these circumstances, the coroner should also be informed.

- Circle one of the numbers adjacent to the correct statement.

    1)   The certified cause of death takes into account the information obtained from the post mortem.

    2)   The information from the post mortem may be available later.

    3)   A post mortem is not being held.

    4)   I have reported the death to the coroner to gain further information.

- Circle one of the letters adjacent to the correct statement.

    a)   Seen after death by me

    b)   Seen after death by another medical practitioner, but not myself

    c)   Not seen after death by a medical practitioner

- Sign the death certificate, fill in my name and give my qualifications (eg BSc, MBChB, MRCS).

- Fill in the date of issue of the death certificate.

- Provide the name of the consultant in charge of the patient.

- Complete the counterfoil, which summarises the information stated.

- If the cause of death cannot be ascertained, the body may need to be sent for a post mortem. This is authorised by the coroner.

- Inform the coroner if there is doubt about the cause of death or if I suspect foul play, (eg suicide or homicide).

Key points

- You can only complete the death certificate if you attended a patient's care during their most recent illness and have seen them at least two weeks prior to their death or soon after their death.

- If you are unsure about the cause of death, speak to your seniors for advice. You should be prepared to refer a death to the coroner.

Medical ethics 5:   Level: *

Palliative care

Throughout your career you will come across patients who are clinically unwell and are often towards the terminal stages of life. As a doctor, you have a duty of care to allow patients in this setting to die with controlled pain relief, be as symptom-free as possible, and with dignity. Palliative care is the branch of medicine which deals with all aspects of care associated with the dying patient. This not only relates to providing suitable analgesia, but also supporting their physical, emotional, spiritual and social concerns and also supporting the patient's family.

QUESTION:

What components of care do you need to be aware of and attempt to address when dealing with a dying patient?

RESPONSE:

- Provide relief from distressing symptoms such as pain, nausea, vomiting and shortness of breath.

- Pain relief can be provided through a variety of routes, this includes oral, intramuscular, intravenous, topical patches and subcutaneous pumps.

- Anti-emetics should be given for nausea and vomiting.

- As a result of the analgesia patients are taking, constipation can be a feature, hence laxatives should also be prescribed.

- A patient's dignity should always be considered; this may be assisted, for example, by providing a side room if one is available.

- A support system should be offered to help patients live as active a life as they are able.

- At all stages, the patient's family should be updated and involved in their care; a support system should be offered to help the family to cope.

- Do not perform routine investigations such as blood tests unless there is a good clinical reason for performing them.

- Depending on the circumstance, consider medical and/or surgical interventions which may have a role to play, eg surgical long-bone fixation for pathological metastatic fractures, or ERCP and insertion of a stent to aid in relieving jaundice in patients with malignancy of the pancreas or gall bladder.

- Consider starting the patient on the Liverpool Care Pathway, in consultation with their family.

- Consider placement in a hospice, also in consultation with their family.

Key points

- Palliative care deals with all aspects of care associated with the dying patient. This not only relates to providing suitable analgesia, but also their other physical, emotional, spiritual and social concerns.

- This care is not only related to how best to manage patients in this setting, but also how to provide the adequate and necessary support for their families.

Medical ethics 6:   Level: *

Deaths to be reported to the coroner

QUESTION:

What scenarios are you aware of which need to be reported to the coroner?

RESPONSE:

A death may be reported to the coroner if:

- The cause of death is unknown.

- The cause of death was sudden and unexplained.

- The death was violent or unnatural.

- The death occurred secondary to alcohol or drugs.

- The death occurred during an operation or anaesthetic.

- The patient was not visited by a medical practitioner during their final illness.

- Death has occurred and no doctor satisfies the attendance requirements for being able to certify death.

- The medical certificate suggests that the death may have been caused by an industrial disease, poisoning or accident.

- Death is suspected to have occurred by suicide or illicit drug usage.

- Death is suspected to have occurred by an illegal abortion.

- Death is suspected to occur from neglect.

Key point

Be able to state a few scenarios where a death needs to be reported to the coroner.

BPP
LEARNING MEDIA

Medical ethics 7:   Level: *

The suicidal patient refusing treatment

You are the medical registrar on call. Your foundation trainee contacts you from A&E to tell you he has just seen a 38-year-old female who has come in by ambulance following a paracetamol overdose.

You discuss the situation with your trainee and find out that the patient clearly has suicidal intention. However, your trainee finds her also to be fully oriented, coherent and apparently rational. The patient does not appear to be psychotic.

Your trainee asks for your assistance. However, you have an emergency to deal with on the ward where you have to treat a critically ill patient.

QUESTION A:

What information do you need from your trainee?

RESPONSE A:

There are a few things that I would need to know:

- The time the overdose was taken

- The quantity of the overdose (in grams)

- What action has been taken up to now by your trainee as well as the A&E staff. This includes finding out what information has been given to the patient.

- Any clear reasons why the patient has refused treatment

QUESTION B:

What would you say to him to advise on dealing with the situation?

RESPONSE B:

- I would try to explain to my colleague what can be done in this setting. Importantly, if the patient is indeed rational, then we cannot force her to have any treatment.

- Also I would stress to him to tell the patient in a direct, but non-confrontational manner, the effects of taking a paracetamol overdose – namely the possibility of irreversible liver damage which can lead to death.

- I would make sure he is aware of the treatment for paracetamol overdose, either for the patient to take oral N-acetylcysteine or its intravenous form, parvolex.

- Even if the patient does not appear to be psychotic, it would be appropriate to seek a psychiatry review for her on the basis of her suicidal intent.

Key points

- When adult patients are deemed as rational and non-psychotic, they cannot be forced to have treatment against their will.

- The antidote for paracetamol poisoning is the drug N-acetylcysteine, the IV version is called parvolex.

Medical ethics 8: Level: *

Deciding on appropriateness of care with limited resources

You are an ITU consultant who has been contacted by your registrar on call. He is faced with a difficult situation:

Ten minutes ago, an 85-year old man was admitted to A&E by ambulance. He was knocked off his bicycle in a hit-and-run incident. He has sustained a severe head injury and was intubated at the scene of the accident by the paramedic crew.

The ITU department has three beds, all of which are occupied at present:

Bed 1: A 67-year-old woman, post-op, following a hip replacement procedure has been admitted to ITU after developing a severe chest infection. She has been intubated and ventilated for the past three days.

Bed 2: A 33-year-old male with known HIV has been admitted with severe systemic sepsis. He is on high-dose intravenous broad-spectrum antibiotics. He is also requiring high levels of inotropic support to maintain his blood pressure. Over the past 12 hours he appears to have developed worsening renal and cardiac function.

Bed 3: A 59-year-old male originally admitted under the care of the medical team with a myocardial infarction. However, he developed severe, pronounced pulmonary oedema, became hypoxic and had to be intubated, ventilated and transferred to ITU to manage his cardiorespiratory status.

QUESTION:

You only have three ITU beds, what factors do you need to take into account when deciding which of the four patients can stay at your unit and which one should be transferred to an ITU bed at a hospital 40 miles away?

RESPONSE:

There are a few factors which need to be considered:

- In this scenario, the patient with the worst prognosis is the 33-year-old male with HIV and multi-organ failure. It could certainly be deemed appropriate to treat this patient, but the question that needs to be asked is how appropriate is it to treat him at the expense of one of the other patients.

- I think it would be right in this setting to discuss with the medical consultant in charge of the HIV patient's care whether ventilation needs to be continued. If the answer is yes, then this patient would not be suitable to be moved as he is the most critically unwell and perhaps the least likely to survive a transfer.

- The 85-year-old male patient who has just arrived in A&E is also unlikely to survive a long transfer.

- Hence one of the two other patients (Bed 1 or Bed 3), should be transferred to the other hospital.

Key points

- This scenario illustrates an important principle regarding the appropriateness of patient care. Often, increasing patient age is regarded as a poor prognostic factor and, in many situations, it may be the only factor that is considered.

- Do not automatically assume that a younger patient should be given priority for treatment. Pre-existing co-morbidities and the resources available at your disposal need to be evaluated.

Chapter 7

Communication skills

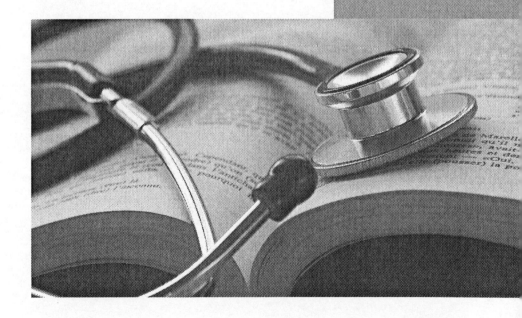

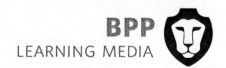

BPP
LEARNING MEDIA

Communication skills 1: Level: *

The multi-disciplinary team (MDT) meeting

Mr Henderson is a 77-year-old male with a new diagnosis of a brain tumour, he has been referred to your consultant from another hospital. You have been asked to discuss his case at the forthcoming neuro-oncology multi-disciplinary team (MDT) meeting.

QUESTION A:

What do you understand by the term 'MDT meeting'?

RESPONSE A:

- This is a meeting which, depending on the specialty concerned, comprises of individuals with different areas of expertise and different grades, the intention being to combine their skillsets in deciding on a management plan for each patient discussed. Members of an MDT will commonly comprise:

    - Consultants in several specialties; in this example, it is likely to include neurosurgeons, oncologists and radiologists

    - Registrars in the same specialties

    - Other senior and junior doctors in the same specialties

    - Physiotherapists

    - Occupational therapists

    - Specialist nurses in the specialty, eg neuro-oncology

    - Ward Sister

    - Administrational staff whose roles include organising the date and time of the meeting, as well as taking the minutes

QUESTION B:

What sort of things are discussed for each patient?

RESPONSE B:

- It is usual to have a management plan for each patient. This would include decisions on further treatment options, such as further surgery, radiotherapy or chemotherapy. Other considerations will include medication changes, as well as the patient's social circumstances (for example, housing circumstances, support from family and friends, and the ability to carry out activities of daily living).

- The MDT meeting allows each specialty team, medical and non-medical, to give their views on how they can best serve each patient's interests, according to their likely prognosis. Collectively a management plan is formulated.

- Each case is discussed in confidence.

Key points

- The MDT meeting is a method of formulating management plans for patients according to the specialty concerned.

- The members of the MDT will usually comprise individuals with different areas of expertise and different grades; this includes both medical and non-medical members of staff.

- It is a formal meeting where the minutes will be logged, usually by administrational staff.

Communication skills 2:   Level: * * *

Discussion with a wife whose husband is to be admitted to your hospital from A&E as a result of a head injury

Mr Banning is a 43-year-old male who has been involved in a road traffic collision (RTC), where he was knocked off his bicycle at a junction by an oncoming vehicle. His Glasgow Coma Score (GCS) is 8 out of 15. He has been intubated and ventilated in the resuscitation room. As the FY2 trainee in A&E you have been asked by your consultant to speak to his wife and inform her of the management plan.

QUESTION A:

What would you do before meeting the patient's wife to prepare yourself?

RESPONSE A:

- To begin with I would familiarise myself with the case; this would involve obtaining and reading the patient's notes, noting his past medical history.

- Review the latest investigations performed in A&E, eg what does the CT head scan show, what are the blood results?

- I would also check his observation charts; these would contain information on his GCS, pupillary response, blood pressure, heart rate, saturations and temperature.

QUESTION B:

What would you say to the patient's wife?

RESPONSE B:

- To begin with I would introduce myself to Mrs Banning and try to establish a rapport.

- I would explain what has happened, namely that as a result of the accident he has become unconscious, and intubated in A&E to maintain his airway.

- Tell her the results of the investigations that have been carried out until now and inform her of any results that are pending.

- Explain that her husband has been referred to another specialty (in this case the neurosurgical team); at this moment in time the intention of this team is to admit to the ITU to manage him conservatively. The neurosurgical team will come to speak to her, the information I have been given is that there is no intention to perform any surgery at present.

- Make sure that she is aware that his condition may deteriorate; if this were the case he may need surgery, and the neurosurgical team would review their management plan accordingly.

QUESTION C:

How would you finish the conversation with Mrs Banning?

RESPONSE C:

- Verify that she has understood what I have told her – ask her to repeat in her own words her understanding of the situation.

- Ask her if she would like to know the hospital and relevant emergency department and ITU telephone number(s).

- Ask if she wants any spiritual support; if so, point her towards the hospital chaplain or priest.

- Inform her that once I have more information, such as test results, I will come back to speak to her.

- Thank her and let her know that she can ask me if there are any specific questions.

Key points

- The intention in this scenario is to remain calm in a difficult environment.

- Remember to inform the patient of the results of any investigations and what investigations are still pending.

- Try to give a realistic opinion on the prognosis.

- There is nothing wrong with stating that the specialty team (neurosurgery in this case) will now be dealing with her husband's care and will be able to give her more details.

- Before leaving the relative give her ample opportunity to ask any questions.

BPP
LEARNING MEDIA

Communication skills 3:   Level: * *

Dealing with an interruption during your consultant ward round

You are a foundation trainee about halfway through a ward round with your consultant. A staff nurse approaches you to insist you need to immediately prescribe some maintenance fluids, normal saline, and rewrite a drug chart for one of her patients. You have informed her that you will do it as soon as you have finished the ward round, but she is very insistent. You are keen not to get involved in a confrontation; talk to her to discuss the problem and try to come to some resolution.

QUESTION A:

What would you do before speaking to the nurse to prepare yourself?

RESPONSE A:

I would want to compose myself, ensuring I am calm; avoid sounding confrontational and making a scene.

QUESTION B:

What would you say to the nurse?

RESPONSE B:

- To begin with, I would apologise.

- Explain that I understand that it is important for the fluids to be prescribed and drug chart to be rewritten. However, I would state that I am with my consultant doing a ward round, that there are a few sick patients that I need to organise further investigations for quite urgently. Once this has been done, I will come straight back and get these jobs done.

QUESTION C:

The nurse tells you that her jobs are equally urgent; she remains persistent you leave the round, what would you do?

RESPONSE C:

- I would try to negotiate with her. I could suggest she ask one of my colleagues to do these jobs (and that I can repay the favour later on).

- Alternatively, if there was no one else available then I would ask her to start the IV fluid infusion for the patient, along with giving the relevant drugs that he would normally take at this time. I would suggest that she signs the chart to say they have been given, and another nurse could also sign to verify this. Once my round is over I would come back and sign the prescription accordingly.

QUESTION D:

The nurse tells you she is not willing to give any fluids or drugs without your signature. What would you do now?

RESPONSE D:

- I would try to compromise and say that I will only rewrite the most urgent drugs that the patient must take at this time, along with a maintenance fluid prescription now. The rest I will be happy to do only after completing my ward round.

- I would do this, thank her, and continue with the consultant round.

Key points

- This scenario is one that you will almost certainly encounter in the first couple of years as a junior doctor. The examiner will be observing your communication skills but also your ability to think on your feet.

- A lot of medicine involves coming to a compromise, particularly when dealing with your peers and other members of the MDT. Have your own strategy for dealing with this type of situation. Remain calm and composed and be clear when you speak.

Communication skills 4:   Level: * *

Dealing with a dispute with a nurse regarding a patient's discharge

You are a foundation trainee working in a medical firm. Mr Ryan is a 78-year-old male who is to be discharged tomorrow. He has been admitted with a chest infection and been treated with a course of antibiotics. He is incontinent of urine, lives alone and has no support at home. The senior nurse on the ward is concerned he is being discharged too early and would like to discuss this with you.

QUESTION A:

What would you do before speaking to the nurse to prepare yourself?

RESPONSE A:

I would want to compose myself, ensuring I am calm; I would avoid sounding confrontational and making a scene. I would review the patient's notes, to make sure I have all the relevant information at hand.

QUESTION B:

The nurse tells you her concerns, namely that she does not think the patient is ready to go home. He is incontinent of urine and has no one at home to help him. She would like him to have an occupational therapy and social service review first. What would you say to the nurse?

RESPONSE B:

- Explain that I understand her concerns. However, the decision to allow the patient to be discharged has been made by the consultant in charge of his care.

- I would advise her to document her concerns in the patient's notes.

- I would speak to more senior members of my team, including the registrar and consultant, informing them of the situation. I would ask whether we can arrange a team meeting comprising the doctors involved in his care – juniors, seniors and consultant. Also the physiotherapists, occupational therapists and senior nurse herself, along with any other nurses who have been involved with Mr Ryan's inpatient care.

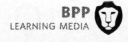

- Once the consultant is aware of the nursing staff's concerns, it will be his decision to either allow the discharge to go ahead or delay it until the patient has been discussed at a MDT meeting.

Key points

- In this scenario you are faced with conflicting decisions between a senior nurse and your consultant. Your role is very much as a mediator. You should relay information between the two, to help them come to some compromise.

- Even though you may only be a junior member of the team, you have a duty of care to your patient. You should not hesitate to speak to your seniors, including your consultant, to help you achieve this.

Communication skills 5:   Level: * *

A gay couple making a complaint about prejudice while on the ward

You are the foundation trainee on a general surgical ward. A male patient and his gay partner have approached a nurse stating they have experienced some prejudice on the ward. You have been asked by the nurse to speak to them.

QUESTION A:

What would you do before speaking to the couple to prepare yourself?

RESPONSE A:

I would review the patient's notes to make sure I have all the relevant information at hand and familiarise myself with his case. I would then ask the nurse to take him and his partner to a quiet room on the ward where I can go to speak to them.

QUESTION B:

What would you say to the couple?

RESPONSE B:

- Initially I would introduce myself to the couple and try to establish a rapport.

- Inform them that I have been told they have raised some concerns, ask them what the problem is.

  The patient informs you that when his partner came to visit with a bunch of flowers, the patient in the bed opposite along with his visiting friends started sniggering at them and started directing homophobic comments towards them.

- Tell the couple that I will speak to the patient concerned, together with his friends when they are next visiting, informing them that this type of behaviour will not be tolerated. I would also tell other members of ward staff to look out for them.

QUESTION C:

The patient and his partner ask you to move him either to another ward or a side room on the same ward. The nurse tells you there are no side rooms available. What do you say to the couple?

RESPONSE C:

- I would tell them that at present there are no side rooms available on this ward. Generally side rooms are reserved for patients with an infective problem such as MRSA or diarrhoea. They are also used for patients who are at the end stage of life, to provide them and their family with some privacy.

- I would also tell them that I will speak to the bed manager, and pass on the couple's concerns; I would request that we move the patient if an appropriate bed becomes available on this or another ward.

QUESTION D:

How would you end your conversation with the couple?

RESPONSE D:

- I would ask them if they have any further questions they would like to ask. Make sure they have understood what I have told them.

- Also make sure they are aware that if this happens again they can ask the nursing staff to contact me directly; if I am available I will speak to the people concerned there and then.

- I would end by making sure I document the conversation in the patient's notes and making sure my seniors (including consultant) are aware of the situation.

Key points

- Try to be diplomatic in this scenario; the patient and his partner should realise that you are fully understanding that this sort of behaviour is unacceptable. Also that you will take reasonable measures to prevent this from happening again.

- The couple's desires to have a side room or be moved to another ward is not inappropriate. You need to be seen to try to do what you can to accommodate this, but make sure that you give a good explanation as to why this may take a while to organise.

BPP
LEARNING MEDIA

Communication skills 6:   Level: * *

A woman requesting a mammogram

You are a foundation trainee seeing patients in your consultant's clinic. Mrs Marple is a 38-year-old female who has come today as a referral from her GP. She tells you that her mother died recently as a result of breast cancer. She is very worried and demands that you arrange a mammogram for her.

QUESTION A:

What would you do before speaking to the patient to prepare yourself?

RESPONSE A:

I would review the patient's notes to familiarise myself with her past medical history.

QUESTION B:

What would you say to the patient?

RESPONSE B:

*   To begin with, I would introduce myself to her and try to establish a rapport.
*   I would speak to her and take a history, directed towards a breast history. This would include asking questions about breast lumps, nipple discharge and family history of breast cancer.

QUESTION C:

The patient tells you that she has had a child around a month ago. As she has been breastfeeding, she feels her breasts are more tender than usual. What would you say to her?

RESPONSE C:

*   I would call a chaperone and perform a breast examination once I have obtained consent.
*   I would inform her that, while someone is breastfeeding, the tissues in the breast may appear dense on a mammogram, hence making it difficult to interpret. For this reason we can offer an ultrasound scan. This is generally not used as a screening tool but rather an investigative method to take a closer look at the breast when there are uncertainties after performing a mammogram as well as a clinical examination.

QUESTION D:

How would you end your conversation with Mrs Marple?

RESPONSE D:

- I would try to reassure her that, because her mother developed breast cancer, it does not mean to say that she will inevitably go on to develop this.

- I would also give her some basic information on breast cancer, by giving out some leaflets that our department has; these outline some of the early symptoms and signs that should be looked out for.

- Finally I would ask her whether she has any further questions. On discharge from the clinic I would arrange for her to be seen again once she stops breastfeeding.

Key points

- This scenario tests your ability to reassure a patient by providing the essential facts relating to the condition at hand and performing a relevant history.

- Breast cancer is an emotional subject for many patients; nearly everyone knows someone who has been affected by this condition. Approach this station with a suitable degree of empathy.

Communication skills 7:   Level: * *

A nurse takes a referral and forgets to let you know

You are the surgical foundation trainee on call. You have been in theatre assisting your consultant with an emergency case, which has now finished. A nurse in theatre who has been answering your pager whilst you have been scrubbed has accidentally forgotten to tell you about a referral. Now you have been informed by the A&E sister that there is a patient who has been waiting six hours for a general surgical review. You go to A&E to see the patient.

QUESTION A:

What would you do before speaking to the patient to prepare yourself?

RESPONSE A:

I would review the patient's notes to familiarise myself with the presenting complaint and the patient's past medical history.

QUESTION B:

What would you say to the patient?

RESPONSE B:

- To begin with I would introduce myself to him. Apologise for the delay in seeing him and let him know I have been in theatre with my consultant dealing with an emergency case. I would try to establish a rapport.

- I would also take a concise history, and perform a relevant clinical examination.

- Then I would arrange for the necessary investigations to be performed.

- I would also inform my registrar (senior) on call about the patient, and request he or she reviews him.

QUESTION C:

You go to see the nurse who took the referral whilst you were in theatre; she appears very apologetic that she didn't tell you about the patient. What would you say to her?

RESPONSE C:

- I would approach her, trying to remain calm.

- I would let her know that she has made a mistake that could have put a patient's life at risk.

- I would ask her to report the mistake to her seniors.

- I would thank her for being honest.

QUESTION D:

Is there any method of reporting the mistake that you could use?

RESPONSE D:

I would fill in a clinical incident form and inform my consultant of the situation as well, letting him or her know about the patient I am waiting for the registrar to review.

Key points

- Be aware that this scenario involves you dealing with two issues: the patient who is waiting in A&E, as well as the nurse who forgot to tell you about the referral.

- Mention that you would remain calm when speaking to the nurse, but be clear and direct when informing her about the seriousness of her mistake.

- Note that a method of reporting errors and near misses in a hospital is by filling in a clinical incident form.

BPP
LEARNING MEDIA

Communication skills 8:   Level: * *

Dealing with a problem colleague

You are a surgical foundation trainee working in a busy acute firm. Your colleague, who is at the same level of training as you and also in the same firm, has been having some difficulty at work; this has resulted in him underperforming. You find him not to be committed to his work; he is frequently late for the morning handover and ward rounds. He has, on a few occasions, also made errors when prescribing drugs on patients' drug charts. On one occasion he prescribed an almost lethal dose of antibiotics.

Previously you have covered for him and corrected his mistakes, but now you have decided to have a word with him directly.

QUESTION A:

What would you do say to him?

RESPONSE A:

I would approach him in a non-confrontational manner and ask him how he is, if he has been having any problems at work or even in his social life.

QUESTION B:

He tells you he is well and has no concerns. What would you say to him now?

RESPONSE B:

- To begin with I would inform him that he has been late for several rounds, which has not gone unnoticed by the registrars and consultants in the firm. The nurses have also noted that some of his prescriptions have errors in the dosing.

- Tell him that I have been having to cover for him, leading to unfair additional work for myself. His mistakes could result in a fatal error by putting patients' lives at risk; it also means that he is putting his career at risk.

- I would also strongly advise that if he is having problems at work or at home he needs to get help. He could speak to one of the registrars, consultants, his own educational supervisor or post-graduate medical officer.

- I would let him know that I am here to support him if he wants to let me know anything in confidence. I do not want him to think I am being disruptive; my priority is to ensure patients are being cared for correctly, as should be his main concern too.

QUESTION C:

Despite all your best efforts, your colleague continues to insist there is nothing wrong. What would you do next?

RESPONSE C:

Well, if I thought nothing I was saying to him appeared to be having any effect, I think I would have to tell one of my consultants about my concerns and seek their advice about how best to deal with the situation.

Key points

- In this scenario, like others where mistakes have or potentially could be made by individuals, it is important to stress that your paramount concern is for patient wellbeing.

- In most hospitals, each trainee will have an educational supervisor (usually a consultant in the firm they are working in) who is responsible for the training of that individual. It is therefore appropriate that concerns should be relayed to this individual in the first instance. If, for whatever reason, this is not suitable, a post-graduate medical officer who is in charge of training for all trainees in a hospital can be informed.

Communication skills 9:   Level: * *

Dealing with a patient who frequently attends for surgical assessment

You are a surgical foundation trainee working in a busy acute firm. Miss Haye is a 35-year-old female who has come to the surgical assessment unit (SAU) direct from A&E. You have been asked by your registrar, who is scrubbed in theatre, to see her.

QUESTION A:

How would you prepare yourself before seeing the patient?

RESPONSE A:

I would try to find out as much as I could about her by reviewing her notes as well as her past medical history.

QUESTION B:

There are no notes for her from A&E, as she has been seen by the surgeons in the past and has been sent directly to the SAU for assessment there by yourself. When you see her she gives a non-specific history of occasional abdominal pain. You perform a history and examination which both appear unremarkable. What would you do next?

RESPONSE B:

- I would ask her if this is a new problem or if it has happened previously. If so, I would ask if she has been to see her GP.

On further questioning you identify that she has not been to see her GP about this or indeed any other complaint for the past five years, but that she has been to A&E on several occasions about the same problem.

- I would then inform her that if there is a problem similar to this again, in the first instance she should visit her GP. If the GP has any concern, I am sure that he or she would organise a general surgical review.

- I would also try to explain my reasoning for this, namely that by coming to A&E, she will probably have to wait a while to see a doctor in the first instance. But she will also inevitably be taking up the time of a doctor who could be dealing with an emergency scenario.

QUESTION C:

Is there anything else you would like to do or say to her before you discharge her?

RESPONSE C:

- Well, while she is in SAU I may request some routine tests – for example, bloods to check her full blood count, Us & Es and CRP result. For reassurance I may also request an abdominal X-ray to make sure there is no bowel obstruction.

- I would also document my conversation, including history, examination and results of investigations in her notes.

Key points

- In this scenario you are trying to reassure a patient that she has no acute surgical problem – but at the same time you are required to be firm, to explain to her that it is not appropriate for her to be utilising the valuable time of staff involved in the emergency care of sick patients.

- If you come across this type of scenario it is important not to be flippant and think this patient clearly has no acute problem as she is a frequent attender – it is still necessary to perform a history, examination and appropriate investigations.

Communication skills 10:   Level: * * *

Dealing with a Jehovah's Witness and blood transfusion

You are a surgical foundation trainee working in a vascular surgery firm. Mrs Carey is a 64-year-old female Jehovah's Witness, who is due to have semi-urgent surgery for repair of a large abdominal aortic aneurysm. Her pre-operative haemoglobin level is 9.4. She is due for her surgery tomorrow and you would like to organise a cross-match of four units of blood for her, as this is a procedure that can result in catastrophic blood loss. Discuss this with her.

QUESTION A:

How would you prepare yourself before seeing the patient?

RESPONSE A:

I would try to find out as much as I could about her by reviewing her notes as well as her past medical history.

QUESTION B:

What specific issues do you need to bear in mind with Jehovah's Witness patients?

RESPONSE B:

- Jehovah's Witness patients do not allow the transfusion of red blood cells or any other blood products from another individual into themselves.

- They will allow the transfusion of their own blood during surgery. This is referred to as an **autologous transfusion**, this involves collection and re-infusion of a patient's own blood.

- The infusion of fluids and drugs are allowed.

- Most Jehovah's Witness patients have a living will in place, along with a Do Not Attempt Resuscitation (DNAR) order.

QUESTION C:

What would you say to her to get your points across?

RESPONSE C:

- To begin with I would introduce myself to her and try to establish a rapport.

- I would explain to her that her haemoglobin level is already a little on the low side, which means that there is already a reduced oxygen-carrying capacity of the blood. The procedure she is about to have can be associated with a significant amount of blood loss.

- If the scenario arose where her haemoglobin levels drop further either intra-operatively (or if this was found out post-op) then the only way to correct this situation would be with a blood transfusion containing whole red blood cells. It is also possible that she may require the addition of clotting factors such as Fresh Frozen Plasma (FFP) and platelets.

- I would make it clear to her that without a transfusion (if it is required) she may end up dying. In this regard I would also have to discuss her DNAR status with her.

- I would also inform the anaesthetist, along with my consultant, of the situation. The anaesthetist will have to make a judgement call, with my consultant, if the procedure should go ahead.

- If the patient continues to refuse to give consent for a blood transfusion, I would inform my seniors accordingly and document my conversation with her clearly in her notes.

QUESTION D:

Is there anyone else you would like to discuss this situation with? What right do you have to overturn her decision?

RESPONSE D:

- I would ask the patient if she has any family or friends she may want to discuss this with, or if she would like me to speak to anyone.

- As Mrs Carey is above 16 years of age and clearly medically competent to make her own informed decision, I would have to respect her wishes.

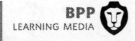

Key points

- This is a difficult scenario, particularly for a junior trainee. Do not hesitate to say that you would need to discuss the patient's wishes with your seniors.

- Jehovah's Witness patients do not allow the transfusion of red blood cells or any other blood products from another individual into themselves, but do allow the transfusion of their own blood during surgery.

- Ensure you emphasise the possibility that without a transfusion the patient may die; also discuss their DNAR status pre-operatively.

Communication skills 11: Level: * *

How to break bad news

Throughout your medical career you will be asked to break bad news to patients. Depending on the type of condition they have, you will have to modify and adjust what you say. However, you should have a strategy to deal with these scenarios, a useful technique and good mnemonic to remember is SPIKES.

What do you understand by the term SPIKES?

RESPONSE:

This is a six-step method or approach that can be used as an aid to breaking bad news:

- SET the scene: Ensure my consultation with the patient is in a quiet area where we will not be disturbed, eg the Sister's office on the ward. Give myself sufficient time for the consultation. Have a member of the nursing staff present with me.

- PERCEPTION: Try to gauge the patient's understanding and perception of their condition, and make a note of any discrepancies between their perceptions and the medical facts.

- INVITATION: Invite the patient to tell me exactly what they wish to know and how much information I should be giving during the consultation, such as 'Are you the kind of person who would like to know everything about your condition in full detail?'

- KNOWLEDGE: Without using medical jargon, give as much detail about the patient's condition as I think they would like to know. Give this information in small pieces. At regular intervals, check their understanding by asking the patient or family to repeat what I have said.

- EMPATHISE: Try to show empathy. Remember that being angry and tearful are normal responses when receiving bad news. Provide the patient with hope – but be realistic. 'I'm sorry to have to give you this bad news, I can assure you we will do everything we can to support you and your family at this time. We will do our best to ensure that you receive the best treatment we have available.'

- STRATEGY: Have at hand a management strategy; explain the options available. At each step, the patient's participation in the decision-making process needs to be encouraged. Summarise the salient points. Invite the patient to ask questions and do my best to answer them as well as I am able. Arrange a time for my next consultation with the patient, giving details of whom to contact in the interim if any urgent questions or clinical deterioration is noted.

Key point

There is no right or wrong way to break bad news; the SPIKES method is a useful way to get your thoughts in order before seeing and giving bad news to a patient. Your thought processes will need to be modified according to the scenario you are faced with.

Communication skills 12:   Level: * *

Breaking bad news: Informing a patient she has breast cancer

You are a surgical foundation trainee working in a general surgery firm. Mrs Potter is a 49-year-old female who has come to the ward following a procedure last week to remove a lump from her breast. The histology results are back, identifying that she has a breast carcinoma with axillary lymph node spread. You have been asked to inform her of the results and the intended management plan.

QUESTION A:

How would you prepare yourself before seeing the patient?

RESPONSE A:

- I would try to find out as much as I could about her by reviewing her notes, as well as her past medical history.

- In order to chase the management plan, I would obtain the outcome from the recent MDT meeting.

QUESTION B:

How would you approach your conversation with her, what would you say to her?

RESPONSE B:

- In the first instance I would ask a senior nurse to find a quiet room where I can speak to the patient and any family who are with her; I would also ask the nurse to sit in on the consultation.

- I would then introduce myself to Mrs Potter and try to establish a rapport.

- I would find out from her what she already knows about her condition and try to identify her understanding of the situation.

- I would tell Mrs Potter that, unfortunately, I have some bad news; the results of the histology are back and they show that the lump is cancerous.

- At this stage I would ask her if she would like someone else to be with her during the consultation (if no one is present already).

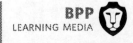

- Then I would tell her that the result shows that cancer has spread to the axillary lymph nodes; it is therefore malignant, but it does not look like it has spread elsewhere.

- I think it would be prudent to give her some time to take in what I have just told her.

QUESTION C:

The patient is understandably very upset and starts to cry. What would you do?

RESPONSE C:

- I would give her some tissues, and tell her that I will be back in a few minutes to talk to her about the diagnosis and management plan. If she has no family or friends with her, then I would ask the nurse to stay with her.

- When I get back, I have to tell her that she will need a mastectomy (removal of the breast) and, following this, a course of chemotherapy.

- I think that it is important that I check that she has been able to take in and understand everything I have told her up until now.

QUESTION D:

Are there any other issues you need to make her aware of?

RESPONSE D:

- Well, we will also be speaking to our oncologists, who are already aware of her (from the MDT meeting) regarding providing chemotherapy; I would briefly outline the side effects associated with chemotherapy. These can include an increased risk of infection, fatigue, blood count disorders that can result in a tendency to bleed. Other associated problems include nausea, vomiting, diarrhoea or constipation and also the possibility of hair loss.

- I could also mention prosthetics to help maintain body shape following the mastectomy.

- Breast reconstruction, including implants, could be discussed if she wants to talk about that at this stage.

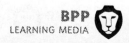

- Before the consultation is over I would give Mrs Potter some literature in the form of leaflets that the department has on breast cancer management; I would also introduce her to our Macmillan nurses.

- I would offer the services of our hospital religious and spiritual services, according to her religious affiliation.

- If she has any family history of breast cancer, or if she belongs to an ethnic group which has an increased genetic disposition to breast cancer (such as Ashkenazi Jews or Afro-Carribeans), I can discuss the screening for breast cancer in any immediate female family relatives.

- Before the consultation is over I would ask her if she has any further questions or concerns that she wants to discuss at this moment. I would end by making sure she is aware that I and the other members of my consultant's team will be available should she have any questions she would like to ask in future.

- I would document my conversation and the management plan as discussed with the patient in her notes.

Key points

- This is a very common scenario when candidates are tested on their communication skills to break bad news.

- Like every scenario in this setting, it is not just your ability to empathise with the patient – but also your background knowledge on the topic at hand that will be assessed. You cannot expect to 'break bad news' to a patient with breast cancer without having satisfactory knowledge to answer questions about types and methods of treatment, support groups available, etc.

Communication skills 13:   Level: * *

Dealing with a difficult patient: A man requests a CT head scan

> You are the medical foundation trainee on call in a small district general hospital. Mr Eden is a 34-year-old male who has come to A&E with a history of headaches. You have been asked by the A&E SHO to see him; apparently he is demanding to have a CT head scan performed.

QUESTION A:

What would you do before speaking to the patient to prepare yourself?

RESPONSE A:

I would review the patient's notes to familiarise myself with the presenting complaint and the patient's past medical history.

In reviewing the notes, you find out that Mr Eden is well known to the neurologists in your hospital, and has been on medication for migraines for several years now.

QUESTION B:

What would you say to the patient?

RESPONSE B:

* To begin with I would introduce myself to him and try to establish a rapport. I would then ask him if there are any differences in the headaches he has experienced recently and those that he is used to when having an exacerbation of his migraines.

Mr Eden tells you that his headaches have increased in frequency over the past few weeks and that a friend of his has recently been diagnosed with a brain tumour after complaining of headaches. For this reason he is convinced there is something more sinister going on, and that he would like to have a CT head scan performed.

You take a history of Mr Eden's presenting complaint and perform a brief examination. Everything points to migraines as being the likely cause for his headaches.

QUESTION C:

Mr Eden, however, remains insistent that he should have a CT head scan; he says that if he had private healthcare he would have had one by now. What would you say to him?

RESPONSE C:

- I would inform him that none of his symptoms point to him having a brain tumour; the likelihood is that he has had a severe exacerbation of his migraines.

- I would also tell him that a CT head scan is better at identifying bony pathology such as fractures, but less good when looking for soft tissue pathology, such as tumours.

- Despite the fact that I don't think he has either a tumour or other acute intracranial pathology, he is obviously very concerned. What I can do to reassure him is to speak to the neurology registrar on call, to refer him for a review by a member of their team. They will then make a decision on the need for further investigations.

The patient appears a little more relaxed on hearing this and agrees to this compromise.

Key points

- The key to this scenario is your ability to negotiate a compromise with the patient.

- There will be many occasions in your practice when patients will ask, or even demand, to be treated or investigated in a certain fashion. You need to be able to communicate effectively – without appearing to be confrontational.

Communication skills 14: Level: *

A parent demanding information about her teenage daughter

You are a foundation trainee doing a rotation in General Practice. Mrs Somer is a parent who has arranged an appointment to see you. When she arrives, she is demanding that you tell her what her 18-year-old daughter Emma, (who is also a patient at the practice) wanted when she saw you yesterday.

QUESTION A:
What would you say to Mrs Somer?

RESPONSE A:
*   To begin with I would introduce myself to her and try to establish a rapport.

Mrs Somer says she is worried about her daughter, and she knows that Emma saw you in the practice yesterday. She asks why she came and wants to know what was discussed yesterday.

*   I inform Mrs Somer that I cannot discuss her daughter, Emma, unless I have Emma's consent.

*   Legally, I can only inform a patient's parents if the patient is less than 16 years of age.

If I am being pushed to give information, I need to give a firm, non-confrontational reply, such as 'Emma did come to see me yesterday, but I am sorry, I am not legally able to divulge any specific matters relating to the consultation. I would suggest you try to speak to her directly. As Emma is older than 16 years of age, she is legally regarded as an adult.'

QUESTION B:
What do you understand by the term 'Gillick competence'?

RESPONSE B:
*   This is a phrase that was introduced following a legal case to identify if a child could give consent to the medical treatment proposed, without the need for parental consent or knowledge. It is based on a decision in the House of Lords in the case Gillick v West Norfolk and Wisbech Area Health Authority. It was first introduced in 1985.

- A member of the House of Lords, Lord Scarman ruled that: 'As a matter of law, the parental right to determine whether or not their minor (child) below the age of sixteen will have medical treatment terminates if and when the child achieves sufficient understanding and intelligence to understand fully what is proposed.'

Key points

- This scenario often occurs in the setting of a child, usually a female wanting a consultation with a doctor for advice on contraception. Alternatively they may be wanting to gain information and advice on termination following an unwanted pregnancy.

- Have an understanding of 'Gillick competence'.

Communication skills 15:   Level: *

Inter-professional communication: Dealing with a senior colleague who leaves you to hold his pager

You are a foundation trainee in general surgery, recently qualified two months ago. You have returned to the ward after a coffee break when the Sister in charge hands you the SHO's pager. She tells you that the SHO has gone to the library to revise for his forthcoming MRCS exams. As far as you are aware, he has not informed anyone else in the firm; certainly you were not previously informed of this. Your consultant is doing an outpatient clinic and the Specialty Registrar (SpR) is on annual leave.

You go to the hospital library, which is not far from the ward, where you see the SHO looking for a book. You approach him.

What would you say to him?

RESPONSE:

- I would use an appropriate introduction and try to establish rapport.

Depending on how you normally address the SHO, it may be acceptable to call him by his first name; however, in an examination scenario it would not be professional to do so.

- Explanation: I would then explain why I have come to see him and say something like: 'There is something I need to talk to you about; could we go somewhere a little more private to discuss the matter?'

The SHO says that's fine; you both go out of the library to a quiet room.

- Relay concerns: I would then relay my concerns. 'I would like to return your pager, as I don't feel comfortable holding it, in case I am asked to deal with a situation beyond my level of experience. As you know I have only recently qualified as a doctor; this is my first job, and I don't feel confident dealing with emergencies without senior support. As you know our SpR is also on annual leave'.

- Show empathy: 'I totally understand these exams are important to you, but patient safety has to be paramount.'

- Offer a suggestion: 'Perhaps you could take some time off for private study to prepare for the exams. We could go together to see the consultant or educational supervisor, to see if study leave could be arranged and some senior cover could be provided'.

- Clarify: By the end of my conversation with the SHO, I would want to clarify what we have discussed and come to some agreement on a plan of action. 'Thanks for the opportunity to speak to you about this; sorry, but on this occasion I can't carry the pager. Later this afternoon we can meet our consultant and request some study leave approved for you and senior cover provided for me.'

Key points

- This type of scenario is not uncommon, in an examination or clinical setting. When communicating with your seniors you should be as professional as you would be when talking to patients.

- Have your own system for dealing with situations of this nature. Using the example here, start by explaining why you wish to talk to your senior; relay your concerns to him or her. Be empathetic to their situation. Offer a suggestion or advice that may be agreeable to both of you. At the end, clarify what has been said and agree on a management plan.

Communication skills 16:   Level: * *

Dealing with an angry patient who is waiting in A&E

> You are a foundation trainee working in Accident and Emergency.
> Mr Wilton is a 46-year-old male who has been in the A&E reception
> for three hours waiting to see a doctor. He is appearing to get
> aggressive and verbally abusive towards members of staff and
> demanding that he see a doctor straight away. There are still two
> patients who have been waiting longer than him who will need to be
> seen first. The senior Sister has requested that you speak to him.

QUESTION A:

How would you approach your conversation with the patient?

RESPONSE A:

- INTRODUCTION: I would introduce myself to him, trying to
  establish rapport with appropriate body language – namely
  maintain some eye contact and an open posture, without
  appearing to be confrontational in any way.

- PROBLEM: I would identify the patient's problems: 'I am one of
  the A&E doctors; I appreciate you have been waiting to see a
  doctor for a while now. What seems to be the problem?'

- CLARIFY UNDERSTANDING: 'Do you know the reason why you
  have been waiting so long?'

- CLARIFY EXPECTATIONS: 'Is there anything you would like to
  know?'

QUESTION B:

What would you say to the patient to reassure him that he will be seen
as soon as is practical?

RESPONSE B:

My intention would be to make sure Mr Wilton realises that I understand
he is angry; I would remain non-confrontational and calm throughout
the conversation.

- 'I apologise that you have had to wait so long and can
  understand that you feel this way. When patients arrive, we have
  a system in place that allows us to deal with patients according

to their medical needs and their time of arrival. I appreciate your understanding at this time; there are two patients who have arrived before you and need to be reviewed sooner than you, but we are seeing and treating patients as quickly as we can. I can assure you that you will be seen as soon as possible.'

Then I would want to check that Mr Wilton has understood what I have told him. Ask him if he has any questions and answer them as best I can.

Before getting on with my work, it would be important to have negotiated some kind of agreement.

- 'I understand that you are in a lot of pain as a result of your accident; whilst you are waiting to be seen I will prescribe, and ask one of the A&E nurses to give you, some analgesia while you wait to be seen by a doctor. Is that OK?'

Key points

- In this scenario you are trying to keep a situation calm through a variety of communication skills. Introduce yourself and establish a rapport early on.

- Be empathetic to the patient's feelings. Listen to the patient's concerns.

- Use appropriate body language throughout, modify your tone and pace of speech accordingly; be non-confrontational with suitable eye contact.

- Reflect to make sure the patient understands what you have said to him and try to come to some kind of agreement.

BPP LEARNING MEDIA

Communication skills 17:

Level: *

Explanation: CT head scan

Mrs Sharmen is a 58-year-old female, who has been referred by her GP to the medical team on call following the development of sudden onset left-sided weakness; the GP is understandably concerned the patient may have had a stroke. As the medical foundation trainee on call, you have been asked to organise a CT head scan for her to identify the cause of her weakness. When she arrives at A&E you need to explain to her what the procedure involves.

QUESTION A:

What would you say to her when she arrives?

RESPONSE A:

- INTRODUCTION: I would start by introducing myself to her, make sure I am speaking to the correct patient, elicit her name, age and occupation. In this way also try to establish a rapport.

- CLARIFY UNDERSTANDING: I would then try to check her understanding of why she has been asked to come to hospital today: 'Mrs Sharmen, I gather that you noticed some weakness of the left side of your body on waking up this morning. In order for us to identify why you have developed this weakness we would like to perform a CT head scan. Can I ask what you understand by the term CT?'

- LISTEN: Listen to the patient about any concerns she has about the CT scan and what she thinks the problem is.

QUESTION B:

How would you explain what a CT scan is?

RESPONSE B:

- 'CT stands for computerised tomography. A CT scan is a process where ordinary X-rays (also known as tomograms) are passed through a computer (computed – hence the term computed tomography) to produce a 2-dimensional or 3-dimensional picture. In this way we can obtain cross-sectional images of a part of the body, just like slices of cheese.'

QUESTION C:

How would you explain in layman terms what the procedure involves?

RESPONSE C:

- I would explain 'Later this afternoon you will taken to the radiology department, where the scan will be performed. You mustn't eat or drink anything for a couple of hours before the scan. The CT scanner itself looks like a large doughnut with a narrow table in the middle. You lie on your back on the table, and this moves through the centre of the machine. Sometimes patients feel a little claustrophobic, but it is a completely painless investigation.'

- 'You will be in the scanner for around 10 to 15 minutes. In the room next to the scanner there will be a radiographer, who operates the machine along with one of his or her assistants. If at any time you want to ask anything, or have any concerns, you can speak to these people through an intercom system.'

Mrs Sharmen tells you she cannot remember ever having a CT scan before and asks you what the risks of the procedure are?

- 'The CT scan is usually a safe procedure, but as mentioned it does involve exposure to X-rays, hence radiation. This is, however, at the lowest dose that is practical to achieve the images we need.'

- 'There are absolutely no health reasons for not having a CT scan, but it is not recommended if, for example, a patient is pregnant. Just to verify, is there any possibility that you may be pregnant?'

Mrs Sharmen tells you she has gone through the menopause, and she is not pregnant.

- 'You may also have an injection of a harmless dye injected into a vein on the back of your hand. This is sometimes used to increase the accuracy of the test. Have you any allergies that you are aware of?'

- 'We do believe that the benefits of having a CT scan outweigh any associated risks, including that of radiation exposure. The information from the scan will help us identify the cause for your weakness and will influence what treatment is required.'

- Once I have answered any further concerns that Mrs Sharmen has, I would reflect on what I have told her and check that she has understood what has been said.

- Once I have obtained her consent for the procedure I would document this in her notes.

Key points

- A CT scan is a very common radiological procedure which could be requested in almost any firm (medical or surgical) that you will be working in.

- Have a good understanding of what a CT scan is and be able to explain the procedure, along with any safety issues that may be asked.

Communication skills 18: Level: * * *

Explanation: MRI knee scan

Mr York is a 22-year-old male, who has been referred by his GP to the Trauma & Orthopaedic (T&O) team on call, following a sporting injury; he had been playing football the previous day and twisted his right knee in a tackle with an opposition player. At the time he carried on playing despite being in pain, but this morning his knee has swollen considerably and he can hardly weight bear. As the T&O foundation trainee on call, you have been asked to organise an MRI scan for him.

QUESTION A:

What would you say to him when he arrives?

RESPONSE A:

- INTRODUCTION: I would start by introducing myself to him, make sure I am speaking to the correct patient, elicit his name, age and occupation. In this way I would also try to establish a rapport.

- CLARIFY UNDERSTANDING: I would then try to check his understanding of why he has been asked to come to hospital today: 'Mr York, I have been informed that you have noticed some swelling on your right knee after having a football injury yesterday. In order for us to identify why you have developed this swelling we would like to perform an MRI scan of the knee. Can I ask what you understand by the term MRI?'

- LISTEN: Listen to the patient about any concerns he has about the MRI scan and what he thinks the procedure is.

QUESTION B:

How would you explain what an MRI scan is?

RESPONSE B:

'MRI stands for magnetic resonance imaging. It is a non-invasive method which allows us to visualise internal structures of the body in detail. It involves exposing the area of the body we are scanning to a strong magnetic field. It does not involve exposure to radiation (X-rays).'

QUESTION C:

How would you explain in layman terms what the procedure involves?

RESPONSE C:

- I would explain 'Later this afternoon you will taken to the radiology department where the scan will be performed. You do not need to stop eating or drinking before the scan. The MRI scanner itself looks like a large tube. You will lie on your back on a bed, which is then moved into the scanning tube. You will be left alone in the scanning room. Sometimes patients feel a little claustrophobic (have a fear of enclosed spaces), but it is a completely painless investigation.'

- 'You will be in the scanner for around 30 minutes. The MRI scanner is controlled by a computer which is in the room next to the scanner. This is to keep it away from the magnetic field generated by the scanner. There will be a radiographer and one of his or her assistants, in that room, operating the computer. If at any time you want to ask anything or have any concerns you can speak to these people through an intercom system.'

- 'You should be aware that at certain times during the MRI scan, the scanner makes a loud clicking sound. This is the sounds of the magnets being turned on and off. For this reason we advise all patients to wear the headphones or earplugs which will be given.'

Mr York tells you he has never had a MRI scan before and asks you what the risks of the procedure are.

- I would say 'The MRI scan is a painless and harmless procedure; it is not associated with any specific risks or side effects. As mentioned it does not involve exposure to X-rays. This means that individuals who may be vulnerable to the effects of radiation such as pregnant women and babies can safely have an MRI.'

- 'However, not everyone can have an MRI scan; for example, it is not recommended for people who have certain types of implants in situ, such as pacemakers, metallic heart valves or surgical clips in their body. Also if there is any possibility a patient may have any metallic fragments in their eyes, we would obtain an X-ray before proceeding to getting the MRI. Can I just check that none of these situations applies to you?'

- 'Although this is unlikely to be the case with your MRI, you may also have an injection of a harmless dye injected into a vein on the back of your hand. This allows us to obtain a contrasted scan and is sometimes used to obtain additional information from the test. Have you any allergies that you are aware of?'

Once I have answered any further concerns that Mr York has, I would reflect on what I have told him and check that he has understood what has been said. I would then obtain his informed consent to proceed with the MRI and document this in his notes.

Key points

- An MRI scan is a very common radiological procedure which, unlike a CT scan, does not involve exposure to radiation.

- Have a good understanding of what an MRI is and be able to explain the procedure, along with any safety issues that may be asked.

BPP
LEARNING MEDIA

Communication skills 19:   Level: * *

Counselling a patient with HIV

You are a foundation trainee doing a rotation in genito-urinary medicine. Mr Woods is 36-years-old male referred by his GP after being recently identified as HIV positive. You have been asked by your consultant to see him, including informing him of methods of support available.

QUESTION A:

What would you say to Mr Woods?

RESPONSE A:

- To begin with I would introduce myself to him and try to establish a rapport. I would review the reasons for the consultation.

- 'Mr Woods, I have a letter from your GP indicating that you have recently been diagnosed as HIV positive. Can you tell me what you understand about the situation?'

The patient tells you that he found out only a few weeks ago, after having some blood tests.

You take a brief but concise history, during which you find out that Mr Woods is a homosexual male in a relationship for the past five years. However, he has been having a few problems and is not sure that he and his partner will be together much longer. He admits to seeing a few other men casually over the past 12 to 18 months.

He tells you that he doesn't want anyone else, including his partner, to know about his HIV status.

QUESTION B:

How would you approach the consultation now?

RESPONSE B:

- Well, I would try to be empathetic and also sympathetic to his situation. However, I would have to stress the necessity for Mr Woods to inform not only his long-term partner, but also his other sexual partners, as he is inadvertently putting their lives at risk.

- I would tell him it is a very natural response for him to be feeling this way, and be worried of what his partner will think.

- I would also recommend him to have HIV counselling, which I should be able to arrange for him with a specialist.

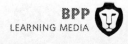

QUESTION C:

What are the salient points you need to get across in your consultation?

RESPONSE C:

- Well, I cannot stress enough to him that all his sexual partners need to be informed.

- I would tell him that there is approximately a 3-month window between being infected with HIV and seroconversion (the time it takes for a person to develop antibodies for HIV, therefore for the immune system to be fully triggered and produce enough antibodies to be reliably detected by an HIV antibody test).

- I would also emphasise that, even though HIV is the virus that causes AIDS, it does not mean that a person with the virus will necessarily develop AIDS.

- He should be told that we will commence him on some antiretroviral medication.

- We will need to monitor the response to medication, by checking certain blood markers, including CD4 count and viral load.

- He should be told that in any future sexual encounters he should use barrier protection (most commonly condoms) in order to reduce the risk of HIV transmission.

- Mr Woods should be aware that if he is having difficulty telling his long-term partner or other sexual partners then I would be willing to speak to them individually, with him, to explain the situation.

- Before the end of the consultation I would give him information on further sources of support, for example leaflets on the Terrence Higgins Trust (a support group which focuses on people with HIV living healthy lives free from prejudice and discrimination).

- Before he leaves I would check if he has any further questions and inform him that I will organise for him to be seen again in the clinic soon – should he have any concerns in the interim he can always ask his GP for an earlier appointment.

Key points

- Essential communication skills in this station comprise the ability to show empathy, but also being firm in your conversation with the patient and making him aware of the necessity to inform other relevant individuals of his HIV status – in this instance, his regular partner, along with those other partners with whom the patient has had casual relations over the past few years.

- Be aware of sources of support for HIV patients, namely the Terrence Higgins Trust. Ensure that the patient does not leave without giving him the opportunity to ask further questions and being aware that you are available for a further consultation should he have any questions.

Communication skills 20: Level: *

An unregistered patient comes to you to ask for a salbutamol inhaler

You are a foundation trainee doing a rotation in General Practice. Mr Storm is a 29-year-old male who is not registered at your practice and has requested an emergency appointment with a doctor.

QUESTION A:

What would you say to the patient?

RESPONSE A:

- To begin with I would introduce myself to him and try to establish a rapport.

- I would speak to him and take a history of the presenting complaint, together with any relevant past medical history and medication history.

Mr Storm informs you that he has come to the region five days ago, on a business trip. He is known to suffer from asthma. He does not use his blue salbutamol inhaler that often, but unfortunately he has left it at home. Over the past couple of days he has felt very wheezy.

QUESTION B:

What would you do now?

RESPONSE B:

- I would examine him and auscultate his chest, listening for a wheeze. I would also measure his peak expiratory flow rate (PEFR).

You identify that he does have an expiratory wheeze on examination. His PEFR is also a little lower than you would expect for his age and height. What would you do next?

- In that circumstance I think it would be appropriate to write him a prescription for a salbutamol (also known as ventolin) inhaler.

- I would also advise him to see his own GP when he returns home. Ask him if he has any questions or if there is anything else he needs.

- I would also document in the notes the outcome of the consultation and make it clear that the patient was seen as an emergency and was not officially registered with the practice.

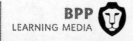

Key points

- This is a relatively straightforward scenario; however, be aware that although this is a communication skills scenario, you are allowed to say that you would examine the patient and allow the examiner to tell you the result.

- Remember that, even though a patient may not be registered with your general practice, if you are requested to see them on an emergency basis, you have a moral obligation to do so.

Communication skills 21:   Level: * * *

Explanation: Gastrointestinal endoscopy

Mr Ramon is a 57-year-old alcohol-dependent male. He has recently been seen in the clinic following a history of passing dark black stools. As a result he has been admitted as a day case to have an endoscopy procedure. As the foundation trainee working for the firm you have been asked to discuss the procedure with him.

QUESTION A:

What would you say to him when he arrives?

RESPONSE A:

- INTRODUCTION: I would start by introducing myself to him, make sure I am speaking to the correct patient, elicit his name, age and occupation. In this way I would also try to establish a rapport.

- CLARIFY UNDERSTANDING: I would then try to check his understanding of why he has been asked to come to hospital today: 'Mr Ramon, I have been informed that you have noticed some passage of dark stools recently. In order for us to identify why this has occurred we would like to perform an endoscopic examination. Can I ask what you understand by this?'

- LISTEN: Listen to the patient about any concerns he has about the endoscopic examination and what he thinks the problem is.

QUESTION B:

How would you explain what an endoscopic examination is?

RESPONSE B:

- Well, the procedure is often abbreviated to an OGD, which stands for oesophagogastroduodenoscopy. We often perform the procedure under sedation to help a patient relax. It comprises having an endoscope, which is a long flexible tube which has a light source at its tip, passed through your mouth into the oesophagus (food pipe), then through the stomach on its way to the duodenum (the first part of the small intestine).

- In this way, it allows the doctor performing the exam a method of looking directly at the lining of these structures. If there is anything that looks like it shouldn't be there, or that requires further investigation, the doctor may take a small piece of tissue, a biopsy, using a set of small forceps passed down the endoscopy tube.

QUESTION C:

How would you prepare the patient for the procedure and what would you tell him it involves?

RESPONSE C:

- I would tell him 'Before the procedure you mustn't eat or drink anything for at least six hours. This will allow the doctor a better view. We will give you an injection or a spray into your nostrils to keep you calm and relaxed during the procedure.'

- 'Before the procedure we will give you a mouthguard, to help keep your mouth open. Then the endoscope tube will be passed through your mouth, through the food pipe on its way into the stomach. Once in the stomach, air will be passed through the endoscope, this will also help to obtain a clearer view. The whole procedure should take around twenty to thirty minutes.'

- 'Following the procedure we would like to keep an eye on you for a couple of hours before letting you go home. Due to some of the medication you are given, it is not uncommon to feel a little lethargic and drowsy after the procedure; for this reason, we do not want you to drive on the same day. We would recommend you try to have someone to drive you back home or get a taxi if required. Most people feel much better the next day. You should be able to carry out your normal activities of daily living at that stage, including going back to work.'

Once I have answered any further concerns that Mr Ramon has, I would reflect on what I have told him and check that he has understood what has been said. I would then obtain his informed consent to proceed with the endoscopic examination and document this in his notes. I would also let him know that we will arrange to see him in clinic in a couple of weeks, to discuss the results when we have them.

Key points

- When explaining this or any other procedure to a patient, your aim is to be as informative as the patient wants you to be; at the same time, you need to allay any concerns they have about how it is performed.

- Remember to mention that following the procedure, due to the medication given, the patient will not be able to drive the same day.

Communication skills 22:   Level: * * *

Explanation: Commencing a patient on thrombolysis

 Mr Lampard is a 54-year-old male who has arrived in A&E with chest pain and has been identified to have a confirmed myocardial infarction. You are the medical foundation trainee on call and have been asked by your registrar to see the patient and obtain verbal consent to carry out thrombolysis.

QUESTION A:

What would you say to him when he arrives?

RESPONSE A:

- INTRODUCTION: I would start by introducing myself to him, make sure I am speaking to the correct patient, elicit his name, age and occupation. In this way I would also try to establish a rapport.

- CLARIFY UNDERSTANDING: I would then try to check his understanding of why he has come to hospital today and explain what has happened: 'Mr Lampard, I understand you have come to hospital today with sudden onset chest pain. The A&E doctors have done a few tests and identified that you have had a heart attack. What has happened is that there has been a blockage or clot in one of the blood vessels (coronary arteries) which supply your heart with blood. This clot results from the rupture of an atherosclerotic plaque in the wall of the artery. The plaque consists of a mixture of fatty substances and white blood cells. This can result in a reduction in the blood supply to the heart – and therefore that part of the heart can become starved of oxygen and can become irreversibly damaged, resulting in death in the worst-case scenario. We would like to commence you on immediate drugs to try to break down and reduce the size of the clot; these drugs are called thrombolytics.'

- LISTEN: Listen to the patient about any concerns he has about thrombolysis.

QUESTION B:

How would you explain how thrombolysis is administered and what side effects should you inform the patient of?

RESPONSE B:

- I would explain 'The thrombolytic drug we use is called streptokinase; it is given intravenously through a cannula in your arm. It works by breaking down the clot and reducing its size. In this way, blood should be able to pass through the artery and oxygen also delivered to the heart.'

- 'There are some side effects associated with the drug used; the more common ones include: nausea, vomiting, dizziness and skin flushing (changes in skin colour). Some of the less common, but more severe, side effects include development of a stroke (bleed in the brain), gastrointestinal bleeding, an allergic response resulting in shortness of breath or wheeze, low blood pressure and the development of a slow or fast heartbeat.'

QUESTION C:

What are the contraindications of giving thrombolysis?

RESPONSE C:

- These can be divided into absolute and relative contraindications. The absolute contraindications include a previous history of intracranial bleeding at any time, uncontrolled high blood pressure (>180 systolic or >100 diastolic), history of active bleeding problems eg from a peptic ulcer, as well as a history of major trauma within the past three months. Relative contraindications include current anticoagulant usage, a history of invasive or surgical procedures in the past two weeks, pregnancy and haemorrhagic or diabetic retinopathies.

- Once I have answered any further concerns that Mr Lampard has, I would reflect on what I have told him and check that he has understood what has been said. At this stage I would ask him for his verbal consent to proceed with thrombolysis and document this in his case notes.

Key points

- Thrombolysis can be a life-saving measure in patients with myocardial infarction; this should be stressed to the patient. Also be informative about the side effects it is associated with.

- It would be foolhardy to proceed with thrombolysis before making sure the patient does not have any of the absolute contraindications. If there are any relative contraindications present, then you should seek senior advice, ie ask your registrar or consultant before giving the go-ahead.

Communication skills 23: Level: *

Dealing with a drug addict who requests a repeat methadone prescription, claiming to have lost his previous one

You are the medical foundation trainee doing an attachment in general practice. The next patient you see is Mr Grant. He is a 29-year-old male known to be an intravenous drug abuser. He has come to ask you for a repeat methadone prescription.

QUESTION A:
What would you do before speaking to the patient to prepare yourself?

RESPONSE A:
- I would review the patient's notes to familiarise myself with the patient's past medical history and, in particular, any relevant history relating to his background of recreational drug usage.

- I would identify how long he has been on a drug rehabilitation programme.

- Also I would find out how much methadone he takes and when his last prescription was.

QUESTION B:
What would you say to the patient?

RESPONSE B:
- To begin with I would introduce myself to him and try to establish a rapport and ask him why he has come to the practice today.

Mr Grant tells you that he has lost his most recent methadone prescription and has come to ask you to re-prescribe one for him.

On review of the patient's case notes you realise that his last prescription was issued only yesterday. It also appears that this is not the first time he has lost his prescription. What would you do next?

- I would ask him why he thinks he keeps losing his prescription. I would also call the patient's pharmacy or chemist to check with them if the most recent prescription has been received and been issued.

On consultation with the chemist, it does not look like the prescription has been handed in on this occasion.

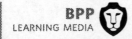

QUESTION C:

What would you do next?

RESPONSE C:

- I would tell the patient that on this occasion I will re-write his prescription. However, I would stress that this cannot keep happening. I would not necessarily be able to re-write another prescription if he loses another one again.

- As an alternative I would give him the option of daily delivery of his methadone to his pharmacist for collection by him daily.

Mr Grant tells you he thinks that is a good idea and agrees with this new plan.

- I would check with the patient's pharmacist as to when they can start delivery of his methadone for daily collection; accordingly, I would write him a new prescription to cover him until then.

- I would end the consultation by asking him if he has any further questions, and advise he arrange another appointment if he has any questions or concerns in the future.

Key points

- Show the examiner you are genuinely trying to identify if the patient has lost his prescription, in this example shown by asking the chemist whether it has been handed in and issued.

- Show your ability to negotiate a suitable alternative with the patient, here illustrated by giving the option of daily delivery of the methadone for the patient to collect on a daily basis.

Communication skills 24:   Level: * *

Explanation: Instilling eye drops

Miss Esha is a 21-year-old female who has come to your general practice clinic today. She tells you that, for the past three weeks, she has noticed her left eye to be itchy and red. As the foundation trainee you have been asked to see and manage her appropriately.

QUESTION A:
What would you say to her when she arrives?

RESPONSE A:

- INTRODUCTION: I would start by introducing myself to her, make sure I am speaking to the correct patient, elicit her name, date of birth and occupation.

- HISTORY: I would then take a brief history from her identifying how long her eye has been affected, and what sort of symptoms she has had. I would ask if there has been any history of trauma or visual problems.

- EXPLANATION: I would explain that the likely diagnosis is conjunctivitis, and explain that this often occurs secondary to a viral infection. However, there is always a possibility of bacterial infection. The condition tends to be associated with an infection of the upper respiratory tract, a common cold and/or a sore throat. It is passed from one individual to another by direct touch or droplets in the air.

- ADVISE ON TREATMENT: I would recommend the use of chloramphenicol eye drops for the involved eye.

  I would say 'Miss Esha, the symptoms you are having affecting your left eye are consistent with an infection called conjunctivitis. This is also a common cause of a red eye. Most often, this is secondary to a virus, but a bacterial cause can also be responsible for the same symptoms. For this reason, I think it would be prudent to start you on some antibiotic eye drops to help with your symptoms.'

QUESTION B:
How would you explain to the patient how to instill the chloramphenicol eye drops?

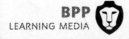

RESPONSE B:

- 'Before you use the drops, wash your hands each time.'

- 'Whilst standing, tilt your head upwards looking towards the ceiling.'

- 'Take the cap off the medication bottle and hold the bottle a few centimetres away from the affected eye (left eye in this case), ensure the bottle itself does not touch the eye.'

- 'With the other hand pull down the affected eyelid, then drop a couple of drops into the lower eyelid.'

- 'Immediately close the eye shut.'

- 'Remember to put the lid or seal back on the medication bottle.'

- I would then want to check if the patient has understood what I have told her, so I would ask her to demonstrate.

- I would tell the patient to do this four times a day. I would also mention that if the symptoms, including the red eye, do not improve after two weeks, or if the symptoms worsen including any change in vision, then she should return to the medical practice to be reviewed again.

QUESTION C:

What advice would you give the patient to limit the spread of conjunctivitis?

RESPONSE C:

- I would say 'Miss Esha, it is important that you take some basic precautions to prevent your other eye from also becoming infected, as well as helping to protect people you come into contact with, including family and friends. This includes washing your hands each time you touch the affected eye; remember to dry your hands, as well as your face, with a towel which is only used by yourself. Another method to help prevent spread is that when you sleep, use a pillowcase that is not shared by anyone else.'

Key points

- After explaining to your patient how to instill the eye drops, check their understanding by asking them to demonstrate on themselves what you have told them.

- Conjunctivitis is a common cause of a red eye, chloramphenicol being one of the most common topical antibiotics used.

Further reading

Useful texts for communication skills:

Parrott, T and Crook, G (2011) *Effective Communication Skills for Doctors*. London: BPP Learning Media.

Silverman, J, Kurtz, S and Draper, J (2005) *Skills for Communicating with Patients*. 2nd edition. Oxford: Radcliffe Publishing.

BPP
LEARNING MEDIA

Appendix

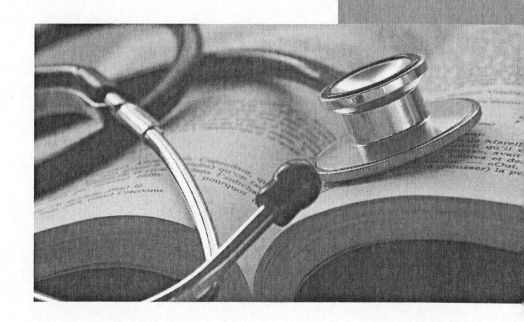

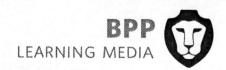

BPP
LEARNING MEDIA

Appendix 1

Normal haematology reference ranges

Index	Range	Unit
White blood cell	4.0-11.0	$X10^9/l$
Differential count:		
Neutrophils	1.7-8.0	$X10^9/l$
Lymphocytes	1.0-4.0	$X10^9/l$
Monocytes	0.2-1.5	$X10^9/l$
Eosinophils	0.00-0.5	$X10^9/l$
Basophils	<0.1	$X10^9/l$
Platelet count	150-450	$X10^9/l$
Red blood cells – male	4.5-6.5	$X10^{12}/l$
Red blood cells – female	3.8-5.8	$X10^{12}/l$
Haemoglobin – male	13.5-18.0	g/dl
Haemoglobin – female	11.5-16.5	g/dl
Haematocrit – male	0.4-0.54	
Haematocrit – female	0.37-0.47	
Mean cell volume (MCV)	80-102	fl
Mean cell haemoglobin (MCH)	26-32	pg
Mean cell haemoglobin concentration (MCHC)	30-36	g/dl
Red cell distribution width (RDW)	11.5-15.0	g/dl
ESR – male	<10	mm/h
ESR – female	<14	mm/h
Serum B_{12}	200-900	pg/ml
Serum folate	3.9-20	ng/ml
Red cell folate	150-630	ng/ml

International normalised ratio (INR)	0.9-1.3	
Prothrombin time (PT)	10-15	sec
Activated partial thromboplastin time (APTT)	25-38	sec
Fibrinogen level	1.5-4.0	g/l
D-Dimer	<0.5	mg/l
Bleeding time (adult)	1.5-8.0	min

Appendix 2

Normal biochemistry reference ranges

Index	Range	Unit
Sodium	133-146	mmol/l
Potassium	3.5-5.0	mmol/l
Urea	2.5-7.5	mmol/l
Creatinine	50-120	μmol/l
Bicarbonate	23-30	mmol/l
Chloride	98-107	mmol/l
C-reactive protein	<5	mg/l
Calcium	2.10-2.65	mmol/l
Phosphate	0.80-1.45	mmol/l
Total protein	60-80	g/l
Bilirubin	3-22	μmol/l
Albumin	35-50	g/l
Globulin	21-38	g/l
Urate – male	<0.42	mmol/l
Urate – female	<0.38	mmol/l
Glucose (fasting)	3.2-6.0	mmol/l
Glucose (random)	3.2-7.8	mmol/l
Enzymes:		
Amylase	30-110	IU/l
ALP (adult)	30-125	IU/l
AST	6-40	IU/l
ALT (male)	21-72	IU/l
ALT (female)	9-52	IU/l
GGT	12-60	IU/l
LDH	300-600	IU/l
CK	30-160	IU/l

Cerebrospinal fluid:

Protein	<0.45	g/l
Glucose	2.2-3.9	mmol/l

(CSF glucose should be half to 2/3 of serum or plasma glucose)

Arterial blood gases:

pH	7.36-7.44	
pO_2	90-100 (12-14.7)	mmHg(kPa)
pCO_2	35-45 (4.5-6.0)	mmHg(kPa)
HCO_3^-	22-28	mmol/l
Base Excess	-2 to +2	

Appendix 3

Helpful mnemonics

SOCRATES: For assessing regional pain

- **S**ite & **S**everity
- **O**nset
- **C**haracter
- **R**adiation and **R**elieving factors
- **A**ggravating factors
- **T**iming
- **E**xercise
- (Associated) **S**ymptoms

MJ THREADS: For taking a medical history, to ensure you cover all the key issues

Myocardial Infarction

Jaundice

Tuberculosis

Hypertension

Rheumatic fever

Epilepsy

Asthma

Diabetes

Stroke

ABCDE: Prioritising trauma treatment

A: Airway and cervical spine control

B: Breathing and ventilation

C: Circulation with haemorrhage control

D: Disability with neurologic evaluation

E: Exposure and environmental control – this requires completely undressing the patient, but also protecting against hypothermia

SCOL: Checking X-ray (osteoarthritis)

- **S**ubchondral sclerosis at the joint margins
- **C**ysts (bone cysts) close to the joint margins
- **O**steophyte formation
- **L**oss of joint space

SPIKES: Six-step method as an aid to breaking bad news

- **S**et the Scene
- **P**erception
- **I**nvitation
- **K**nowledge
- **E**mpathise
- **S**trategy

EC PQRST: Causes of a raised jugular venous pressure (JVP)

- Pulmonary **E**mbolism/Pericardial **E**ffusion
- **C**annon waves
- Constrictive **P**ericarditis
- **Q**uantity of fluid increased (resulting in a fluid overload)
- **R**ight heart failure
- **S**uperior vena caval obstruction
- **T**ricuspid stenosis/Tricuspid regurgitation/Cardiac tamponade

5Fs: Signs of abdominal distension

- **F**at
- **F**luid
- **F**oetus
- **F**latus
- **F**aeces

6Ps: Signs and symptoms of acute ischaemia

- **P**ain
- **P**araesthesia (numbness)
- **P**allor (pale)
- **P**ulseless
- **P**aralysis
- **P**erishing cold

APGAR: Test for neonates

- **A**ppearance
- **P**ulse rate
- **G**rimace
- **A**ctivity
- **R**espiratory effort

The following websites have been selected by the author as containing further suitable mnemonics which may provide candidates with more useful learning aids during their exam preparations:

http://www.medicalmnemonics.com

https://www.facebook.com/MedicalPneumonics

http://www.valuemd.com/mnemonics.php

Appendix 4

Common medical abbreviations

A1AT	α-1-antitrypsin
AAA	abdominal aortic aneurysm
ABG	arterial blood gas
ABPI	ankle brachial pressure index
ACTH	Adrenocorticotropic hormone
ADH	Antidiuretic Hormone
ADL	activities of daily living
APGAR	Appearance, pulse rate, grimace, activity, respiratory effort (test for neonates)
AP	anteroposterior
APTT	activated partial thromboplastin time
ASIS	anterior superior iliac spine
BLS	basic life support
BM	blood (sugar) meter
BMI	body mass index
BNF	British National Formulary
CIN	cervical intra-epithelial neoplasia
COPD	chronic obstructive pulmonary disease
CPN	community psychiatric nurse
CRP	c-reactive protein
CRT	capillary refill time
CSF	cerebrospinal fluid
CT	computed tomography
CTR	cardiothoracic ratio
CVA	cerebrovascular accident
CXR	chest X-ray
DIP	distal interphalangeal
DNAR	Do Not Attempt Resuscitation

DPL	diagnostic peritoneal lavage
DRE	digital rectal examination
DVT	deep vein thrombosis
EGFR	Estimated Glomerular Filtration Rate
ERCP	Endoscopic retrograde cholangiopancreatography
FAP	familial adenomatous polyposis
FBC	full blood count
FFP	Fresh Frozen Plasma
G&S	group and antibody screen
GCS	Glasgow Coma Score
GFR	Glomerular Filtration Rate
GI	gastrointestinal
GTN	Glyceryl trinitrate
Hb	Haemoglobin
HNPCC	hereditary non-polyposis colorectal cancer
HOCM	hypertrophic cardiomyopathy
HPC	history of presenting complaint
HRT	hormone replacement therapy
IBD	inflammatory bowel disease
IHD	Ischaemic Heart Disease
INR	international normalised ratio
IV	intravenous
JVP	jugular venous pressure
LFTs	liver function tests
LIF	left iliac fossa
LLQ	left lower quadrant
LMP	last menstrual period
LRTI	lower respiratory tract infection
LUQ	left upper quadrant
LVF	left ventricular failure

LVH	left ventricle hypertrophy
M,C&S	microscopy, culture and sensitivity
MCH	mean cell haemoglobin
MCHC	mean cell haemoglobin concentration
MCP	metacarpophalangeal
MCV	mean cell volume
MDT	multi-disciplinary team
MMSE	mini-mental state examination
MRC	Medical Research Council
MRI	magnetic resonance imaging
MRSA	methicillin-resistant staphylococcus aureus
MS	multiple sclerosis
NKDA	No Known Drug Allergies
NSAIDs	non-steroidal anti-inflammatory drugs
OGD	oesophagogastroduodenoscopy
PA	posteroanterior
PC	presenting complaint
PCV	packed cell volume
PEFR	peak expiratory flow rate
PID	pelvic inflammatory disease
Plt	platelets
PMH	past medical history
PPI	proton pump inhibitor
PUO	pyrexia of unknown origin
RDW	red cell distribution width
RLQ	right lower quadrant
RIF	right iliac fossa
RTA	renal tubular acidosis
RTC	road traffic collision
RUQ	right upper quadrant

SAU	Surgical Assessment Unit
SIADH	Syndrome of Inappropriate Antidiuretic Hormone
SOB	shortness of breath
SpR	Specialty Registrar
TFTs	thyroid function tests
T&O	Trauma & Orthopaedic
TSH	thyroid stimulating hormone
TTA	To Take Away – discharge form
TTO	To Take Out – discharge form
URTI	upper respiratory tract infection
Us & Es	urea and electrolytes
WCC	white cell count

Appendix 5

Common abbreviations encountered within prescriptions

od	once daily
bd	twice daily
tds	three times a day
qds	four times a day
PRN (pro re nata)	as required
mg	milligram
mcg/µg	microgram
gm	gram
p.o. (per os)	by mouth
i.v.	intravenous
i.m.	intramuscular
s.c.	subcutaneous

Index

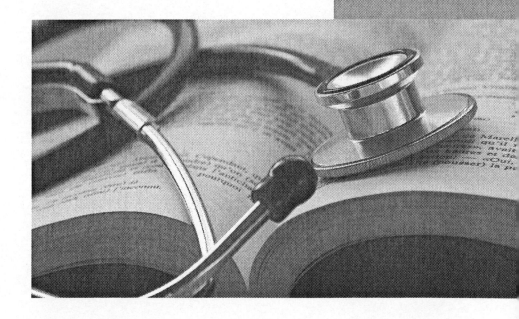

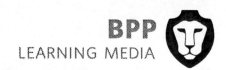

M

N

O